THE BIOLOGY
OF DISEASE

The Biology of Disease

EDITED BY

JONATHAN PHILLIPS BSc PhD
Senior Lecturer in Biomedical Science
School of Health Sciences
University of Wolverhampton

PAUL MURRAY MSc
Senior Lecturer in Biomedical Science
School of Health Sciences
University of Wolverhampton

ASSOCIATE EDITOR

JOHN CROCKER MA MD MRCPath
Consultant Histopathologist
Department of Histopathology
Birmingham Heartlands Hospital
and Visiting Senior Clinical Lecturer
University of Warwick

b
Blackwell
Science

© 1995 by
Blackwell Science Ltd
Editorial Offices:
Osney Mead, Oxford OX2 0EL
25 John Street, London WC1N 2BL
23 Ainslie Place, Edinburgh EH3 6AJ
238 Main Street, Cambridge
    Massachusetts 02142, USA
54 University Street, Carlton
    Victoria 3053, Australia

Other Editorial Offices:
Arnette Blackwell SA
    224, Boulevard Saint Germain
    75007 Paris, France

Blackwell Wissenschafts-Verlag GmbH
    Kurfürstendamm 57
    10707 Berlin, Germany

    Zehetnergasse 6
    A-1140 Wien, Austria

First published 1995
Reprinted 1997

Set by Excel Typesetters, Hong Kong
Printed and bound in Great Britain
at the University Press, Cambridge

The Blackwell Science Logo is a
trade mark of Blackwell Science Ltd,
registered at the United Kingdom
Trade Marks Registry

DISTRIBUTORS

Marston Book Services Ltd
PO Box 269
Abingdon
Oxon OX14 4YN
(*Orders:* Tel: 01235 465500
             Fax: 01235 465555)

USA
Blackwell Science, Inc.
238 Main Street
Cambridge, MA 02142
(*Orders:* Tel: 800 215-1000
             617 876-7000
             Fax: 617 492-5263)

Canada
Copp Clark Professional
200 Adelaide Street, West, 3rd Floor
Toronto, Ontario M5H 1W7
(*Orders:* Tel: 416 597-1616
             800 815-9417
             Fax: 416 597-1617)

Australia
Blackwell Science Pty Ltd
54 University Street
Carlton, Victoria 3053
(*Orders:* Tel: 3 9347 0300
             Fax: 3 9347 5001)

A catalogue record for this title
is available from the British Library

ISBN 0-632-03855-1
International Edition 0-86542-968-5

Library of Congress
Cataloging-in-Publication Data

The biology of disease / edited by
    Jonathan Phillips, Paul Murray,
    associate editor John Crocker.
        p.   cm.
    Includes bibliographical references and index.
    ISBN 0-632-03855-1
    1. Pathology.   2. Physiology, Pathological.
    3. Diseases.   I. Phillips, Jonathan, PhD.
    II. Murray, Paul, MSc.   III. Crocker, J.
    [DNLM: 1. Disease.   QZ 140 B6145 1995]
    RB111.B48 1995
    616.07—dc20
    DNLM/DLC
    for Library of Congress   94-46340
                                            CIP

Contents

Contents

List of Contributors

R. F. AMBINDER, MD PhD, *Associate Professor of Oncology, Oncology Center, Johns Hopkins University, 418N Bond Street, Baltimore 21205, USA* [31.2]

J. G. AYRES BSc MD FRCP, *Consultant Chest Physician, Birmingham Heartlands Hospital, Birmingham B9 5SS* [2]

A. E. BENDER, PhD DSc (Hon), *Emeritus Professor of Nutrition, 2 Willow Vale, Fetcham, Leatherhead, Surrey KT22 9TE* [16]

D. BURNETT PhD FRCPath, *The Liver Research Laboratories, Queen Elizabeth Hospital, Edgbaston, Birmingham B15 2TH* [4]

C. K. CAMPBELL BSc MSc PhD, *Deputy Head, Mycology Reference Unit, Public Health Laboratory, Myrtle Road, Kingsdown, Bristol BS2 8EL* [9]

R. CRAMB, MB ChB MSc MRCPath, *Consultant Chemical Pathologist, Department of Clinical Biochemistry, Queen Elizabeth Medical Centre, Edgbaston, Birmingham B15 2TH* [22, 24.1]

C. B. CROCKER MRCGP, *General Practitioner, The Surgery, 30, Westfield Road, Birmingham, B27 7TL* [19.3, 31.3]

J. CROCKER MD MRCPath, *Consultant Histopathologist, Department of Histopathology, Birmingham Heartlands Hospital, Bordesley Green East, Birmingham B9 5ST* [3]

C. DAVENPORT PhD, *Research Assistant in Immunology, Medical School, Queen's Medical Centre, Nottingham NG7 2UH* [13]

P. G. de TAKATS, PhD MRCP, *CRC Institute for Cancer Studies, Clinical Research Block, Queen Elizabeth Hospital, Edgbaston, Birmingham B15 2TH* [30]

D. EDGAR BSc MRCP DipRCPath, *Department of Immunology, Queen's Medical Centre, Nottingham NG7 2UH* [12, 15.2]

A. HADDON, MB ChB, *Registrar in Chemical Pathology, Department of Clinical Biochemistry, Queen Elizabeth Hospital, Edgbaston, Birmingham B15 2TH* [22]

J. M. JEWSBURY PhD, *29 Melloncroft Drive, Caldy, Wirral, Merseyside L48 2JA* [10]

E. M. JOHNSON BSc PhD, *Clinical Scientist, Mycology Reference Unit, Public Health Laboratory, Myrtle Road, Kingsdown, Bristol BS2 8EL* [9]

D. KILLINGTON PhD, *Senior Lecturer in Microbiology, Microbiology Department, Leeds University, Leeds LST 9JT* [8]

J. R. KING BSc MB ChB LRSC, MRCPsych, *Consultant Psychiatrist, N. E. Worcestershire Community Healthcare, Hill Crest, Quinneys Lane, Redditch, Worcestershire, B98 7WG* [34.1]

P. R. KIRK MSc DPhil, *Head, Biomedical Science Human Biology Division, School of Health Sciences, University of Wolverhampton, 62–68 Lichfield Street, Wolverhampton WV1 1DJ* [5]

H. LEDERMAN MD PhD, *Associate Professor of Paediatrics, Department of Paediatrics, School of Medicine, CMSC 1103, Johns Hopkins Hospital, Baltimore 21205, USA* [14]

List of Contributors

D. MAXTON MD MB BS MRCP, *Consultant Physician and Gastroenterologist, Department of Gastroenterology, Royal Shrewsbury Hospital, Mytton Oak Road, Shrewsbury, Shropshire SY3 8XF* [18, 19.1, 19.2]

F. McDONALD PhD, *Principal Molecular Geneticist, DNA Laboratories, West Midlands Regional Genetics Service, Birmingham Heartlands Hospital, Birmingham, B9 5SS* [25, 27.1]

P. G. MURRAY MSc FIBMS, *Senior Lecturer in Biomedical Science, University of Wolverhampton, 62–68 Lichfield Street, Wolverhampton, WV1 1DJ* [1, 6, 8, 15.1, 28, 29]

D. H. MYERS BM MRCP FRCPsych FRCPE, *Consultant Psychiatrist, Shropshire's Mental Health Trust, Bicton Heath, Shrewsbury SY3 8XF* [33, 34.2]

C. NYE MB ChB MRCPath, *Consultant Microbiologist, Birmingham Heartlands Hospital, Bordesley Green East, Birmingham B9 5ST* [7]

J. PALEFSKY, MD PhD, *Assistant Professor, Department of Laboratory Medicine, University of California, San Francisco, USA* [11.2]

S. A. PERERA, MSc PhD, *Senior Lecturer in Biomedical Science, School of Health Sciences, University of Wolverhampton, 62–68 Lichfield Street, Wolverhampton WV1 1DJ* [6]

J. D. PHILLIPS, BSc PhD FIBMS, *Senior Lecturer in Biomedical Science, School of Health Sciences, University of Wolverhampton, 62–68 Lichfield Street, Wolverhampton WV1 1DJ* [1, 17, 19.1, 19.2, 20, 21, 31.1, 32]

P. B. RYLANCE BSc MB MRCP, *Consultant Physician, The Renal Unit, New Cross Hospital, Wednesfield Road, Wolverhampton WV10 0QP* [23, 24.1, 24.2]

B. M. SINGH, MD MRCP, *Consultant in Diabetes and Endocrinology Wolverhampton Diabetes Centre, New Cross Hospital, Wolverhampton WV10 8QP* [24.3]

M. J. TARLOW MB MSc FRCP, *Senior Lecturer in Paediatrics & Child Health, Birmingham Heartlands Hospital, Bordesley Green East, Birmingham B9 5ST* [11.1]

I. TODD PhD, *Lecturer in Immunology, Medical School, Queen's Medical Centre, Nottingham NG7 2UH* [13]

J. J. WATERS BSc PhD DipRCPath, *Principal Cytogeneticist, Regional Cytogenetics Laboratory, West Midlands Genetics Service, Birmingham Heartlands Hospital, Birmingham B9 5SS* [26, 27.2]

S. M. WHEELEY MSc MBBS, *Department of Respiratory Medicine, Birmingham Heartlands Hospital, Bordesley Green East, Birmingham B9 5SS* [2]

L. S. YOUNG PhD MRCPath, *Professor of Cancer Biology, CRC Institute for Cancer Studies, Cancer Research Campaign Laboratories, University of Birmingham, Birmingham B15 2TT* [30]

Preface

The Biology of Disease aims to present the basic principles of disease processes in a form readily accessible to students trying to assimilate large volumes of information from a variety of sources. In conceiving this book, we recognized a need for a succinct volume that would give a broad yet sufficiently detailed account of the biology of disease. Acknowledging the expertise which lies in our medical and scientific colleagues (some working in education, some in research and others in clinical practice), we have drawn upon the experience and enthusiasm of a wide range of authoritative contributors. We feel that the book has benefited from this diversity of expertise, which has enabled us to cover many of the important topics in medicine today. Equally importantly, we were keen to adopt an accessible style of presentation and a common writing style, and we are grateful to all our contributors for their help in enabling us to achieve this aim.

From the outset, we felt it important to integrate the biological principles of disease processes with their clinical manifestations—the signs and symptoms which enable a diagnosis to be made. We have achieved this by ensuring that the principal chapters are clinically relevant and, where possible, that they bridge any gap between the biological and clinical features of disease. In addition, we have included clinical case studies in all the major sections of the book, each of which emphasizes the link between our current understanding of the basic science of the relevant condition and its clinical presentation. There is inevitable overlap and integration of topics in different sections of the book, so we have indicated cross-references where appropriate.

We anticipate that this book will be of use to a wide range of readers, particularly medical students approaching their clinical studies, students of clinical and biomedical sciences, and students of other paramedical subjects. Sections of the book cover major areas of clinical science including epidemiology, immunology, infection, disorders of the blood, genetic diseases, oncology and mental health. Each section is complete in itself, enabling the book to be used selectively for the study of individual topics. We have tried to provide a succinct, yet comprehensive, overview of each topic and we hope that readers will be stimulated to seek out further, more detailed information. For this reason each chapter concludes with key points and suggestions for further reading.

We are most grateful to all our contributors whose cooperation and expertise has been invaluable in achieving the aims of the book. We also thank our Associate Editor, John Crocker, for his help and guidance in the early stages of the editing process. Finally, we wish to acknowledge the support of our colleagues in the School of Health Sciences, of the editorial team at Blackwell Science and not least, that of our respective families, all of whom have helped us to nurture this venture to fruition.

Jonathan Phillips
Paul Murray

Part 1
Introduction

The Nature of Disease

Definitions of health and disease

Health and disease are difficult concepts to define. Health is often defined as the absence of disease and an individual may be in good health if there are no impediments to his functioning or survival. The World Health Organisation (WHO) defines health as '. . . a state of complete physical, mental and social well being and not merely the absence of disease or infirmity'. This latter definition is obviously much broader and it is likely that most of us would not be considered 'healthy' on the basis of these criteria.

Nevertheless, the WHO definition is useful since it acknowledges the importance of psychological and social well being in the maintenance of health. Perhaps a more realistic definition considers that health is a condition or quality of the human organism which expresses adequate functioning under given genetic and environmental conditions. This definition allows room for manoeuvre since it implies that an individual may be considered healthy even if compromised in some way. An example here would be an individual with Down's syndrome who might well be considered healthy under the latter definition but not under the former.

Implicit in many of these definitions of health is the concept that efficient performance of bodily functions takes place in the face of a wide range of changing environmental conditions. Health in this context may be regarded as an expression of adaptability and disease a failure thereof. Disease can also be defined as a pattern of responses to some form of insult or injury resulting in disturbed function and/or structural alteration.

Concepts of normality

Individuals who are free from disease are often described as being 'normal'. It is important to recognize that normality does not always indicate health but is merely an indication of the frequency of a given condition in a defined population. Some diseases occur with such frequency in the population that they might be considered to be normal e.g. dental caries. If we examine the distribution of an indicator of health, let us say blood haemoglobin levels (Fig. 1.1), we can see that they *usually* follow a *normal distribution* in the population. Applying limits to the distribution curve produces two cut off points. Below and above these points haemoglobin levels may be considered abnormal. However, the borderline between the normal and abnormal is not so clear cut. For instance, a value within the normal range may be considered pathological in a particular individual or under certain circumstances. Likewise, a small percentage of individuals falling within the abnormal zones will remain healthy and suffer no consequences as a result of their slightly 'abnormal' haemoglobin values. Furthermore, in females the haemoglobin concentration tends to be lower than in males. Taking another example, that of blood cholesterol concentration, the normal distribution in Western countries may not reflect ideal levels for the maintenance of health. For this reason we prefer the term *reference range* instead of *normal range* when defining the desired level of an analyte.

The onset of disease

It can be difficult to be precise about the transition from health to disease because pathological

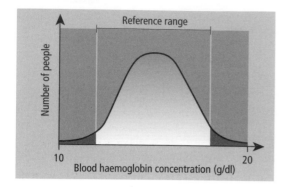

Fig. 1.1 Normal distribution of blood haemoglobin concentrations in the UK population. Application of limits gives a reference range outside which haemoglobin levels may be considered abnormal.

changes with the potential to cause disease are present in many apparently healthy people. For example, early atheromatous (fatty) deposits (see Chapter 22) are present in the arteries of a substantial proportion of symptom-free middle-aged adults in Western societies, increasing their risk of cardiovascular disease (diseases of the heart and blood vessels). Most patients with coronary heart disease would date the onset of their illness from the first clinical manifestation (for example chest pain), rather than from the blood lipid changes or hypertension (increased blood pressure) which may have begun many years before and which predisposed them to heart disease.

Causes of disease

A myriad of agents and stimuli are implicated in the causation (*aetiology*) of human disease. In the majority of cases it is not possible to discover a single causative agent which always causes disease when present. For example, exposure to the micro-organism *Mycobacterium tuberculosis* does not invariably result in tuberculosis. A variety of other factors are also important for establishment of infection, including the status of the host immune system and the size of the infective dose. However, tuberculosis cannot occur in the absence of the organism. Exposure to *M. tuberculosis*

is therefore the necessary causal factor and the other factors may be defined as subsidiary causal factors.

Tuberculosis represents an example of a disease for which the causal factors involved are well established. For other diseases, identification of the causal factors has proved more difficult and the search for these factors continues to represent a significant challenge to medical science. Often the initial search for a causal factor begins by the examination of the patterns of disease within human populations. This is *epidemiology* and is the subject of Chapter 2. Epidemiological studies often involve analysis of mortality and morbidity rates.

Types of aetiological factors

There is a widespread perception that a disease is an entity that is able to attack humans from the outside rather than a failure of adaptive responses from within. In fact, the types of aetiological factors implicated in disease may be broadly divided into *endogenous* factors (those which create a disturbance or imbalance from within) and *exogenous* factors (factors which threaten existence from the outside). Chromosome abnormalities giving rise to genetic disorders may be regarded as endogenous factors, whereas micro-organisms are good examples of exogenous aetiological agents. However, there is overlap between these two groups. For example, some chromosome abnormalities have been shown to be the result of parental exposure to mutagens in the environment e.g. ionizing radiation. Some genetic disorders then, may ultimately be attributed to exposure to exogenous factors.

Classification of disease

Diseases are either classified on the basis of the outward signs produced by disease (manifestations) or on the existence of a common aetiological agent. Most diseases are classified on manifestational criteria irrespective of the causative agents involved. Thus, a number of causal factors are implicated in the development of various types of carcinoma of the lung including cigarette smoke, asbestos, coal smoke and other atmospheric pollutants, but patients with the manifestations of lung cancer are often grouped together irrespective of the involvement of one or more of these agents. On the other hand, disease caused by *M. tuberculosis* may produce different clinical manifestations in different individuals, yet all are classified as forms of tuberculosis.

Classification of disease on the basis of shared aetiology may follow identification of a new and important aetiological agent, particularly if this offers promise of major therapeutic or preventive advantage. However, this is not always so. The identification of cigarette smoke as the most important cause of lung cancer, for example, did not promote a revision of the classification of lung cancer or of other diseases known to be associated with smoking (e.g. emphysema, bronchitis, atherosclerosis).

The classification of disease into discrete entities enables patients to be assigned to specific groups. The patient may then be treated in a similar fashion to other patients assigned previously to the same group, thus, at least in theory, improving the clinical outcome based on past experience. However, this rather simplistic statement does not acknowledge the view that the development of disease, its progression and response to treatment should be regarded as unique to the individual.

Identifying disease

We have seen how diseases are classified but have not yet considered how a particular set of features is first designated as a disease state. Doctors use *signs* (what the doctor sees or feels when carrying out a physical examination), *symptoms* (what the patient complains of) and a range of laboratory and clinical tests to determine whether a patient has a disease. Thorough history-taking will determine whether there has been exposure to any potential aetiological agents. The existence of certain predisposing conditions may make the develop-

ment of a disease more likely. Examples of these risk factors include certain genetic disorders, lifestyle, psychological and personality profile, age and environmental factors such as climate and pollution.

One of the early steps in identifying a disease is to establish a range of diagnostic possibilities from which the eventual diagnosis will be selected. The final diagnosis may be established shortly after clinical presentation, perhaps only after extensive use of laboratory and clinical tests, or may never be identified during the lifetime of the patient. It must be remembered that disease is a dynamic process and the indicators of disease may vary as the disease progresses. Furthermore, in some patients different diseases may co-exist, confusing the diagnostic process.

Prognosis is the likely future for the patient in terms of length and quality of life. Prognosis depends on many factors, including the stage the disease has reached and the likely impact of therapy. Once a disease has been identified, treatment aimed at cure or relief of symptoms is usually initiated. Patients may be cured of the disease, enter *remission* (a symptom free period) from which they may either *relapse* (symptoms of disease return) or be cured. Some diseases are not amenable to cure, but can be controlled by the administration of drugs, hormones or by surgery. Some patients with advanced disease may receive palliative treatment only.

Mechanisms of disease

Understanding the way in which disease begins and develops is the major focus of research within the medical sciences. The assumption is made that an understanding of the biology of disease will contribute to an improvement in health care, both in terms of the prevention of disease and its treatment. In many cases this has proved to be satisfyingly correct. For example, the recognition that type I diabetes mellitus results from damage to insulin-secreting cells in the pancreas led to the development of insulin replacement therapy. However, an understanding of the biology of many important diseases (e.g. cancer) is only beginning to emerge and for the most part this has not yet contributed greatly to a decline in mortality rates.

The aim of this book is to instil an appreciation of the biological basis of disease. It does not attempt to be a comprehensive textbook of pathology, but seeks to draw attention to the important biological features resulting in disturbed homeostasis. Subsequent chapters in this book address the fundamental biological aspects of important groups of human disease, while case studies consider the clinical aspects of selected disease states relating these, where possible, to their underlying biology.

Principles of Epidemiology

Introduction

Epidemiology is the study of patterns of disease occurrence in relation to possible causal factors. Once a pattern has been observed, it is the task of the epidemiologist to establish whether or not the factors implicated are truly causal.

Epidemiological terms and measures

Exposure: this defines factors to which individuals in a population may be exposed, which may affect a disease process either adversely (e.g. cigarette smoke) or beneficially (e.g. vaccine).

Outcome: this defines the resulting disease (or disease free) state in the population at the termination of the study.

Prevalence: this is the proportion of a population with a particular condition at a specific time. For example, in a survey in the USA, 310 individuals (the numerator) were found to have cataracts out of a population of 2477 (the denominator).

Thus prevalence $= \dfrac{310}{2477} \times 100 = 12.5\%$

Risk: this is the likelihood of an individual in a population having a disease. The risk of having a disease can be compared between sub-groups in the population, for example, those exposed to a potential causal factor and those not exposed. Data on risks in such comparative groups are classically summarized in a '2 by 2' table (Table 2.1):

Table 2.1 Assessment of risk

	Exposure		
Disease	Yes (+)	No (−)	**Totals**
Yes (+)	a	b	m
No (−)	c	d	n
Totals	p	q	T

The overall numbers of those with the disease are $a + b = m$; the numbers of those exposed are $a + c = p$; the numbers of those exposed with the disease $= a$; the numbers of those not exposed and disease free $= d$.

Consequently: the risk of developing disease in those exposed is $a/p = R1$; the risk of developing disease in those not exposed is $b/q = R2$.

The *risk ratio* or *relative risk* expressed as $R1/R2$ then gives a measure of the strength of the effect of an exposure on the development of a disease.

A *relative risk* of 1.0 means there is no increased risk from exposure whereas a *relative risk* of 6.0 denotes a six-fold risk of developing disease if exposed. On the other hand, the *risk difference* or *attributable risk*, R1−R2 is a better guide to the overall impact of an exposure on a population and has important public health implications.

Incidence: this term refers to the numbers of new events or cases of disease that develop over a specified span of time. Examples of incidence rates are mortality rates, rates of hospital admission and attendance rates at family doctor surgeries. Rates calculated for a total population are called *crude rates*. These can be refined for subject characteristics and expressed as age-, sex- or race-specific rates. A further refinement to facilitate comparison between populations is the *standardized mortality/morbidity rate* (SMR) which takes into account demographic structure.

Epidemiological studies

Epidemiological studies can be divided into two types: descriptive and analytical.

Descriptive studies

These are fundamental in defining the incidence and/or prevalence of disease in a population. The questions always to be asked are: *who* is affected and *when* and *where* they are affected. When it is not possible to study an entire population *cross-sectional surveys* may be carried out, in which case sampling methods must be used. These are designed to produce statistical results which will be representative of the entire population. Such studies are economical in terms of time and expense, but do not assist in unravelling the relationship between cause and effect, as information on both is gathered at the same time.

Analytical studies

Once a disease pattern has been described, analytical studies are required to determine causation. The types of analytical study chosen to address a particular problem will often depend on such logistical considerations as time, money and access to the required information. The commonly used analytical study types are:

Case control studies: cases (affected individuals) are identified along with controls (individuals unaffected by the disease). Exposure to potential disease causes can then be compared between the two groups. Such studies are particularly useful for rare conditions and are efficient in terms of time and cost.

Cohort studies: specific populations with defined characteristics (e.g. children born in the same calendar year, i.e. a birth cohort) are followed through time, often for years. Such studies are expensive and take a long time to produce a result but allow examination of the temporal relationship between exposure and disease. They are also useful in studying the relationship between rare exposures and disease and can take into consideration the effects of multiple exposures.

Intervention studies: in an intervention study, a positive step is taken to eliminate or control exposure to a supposed causal agent. Statistical analysis can then be used to demonstrate any improvement in outcome when the exposure (or causal agent) is removed. The intervention study is often the final stage in testing a hypothesis and proving a causal link. A special application of the intervention study using epidemiological principles is the clinical trial where affected individuals are allocated randomly to one of two (or more) treatment regimes to determine which is more beneficial.

Statistical associations

When a statistically significant association is shown between an exposure ('cause') and an outcome ('effect') it does not necessarily mean that there is a true cause and effect relationship. For example, in the summer months, sales of ice cream rise as does the incidence of sunburn. These two can be shown to be associated statistically and yet, of course, it would be quite ridiculous to consider the sale of ice cream as a cause of sunburn! If a statistical association is found, the following three factors must be considered before accepting that the association is truly brought about by 'cause and effect'.

Chance

A statistical association may arise by *chance*, i.e., a purely fortuitous coincidence. For instance, when trying to determine the frequency with which a disease occurs in a community, to be absolutely sure of the true rate, every individual would need to be assessed over a period of time. This is often not possible and so a sample of the population is studied. The technique used for choosing the sample should ensure that this smaller group is representative of the overall population. However, because of random variation there is a possibility that the characteristics of the sample will vary slightly from the overall population and give misleading results. Good study design should ensure that the possibility of chance affecting the results will be kept to a minimum.

The contribution of *chance* to an association can be estimated by a test of statistical significance (e.g. Student's *t* test or the chi square test). Detailed discussion of these tests will be found in any standard statistical textbook. These tests are designed to produce a *probability value* (P), a measure of the likelihood that an observed effect/association could have occurred by chance alone. *P* values are given as a probability, i.e., $P = 0.05$ means that there is a 5% (or 1 : 20) likelihood of an association occurring by chance. This 5% level is usually interpreted as the cut off point for achieving statistical significance.

When working with a statistical result from a sample, the range within which the true value for the whole population is likely to fall can be calculated. The upper and lower levels of this range are known as *confidence intervals*. The larger the sample size, the narrower the confidence intervals.

Bias

If there is a bias in the way a study is designed or in the way in which it is carried out, a systematic or regularly repeated error can be introduced and cause an apparent statistical association when findings are analysed.

Selection bias: this occurs where the criteria used for selection of study subjects lead to the sample under study being poorly representative of the total population. Different characteristics may be either over-, or under- represented.

Observation bias: this occurs either when data are acquired in a biased fashion by the investigator (observer bias) or given in a biased manner by the patient as he or she recalls details of his or her illness (recall bias). For example, a study in South Africa exploring the health effect of air pollution showed that those subjects who believed that air pollution was detrimental to health were more likely to report respiratory symptoms than those who had no strong feelings on the subject.

Confounding

Confounding occurs when the apparent statistical association between the exposure and outcome is attributable to an entirely different exposure, known as the *confounder*.

The confounder is independently associated with both the exposure under study and the outcome. In the previous example of ice cream sales and sunburn, the confounding factor is sunny weather which independently causes both sunburn and a rise in ice cream sales.

Cause and effect

When chance, bias and confounding have been ruled out as explanations of a statistical association, then the possibility that the association is truly causal must be considered further. Bradford-Hill (1965) identified nine criteria which act as useful guidelines in this regard.

1 Strength: the strength of the association can be measured by the size of the relative risk. For example, regular smokers of cigarettes have a nine–10-fold increase in risk of lung cancer compared to non-smokers, indicating a strong association.

2 Consistency: an association is more likely to be causal if differently designed studies by different workers from different centres produce the same results.

3 Specificity: this is present if the disease under study is seen almost uniquely in those exposed to a particular causal factor.

4 Temporality: the time sequence must be appropriate, i.e., the exposure to the 'cause' must always precede the onset of disease.

5 Biological gradient: this is otherwise known as the dose – response effect. For example, there is a linear rise in the risk of dying from lung cancer with increasing exposure to cigarette smoke. The risk is 0.07 per 1000 non-smokers, increasing through light and medium smokers to a risk of 3.15 per 1000 in men smoking 35 or more cigarettes per day.

6 Biological plausibility: it is easier to accept an association as causal if there is a plausible mechanism to explain the effect in the light of scientific knowledge at the time.

7 Coherence: the association should not conflict with the generally known and accepted facts of the natural history and biology of the disease.

8 Experiment: if removing or reducing exposure leads to a reduction in, or disappearance of, the disease, this gives strong support for an association being causal.

9 Analogy: if there is already an established pattern of cause and effect in a specific situation. For example, fetal damage arising from maternal use of thalidomide during pregnancy is well-described. Therefore, damage arising from other drugs administered during pregnancy may be more readily recognized.

None of these criteria, except the temporal relationship between cause and effect, should be regarded as an absolute requirement.

A worked example

In Barcelona in the 1980s on a number of isolated days there were unprecedented numbers of hospital admissions for acute asthma (Fig. 2.1). Investigators considered the possibility of an airborne cause for these 'epidemic days' and were suspicious that emissions from the industrial area to the west of the city might be the cause.

The first step in the investigation was a descriptive study mapping the distribution of the attacks (Fig. 2.2). The attacks were seen not to cluster round the industrial area as suspected but round

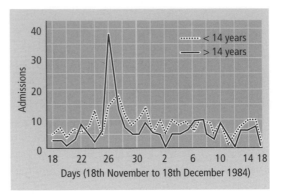

Fig. 2.1 Daily number of adult and children asthma emergency room admissions from November 18 to December 18, 1984. From Anto *et al.* (1989) © by the Lancet Ltd, 1989.

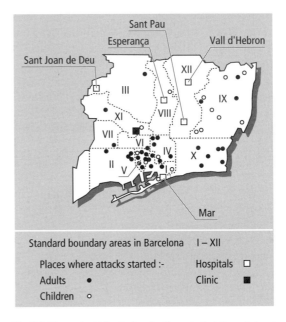

Fig. 2.2 Places at which attacks of asthma started. From Anto *et al.* (1989) © by The Lancet Ltd, 1989.

the docks. In the next stage the investigators considered what goods were being unloaded on epidemic and non-epidemic days. Initial analysis pointed to two types of goods; soya bean products and wheat, being unloaded significantly more frequently on epidemic days. Statistical analysis using a 2 × 2 table (Table 2.2) showed that an epidemic day *never* occurred when soya products were *not* being handled. The relative risk is thus unquantifiably high, indicating a very strong association. The epidemics were *temporally* related to soya bean unloading; the mechanism was *biologically plausible* and an *analogous* situation already existed as castor bean dust was known to be a potent aero-allergen.

A case control study was undertaken and this confirmed the hypothesis that patients admitted with acute asthma on epidemic days were more likely to show evidence of allergy to soya than patients admitted with asthma on non-epidemic days.

Soya had been unloaded into two dockside silos, one with and one without a cap. When dust released from the uncapped silo was effectively eliminated by the addition of a cap (in epidemiological terms an *intervention* to remove an *exposure*) no further epidemic days occurred (Table 2.3), providing ultimate proof of a causal relationship.

Table 2.2 Unloading of soya bean on epidemic and non-epidemic days. Figures are given as numbers of days

SOYA	Unloading	Not unloading	Total
Epidemic days	13	0	13
Non-epidemic days	262	468	730
Totals	275	468	743

The relative risk of an epidemic day occurring when soya was being unloaded is unquantifiably high.

Table 2.3 Effect of intervention on soya bean epidemic asthma (only days on which soya bean was unloaded are included)

	Total days	Days with high no. of asthma admission	Epidemic days	Admissions to intensive care/day
Before cap installation	167	29	18	0.26 ± 0.9
After cap installation	133	6	0	0.01 ± 0.12
P value		<0.001	<0.001	<0.001

Summary

For the investigation of the influence of various factors on the causation of disease, rigorous, statistical epidemiological analysis is essential. This process may be beset by numerous difficulties but can reveal important information about disease aetiology.

Key points

1 Epidemiology is the study of patterns of disease occurrence.
2 A variety of epidemiological approaches may be employed. These include descriptive and analytical studies.
3 Descriptive studies are able to help establish the incidence and/or prevalence of a disease within a population.
4 Analytical epidemiological studies give information about the importance of causal factors. An intervention study is a special type of analytical study in which a positive step is taken to eliminate exposure to a potential causal agent. Failure to develop the disease after such intervention suggests a causal link.
5 Sophisticated statistical techniques are often required to analyse the results of epidemiological studies. Care is required in the interpretation of statistical associations since these do not necessarily indicate a true cause and effect relationship.

Further reading

Hennekens C.H. & Bury J.E. (1987) In *Epidemiology in Medicine*, 1st edn., ed. Mayrent S.L. Little, Brown, Boston.

References

Anto J.M., Sunyer J., Rodriguez-Roisin R., Suarez-Cervera M. & Vazquez L. (1989) Community outbreaks of asthma associated with inhalation of soyabean dust. *New Engl. J. Med.* **320**, 1097–1102.
Bradford Hill A. (1965) The environment and disease: association of causation? *Proc. Roy. Soc. Med.* **58**, 295–300.

Part 2
Host Responses to Injury

Cell Injury and Death

Introduction

The ultimate form of response to noxious or harmful stimuli is death of the affected cell; however, before this can occur, various changes take place in the cell and these are known collectively as 'cell injury'. The morphological and biochemical features of cell injury are given below, together with an account of their causes and mechanisms. Many agents and stimuli can lead to cell damage; these include ionising radiation, toxins and chemicals, heat and cold, immune and inflammatory attack and infectious agents.

The morphology of cell injury

The nucleus

Injured nuclei commonly shrink and become irregular in outline and with more severe insult may swell and disrupt. In response to the osmotic damage which affects the endoplasmic reticulum, the nuclear envelope (which is in continuity with the endoplasmic reticulum) separates and forms dilated areas (*cisternae*). When this occurs, with eventual nuclear dissolution, the damage is irreversible. Inclusions can also form in the injured nucleus; these include portions of cytoplasmic organelles, glycogen, viral particles and deposits of heavy metals. Also, the nucleoli themselves may become disorganized, with separation of the fibrillar centres from the outer nucleolar components.

The cytoplasm

The changes observed in the cytoplasm in cell injury are often encountered earlier and may be more subtle than those in the nucleus.

The *cell surface* is, of course, the first part of the cell to encounter any noxious stimulus; accordingly, superficial structures such as microvilli and cilia become swollen or even lost early in cell damage. Furthermore, the cell membrane may exhibit *'blebs'* and, ultimately, severe defects and disruption. Cell–cell relationships are also affected. For example, ciliate cells may lose their continuity and eventually even change the commitment of their differentiation, for example to squamous cells.

Mitochondria exhibit some of the earliest and most subtle changes in response to cell abuse. Initially, the mitochondria show an increase in electron density and an increase in size. This is associated with impairment of the cation pump, as a result of defective oxidative metabolism. Calcium-rich bodies may accumulate and the mitochondria may even burst. In addition, a common change lies in alteration to or disruption of the mitochondrial cristae.

The *Golgi complex* is affected by many chemical substances, notably chemotherapeutic agents such as puromycin and cycloheximide, which result in diminution of the cisternae. Nutritional deficiency has a similar effect. Conversely, certain agents can lead to an increase in sizes of the cisternae.

The *endoplasmic reticulum* (ER) is, not surprisingly, a highly susceptible target for many agents inducing cell injury. The surface area of the ER is relatively enormous and the complex runs through most of the cytoplasm. Thus, most noxious agents induce cisternal swelling, especially if protein accumulates within the cell. Furthermore, the ribosomes may detach from the rough ER and polyribosomes may disaggregate, indicating disordered protein synthesis. Proliferation can also occur in the ER in some circumstances, with the formation of large concentric lamellar bodies.

Lysosomes are an essential part of the cell injury process, by virtue of their involvement in phagocytosis. Accordingly, they are vulnerable to damage by material they are involved in processing. Lysosomes play an essential role in the removal of whole eukaryotic cells or their fragments (for example in apoptosis) as well as microbial agents. Lysosomal enzymes released from injured cells can lead to further tissue damage.

Peroxisomes may increase or decrease in relation to numerous substances, notably those which interfere with oxidative and fat metabolism. *Cytoskeletal elements*, including microfilaments and microtubules are rather difficult to study as they are structurally labile. At the electron microscope level, therefore, little is understood of the pathological changes in these elements, beyond their involvement in the cell cycle. Disorganization has, however, been observed in certain degenerations of neurones and muscle cells.

Cytoplasmic inclusions

A large range of inorganic or organic inclusions can be deposited in the cytoplasm, in a diffuse series of conditions. These may have morphological appearances which are distinctive at the light or electron microscope level. Many are lysosomal, as described above. Others are outlined in Table 3.1.

Table 3.1 Cytoplasmic inclusions in disease

	Substance	Disease or cause
Inorganic inclusions	Silica	Silicosis
	Asbestos	Asbestosis
	Barium sulphate	Radiological contrast medium
	Iron compounds including ferritin	Haemochromatosis
	Copper compounds	Wilson's disease
	Calcium compounds	Calcification
	Carbon	Anthracosis
Protein inclusions	Immunoglobulin	Overactive or malignant plasma cells
	α_1–Antitrypsin	α_1–Antitrypsin deficiency
Lipid inclusions	Triglyceride	Numerous, including alcoholic liver damage, myocardial ischaemia, fat necrosis and histiocytic neoplasms
Filament inclusions	Intermediate filaments	Mallory's (alcoholic) hyaline in liver
	Cytokeratin filaments	Crooke's hyaline in pituitary over-stimulation

Mechanisms of cell injury

A vast number of agents or stimuli can cause cell injury, yet most act in a fundamentally similar way at the biochemical level. Thus, cell membrane permeability is first affected, usually by damage to stabilizing processes such as synthesis of ATPase. Consequent upon this, water, Na^+ and Ca^{2+} ions flood into the cell and provoke further release of Ca^{2+} from organelles, notably the mitochondria and ER. This in turn stimulates the Na^+- and Ca^{2+}-dependent ATPases and thus the levels of ATP fall further, leading to activation of phosphofructokinase then pyruvate kinase with consequent build-up of pyruvate. With the resulting fall in pH, numerous enzyme activities become deranged and continuing biochemical and morphological disruptions ensue. A vicious cycle of injury can therefore follow.

Cell death

Two principal modes of cell death are now recognized, namely *necrosis* and *apoptosis*. Both may follow cell injury but the nature of the two types of death are quite different.

Cell necrosis

The changes in cells undergoing necrosis are essentially a continuation of those described above, in cell injury. However, they are, of course, more profound and are irreversible. It has thus been proposed that there is a 'point of no return', beyond which the process of cell injury cannot be revoked. While moderate mitochondrial swelling, the formation of cell surface 'blebs' and ribosomal disaggregation appear to be reversible, there are certain changes which will inevitably lead to cell necrosis. These include extreme 'blebbing' at the cell surface, together with much greater dilation of the mitochondria ('high amplitude swelling') and the formation of electron dense areas in the mitochondrial matrix. Eventually, there is cell membrane disruption, dissolution of organelles, including the nucleus, and lysosomal degeneration with activation of an inflammatory response. The latter is probably induced by complement-activation by fractions from mitochondria and by leukotrienes formed by lipid peroxidation (see Chapter 4).

Apoptosis

Apoptosis or 'programmed cell death' has been described for over 20 years but only comparatively recently has its fundamental importance been recognized. It is known to be central to many developmental processes where cells have to be lost as part of the organization of tissues or organs. Examples lie in the loss of tadpole tails, the loss of interdigital webs, the control of B lymphocyte proliferation and the removal of excess cells in nervous system maturation.

In pathological terms, apoptosis is fundamental to the process of atrophy, where cells are lost from mature organs or tissues as a result of endocrine or physical means. For example, hormones may suppress target glands by this route and surgical ligation of the draining ducts of, for example, the pancreas can lead to cell loss by apoptosis.

One great 'advantage' of apoptosis versus necrosis is that there is no induction of acute inflammation and thus further tissue damage is not incurred. This is of particular importance in the removal of neutrophils, whose lysosomal enzymes could continue to cause tissue disruption if left unchecked. Apoptosis also appears to be a major mechanism by which malignant cells are removed and imbalances between apoptotic and mitotic rates could lead to tumour progression or regression. The observation that some chemotherapeutic drugs used for treating cancer can act by inducing apoptosis may be of great therapeutic importance and estimates of apoptotic rates may be of value in assessing the efficacy of therapeutic regimes.

The morphological changes accompanying apoptosis are quite different to those seen in necrosis. First, there is loss of cell–cell adhesion and *in vitro* the affected cells 'float' above their normal counterparts. The cells also become rounded and smaller, sometimes with lobulation, although some organelles, including mitochondria, remain intact. This shrinkage results from loss of Na^+ and water. The nuclear chromatin condenses to form 'half-moon'-shaped structures just within the nuclear membrane (Fig. 3.1) and the nucleoli appear disorganized. The nucleus may also break up into multiple portions (Fig. 3.2). There is an increase in transglutaminase activity in the cell, leading to insolubilization of proteins, which form a 'shell' round the inner surface of the cell membrane. There is also a rise in Ca^{2+},

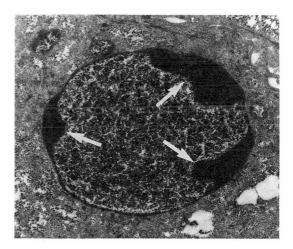

Fig. 3.1 An electron micrograph of an apoptotic nucleus, showing crescentic areas (arrowed) of condensed chromatin beneath the nuclear membrane. (Preparation by courtesy of Prof. George Antonokopolous, Department of Pathology, University of Athens.)

17

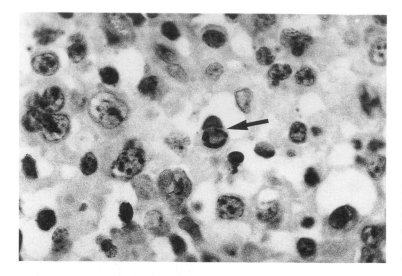

Fig. 3.2 An apoptotic cell (arrowed) in a malignant lymphoma (a cancer of lymphoid cells) exhibiting partitioning of the nucleus with dense, heavily stained chromatin. These appearances correspond well with those in Fig. 3.1.

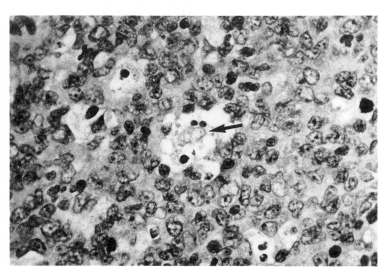

Fig. 3.3 A macrophage (arrowed) containing apoptotic debris, seen as dense, round bodies (so called 'tingible bodies'). This cell is in a secondary lymphoid follicle of a lymph node. The macrophage has phagocytosed a B lymphocyte deleted by apoptosis as part of the process of affinity maturation. (Chapter 5.) This is an example of physiological apoptosis.

Mg^{2+}-dependent endonuclease, which is responsible for the chromatin condensation and the nuclear fragmentation.

Finally, the apoptotic cells are rapidly recognized by macrophages, which phagocytose them, with the formation of apoptotic bodies within the cytoplasm of the consuming cells (Fig. 3.3), where they may be seen for up to about 9 hours following phagocytosis. The binding of macrophages to apoptotic cells appears to be mediated by the macrophage *vitronectin receptor*, which is also a cell adhesion molecule. Binding is also facilitated via a lectin-type receptor on the macrophage surface.

Apoptosis is a genetically regulated phenomenon and has been studied extensively in the nematode worm *Caenorhabditis elegans*, where mutations of certain gene loci are related to programmed cell death. Thus, mutations of the loci *ced-3* and *ced-4* lead to the blockage of the apoptosis known to be necessary during development of this organism. A further gene, *ced-9*, appears to have some control over the process and it appears that its gene product may either enable

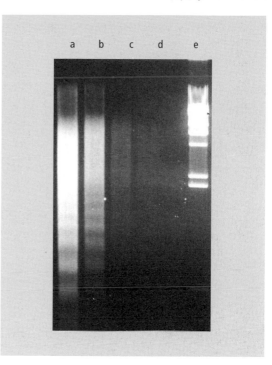

Fig. 3.4 A 'DNA ladder' showing the characteristic appearances of fragmented DNA from apoptotic cells. The vertical channels represent oligonucleotide fragments which have been spread by means of electrophoresis then visualized in ultraviolet light. Channels a and b show multiple bands ('ladders') representing fragmented DNA from apoptotic leukaemic cells. Channels c and d are from normal, control cells and show no such ladder effect and Channel e shows molecular weight markers. (Preparation by courtesy of Dr. David Burnett, Liver Research Laboratories, Queen Elizabeth Hospital, Birmingham.)

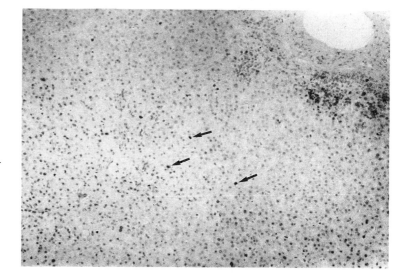

Fig. 3.5 A histological section of a rejecting liver transplant specimen under low power microscopy, showing several apoptotic cells (arrowed) stained by means of *in situ* end-labelling of fragmented DNA. (Preparation by courtesy of Dr Simon Afford, Liver Research Laboratories, Medical School, Birmingham.)

or disenable the apoptotic system. Furthermore, *ced-9* has been shown to possess homology with the human oncogene *bcl-2* (see also Chapter 29). This gene is one of several known to regulate apoptosis in human cells.

Techniques for the detection of apoptosis

The simplest method for the detection of apoptotic cells is observation of the characteristic bodies in tissue sections at either light or electron microscope level. *In vitro*, the apoptotic cells can be visualized by means of phase or interference contrast microscopy, where they can be seen to be rounded and lying above the cell monolayer. However, the 'gold standard' lies in the demonstration of 180–200 base pair oligonucleotide fragments resulting from nuclear damage. These fragments can be separated by gel electrophoresis and viewed under ultraviolet (UV) light, where they produce a characteristic 'ladder' effect (Fig. 3.4). This method is applied to cell extracts and has the disadvantage that it is not quantitative. Other approaches include the use of cell suspensions stained with fluorescent DNA-binding dyes which are then analysed in a DNA flow cytometer. A novel approach is that of DNA end-labelling, in which nucleotides, tagged with a suit-

Table 3.2 Differences between necrosis and apoptosis

	Necrosis	Apoptosis
Appearances	Large swathes of cells die	Individual cells die
	Cells (and nuclei) swollen	Nuclei and whole cells shrunken, rounded and darkly stained
	Plasma membranes disrupted	Chromatin condensed in demilunes and caps
Causes	Always pathological	Can be physiological, developmental or pathological
Inflammatory effect	Wide range of cells attracted	Only phagocytic macrophages attracted

able marker, are bound to the broken ends of DNA fragments in apoptotic cells (Fig. 3.5). This method has the advantage that it enables the enumeration of affected cells.

Differences between apoptosis and necrosis

The numerous differences between the two processes are outlined in Table 3.2. In summary, the principal difference at the level of the light microscope is that necrosis occurs in broad swathes

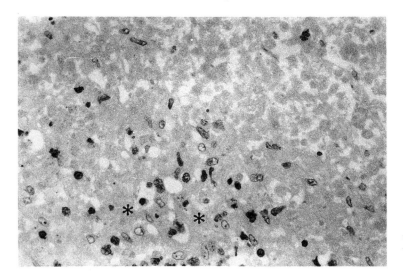

Fig. 3.6 A section of a malignant tumour, showing necrosis, with destruction of tissue architecture and a mixed inflammatory infiltrate (asterisks).

Key points

1 Cell injury can occur in many ways, under the influence of many agents, but may have similar morphological appearances.
2 Cell injury may or may not lead to cell death.
3 Cell death occurs in two forms: necrosis and apoptosis.
4 Necrosis affects swathes of cells, causes extensive cell loss and incurs a mixed inflammatory response.
5 Apoptosis is more specific than necrosis. It affects individual cells, has characteristic biochemical features and unlike necrosis, may occur as a normal physiological event.

(Fig. 3.6), affecting many contiguous cells, whereas in apoptosis, cell death occurs in individual cells which are often far apart. Furthermore, in necrosis there is a mixed inflammatory response but in apoptosis only macrophages appear to engulf apoptotic debris.

Summary

Cells and tissues can be damaged or killed in a large number of circumstances. These insults often have common pathways both morphologically and biochemically. Death of cells can occur in two main ways, namely by means of necrosis, where nutrients are deficient or where the cell is exposed to other stimuli causing cell damage, or by apoptosis ('programmed cell death'), where individual cells die and are consumed by macrophages.

Further reading

Arends M.J. & Wyllie A.H. (1991) Apoptosis: mechanisms and roles in pathology. *Int. Rev. Exp. Pathol.* **32**, 223–254.

Arends M.J. & Harrison D.J. (1994) Apoptosis: molecular aspects and pathological perspective. In *Molecular Biology in Histopathology*, ed. Crocker J. Wiley, Chichester, pp. 153–172.

Boobis A.R., Fawthrop D.J. & Davies D.S. (1994) Mechanisms of cell injury. In *Oxford Textbook of Pathology*, eds. McGee J.O.D., Issaacson P.G. & Wright N.A., pp. 181–191. Oxford University Press, Oxford.

Ghadially F.N. (1988) *Ultrastructural Pathology of the Cell and Matrix*. Butterworths, London.

Wyllie A.H. & Duvall E. (1992) Cell death. In *Oxford Textbook of Pathology*, eds. McGee J.O.D., Issaacson P.G. & Wright N.A., Oxford University Press, Oxford. pp. 141–157.

Inflammation

Introduction

Inflammation is the body's normal response to tissue injury, although it can sometimes lead to pathological tissue damage, including that seen in the *hypersensitivity reactions* (see Chapter 12). The 'purpose' of inflammation is:

1 to contain and control infection or injury;
2 to eliminate pathogens;
3 to initiate healing and tissue repair;

Inflammation represents a complex interaction of many components including blood vessels, tissue-derived *mediators*, white cells (leucocytes), fibroblasts, endothelial cells, epithelium, the coagulation and fibrinolytic systems, the kinin system and the complement system. Inflammation is characterized by local tissue signs, first described in about 30 BC by Celsus, which are *tumor* (swelling), *rubor* (redness), *calor* (heat) and *dolor* (pain). Systemic effects include fever, increased production of leucocytes by the bone marrow (*leucocytosis*) and increased synthesis of some plasma proteins by the liver. The purpose of this chapter is to summarize briefly the tissue changes associated with inflammation.

Tissue changes associated with inflammation

Inflammatory responses are classified as *acute* or *chronic* reactions, depending upon the histological and morphological features, although these are not always exclusive. The nature of the inflammatory response and its detailed appearance depend on the type of injury and the tissue involved. For instance, acute inflammation in the skin has a different macroscopic appearance to that in internal organs or mucous membranes. Chronic inflamma-

tion sometimes follows acute inflammation if, for instance, the acute response fails to eliminate a pathogen. However, chronic inflammation can occur without an acute response.

Acute inflammation

The acute inflammatory response occurs rapidly (minutes to hours) after injury or infection. Initially, there is dilatation of small blood vessels (*venules* and *arterioles*) with an increased local blood flow (*hyperaemia*), which then decreases or stops (*stasis*). The vessels become more permeable, leading to movement of blood plasma and platelets into the tissues (this is often referred to as a *serous exudate*), causing *oedema* (an excess of intercellular fluid in the tissues). A serous exudate below the epidermis is what causes a blister. Fibrinogen in the exudate is converted to fibrin, which is deposited and helps to localize tissue damage and control bleeding. Blood cells, especially *neutrophils*, migrate into the tissue. Sometimes, typically in response to *pyogenic* (pus-forming) bacterial infection, a *purulent exudate* or *pus* is formed, consisting of dead cells, neutrophils and bacteria. When large numbers of neutrophils are present the pus appears yellow or green, because of the presence of *myeloperoxidase*, a green-coloured protein in neutrophil granules. Localized pus accumulation causes an *abscess*.

Chronic inflammation

Chronic inflammation, lasting from weeks to years, may result from unresolved or recurrent acute inflammation; alternatively it may follow exposure to insoluble agents, foreign bodies, intracellular pathogens (e.g. *Mycobacterium tuberculosis* or *M. Leprae*) or unknown aetiological factors, as in rheumatoid arthritis (see Chapter 13). Whereas the cellular infiltrate in acute inflammation consists mainly of neutrophils, in chronic inflammation it is composed of a mixed cell population including macrophages. The macrophages are derived from blood monocytes which migrate to the site of inflammation, become activated (see below) and proliferate. Lymphocytes and plasma cells (Fig. 4.1a) are usually also present at the sites of chronic inflammation. In some forms of chronic inflammation (e.g. tuberculosis) *granulomas* are formed. These consist of collections of *epithelioid* (epithelial-like) macrophages (Fig. 4.1b) and lymphocytes, sometimes with much necrotic tissue. Often these necrotic granulomas have the appearance of 'soft cheese' and this has led to the alternative designation of 'caseating granulomas'. The epithelioid macrophages are sometimes very large, with multiple nuclei and are often referred to as *giant cells*.

Mediators of inflammatory reactions

The inflammatory process is initiated, maintained and controlled by many factors, which often have multiple and interacting effects.

Vasoactive amines

The early vasodilatation and increased vascular permeability of acute inflammation are caused largely by the release of *vasoactive amines* such as *histamine* and *5-hydroxytryptamine (serotonin)*. These are secreted by a variety of cells including platelets, mast cells and basophils.

Arachidonic acid metabolites

Arachidonic acid metabolites (Fig. 4.2) are pro-inflammatory factors which are expressed early, are short-lived and have a wide range of activities. Prostaglandins cause vasodilatation and pain; thromboxanes cause platelet aggregation and vasoconstriction (see Chapter 21). Leukotrienes increase vascular permeability and leukotriene B4 (LTB4) is a *chemotactic* and activating factor

for leucocytes, especially neutrophils (see below). *Chemotaxis* is the process by which cells, for example neutrophils, are attracted to sites of injury or infection by the release of a specific chemical agent.

Coagulation, fibrinolytic, kinin and complement systems

The serous exudate at an inflammatory site contains the components of these systems (see Fig. 4.3), which interact and co-activate through a number of initiation stimuli. Thus, activation of *Hageman factor (factor XII)* of the coagulation system by surface active agents such as damaged connective tissues or microbial components, results in the conversion of fibrinogen to fibrin through the activation of several proteinases including *thrombin* (see Chapter 21). Hageman factor also activates the *kinin* system, which results in the production of the vasoactive peptide *bradykinin* from the precursors *prekallikrein* and *kininogen*. The complement system, like the clotting/fibrinolytic and kinin systems, includes proteolytic enzyme activities in a *cascade* of events. Because all these systems rely on the proteolytic activation of latent pro-enzymes (*zymogens*), there is often cross-activation. In addition, they all contain positive feedback loops which amplify the activation of each system. Complement is activated through the *classical pathway* by antibodies attached to a target pathogen, or through the *alternate pathway* by contact with a variety of agents, including bacteria (Fig. 4.4). The products of complement activation are designed largely to eliminate pathogens and include the following.

1 The release of *anaphylatoxins*, the small peptides derived from the cleavage of complement factors C3, C4 and C5. These peptides initiate increased blood vessel permeability and smooth muscle contraction, probably by causing histamine release from mast cells. In addition, C5a is a chemotactic factor and an activator of neutrophils.

2 Production of *opsonins*. Some products of activated complement factors e.g. (C3b) on pathogen surfaces stimulate phagocytosis by effector

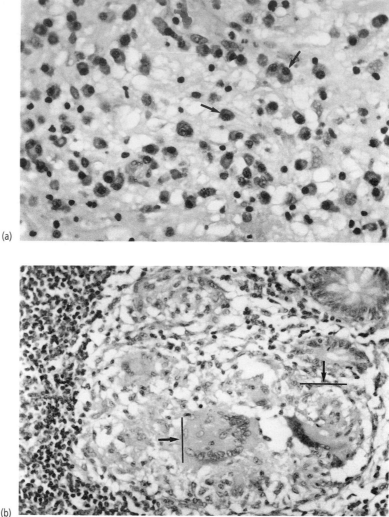

(a)

(b)

Fig. 4.1 Histological examples of acute and chronic inflammation. (a) B lymphocytes within tissue during chronic inflammation. Two mature antibody-secreting B lymphocytes (known as plasma cells) are arrowed. (b) Granuloma with giant cells, typical of the chronic inflammation that follows infection with *Mycobacterium tuberculosis*. The macrophages take on a characteristic 'epithelioid' (epithelial cell-like) appearance and may fuse to form giant cells. Two representative giant cells are arrowed.

cells such as neutrophils and macrophages (see also Chapter 5).

3 Lysis of cells by the formation of the *lytic* or *membrane attack complex (MAC)* of complement proteins on the target cell membrane.

Cytokines

Cytokines (including the *interleukins, colony-stimulating factors,* and *tumour necrosis factors*) are proteins produced by many cell types. A cell

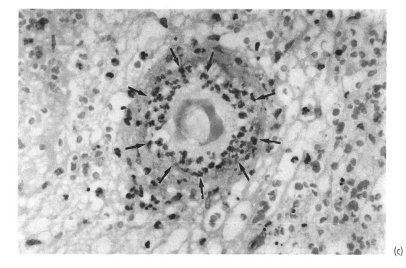

Fig. 4.1 (c) Adherence of neutrophils (arrowed) to a blood vessel wall ('pavementing') during acute inflammation.

(c)

responds to cytokines for which it bears specific surface receptors; the response depends on the concentration of the cytokine and the numbers or 'affinity status' of the receptors. Cytokines modulate a large range of tissue functions, including chemotaxis and activation of inflammatory cells (e.g. leucocytes), morphogenesis, differentiation, proliferation, apoptosis, (see Chapter 3), haemopoiesis and metabolism. Some cytokines activate cell functions directly, others 'prime' cells, making them more sensitive to other stimuli. Cytokines should not be viewed as acting in isolation; cytokines affect cells in cascades or *networks*.

Leucocyte recruitment and activation

Cell recruitment

Changes in blood flow during acute inflammation favour the conditions for the first stages in migration of leucocytes from the blood to the tissues (Fig. 4.5). Cell migration is *selective* since particular leucocytes are seen in different forms and stages of inflammation. The first stage in migration of blood cells from the blood to the tissues is adherence to the endothelium (*margination* or *pavementing*, see Fig. 4.1c).

Vascular endothelium expresses receptors for adhesion molecules present on the leucocyte surface. The expression of specific receptors on endothelium is induced by the presence of inflammatory mediators. The process of cell adhesion to endothelium and migration is now recognized as representing an *adhesion cascade*, which has the following four distinct stages.

1 *Tethering*, where leucocytes 'roll' along the vessel wall, being slowed or 'tethered' by low-affinity receptors called *selectins*; L-selectin is expressed constitutively on leucocytes; E-selectin and P-selectin are expressed on the endothelial cells when activated by cytokines.

2 *Triggering*, involves the induction of adhesion molecules, known as *integrins*, on the leucocytes following their activation by complement proteins, bacterial products and a variety of cytokines, including platelet-activating factor and interleukin-8 (IL-8).

3 *Strong adhesion*, where integrins on the leucocytes bind strongly to endothelial cells. Strong adhesion is mediated by activation of the leucocytes and endothelium.

4 *Migration* of the leucocytes through endothelium, a process known as *diapedesis*. This is mediated by chemotactic factors including: LTB4, bacterial products such as formylated peptides (e.g. formyl-met-leu-phe), complement peptides, chemokines and soluble peptides derived from damaged connective tissue constituents such as elastin, collagen and laminin. Many chemotactic

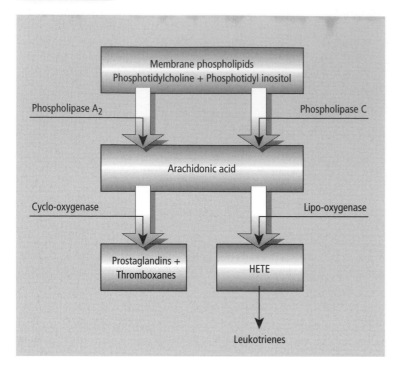

Fig. 4.2 Simplified pathways in the production of mediators from membrane phospholipids. Arachidonic acid is a fatty acid derived from the phospholipids of cell membranes under the influence of phospholipase A_2 or phospholipase C depending on the cell and type of stimulus. The arachidonic acid is metabolized by the lipo-oxygenase pathway to produce hydroxy eicosatetraenoic acid (HETE) and leukotrienes or by the cyclo-oxygenase pathway to produce prostaglandins and thromboxanes (see also Chapter 21).

factors also 'activate' leucocyte functions such as phagocytic activity and production of the *respiratory burst* (see below).

The importance of cell recruitment during inflammation is illustrated by deficiencies such as *leucocyte adherence deficiency* (LAD, see Chapter 14), where components of adhesion molecules are absent or reduced, resulting in recurrent infections in the affected individual.

Leucocyte functions

Lymphocytes recruited during chronic inflammation contribute to the specific immunological component of pathogen elimination (see Chapter 5). Neutrophils and macrophages are *phagocytic* cells, capable of engulfing micro-organisms and, particularly in the case of macrophages, apoptotic or damaged cells and non-living particulate material. Phagocytosis is enhanced if the target is coated by antibodies (opsonized), complement proteins, or both. Phagocytes have receptors for

immunoglobulin (Ig) and complement. Following their activation phagocytic cells produce a *respiratory* (oxidative) *burst* in which the membrane-bound *NADPH-oxidase system* produces *reactive oxygen intermediates* such as superoxide radicals (O_2^-), hydrogen peroxide, hypochlorous acid and chloramines. These oxidative products are toxic to micro-organisms. Individuals with *chronic granulomatous disease* (see Chapter 14) suffer from recurrent infections because their cells cannot produce these oxidative products. Phagocytosed material is enclosed in a *phagocytic vacuole* which fuses with lysosomes to form *phagolysosomes*. Lysosomes contain proteins and peptides which create 'holes' in the membranes of phagocytosed cells, causing lysis, and enzymes which can degrade peptides and proteins, carbohydrates and lipids. Thus there is complete degradation of phagocytosed organic material. Macrophages, eosinophils and mast cells also secrete enzymes and proteins that are damaging to foreign organisms and other cells.

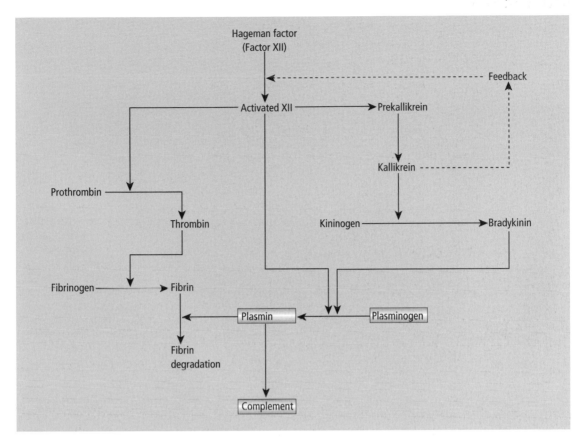

Fig. 4.3 Activation of the 'contact' factors of the blood coagulation cascade is accompanied by concurrent activation of fibrinolysis, complement and a range of inflammatory mediators (see also Chapter 21).

Healing and tissue repair

The main purpose of healing is to replace damaged tissue with functional cells, a process involving migration, proliferation and differentiation of surviving or nearby cells, contraction of the wound by *myofibroblasts* and production of appropriate connective tissues by cells including *fibroblasts* and *chondrocytes*. Healing begins with the proliferation of fibroblasts and small blood vessels (producing so called *granulation tissue*). The success of regeneration depends on the type, degree and duration of inflammation and the integrity of remaining tissue. Some tissues, such as skin and liver, regenerate relatively well whereas others (e.g. nervous tissue) do not. In the absence of regeneration, functional tissue is replaced by *fibrotic (scar)* tissue composed of large amounts of connective tissue proteins, especially *collagen*.

The healing process is mediated by a number of hormones, cytokines and growth factors, (including *platelet-derived growth factor, epidermal growth factor*, and *transforming growth factors α and β*) which interact in complex networks. They can act in synergy and some are inhibitory.

The resolution of the inflammatory process depends on the removal of the initial insult and changes in the pattern of mediators from those which are pro-inflammatory to those which induce healing. Remaining inflammatory cells appear to undergo apoptosis (see Chapter 3) and are recognized and phagocytosed by macrophages.

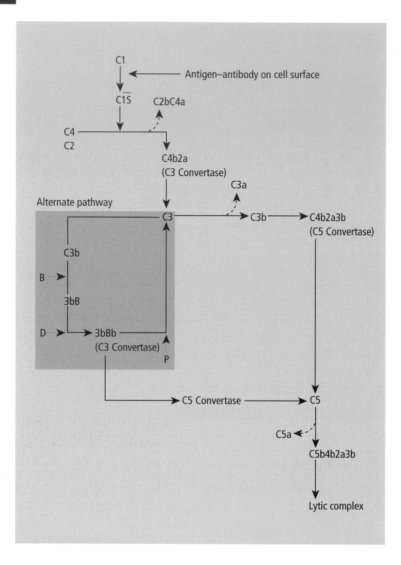

Fig. 4.4 An overview of the complement system (showing the role of the alternate pathway as a positive feedback loop enhancing the activity of the classical pathway). Stimulation of the complement cascade by antibody binding to antigen on a target cell (e.g. bacterial cell) begins with the activation of the C1 subunit (C1s). C1s acts upon C4 and C2, splitting off small, soluble fragments (C2b, C4a) from each, leaving a complex known as C4b2a (C3 convertase) on the target cell membrane. In the classical pathway C3 convertase acts on C3, splitting off another small fragment (C3a) leaving the larger complex (C4b2a3b) which has C5 convertase activity. C5 convertase then cleaves C5, following which complement components C6–C9 form the membrane attack (lytic) complex which lyses the target cell. Many of the soluble products of complement activation (e.g. C3a and C5a) are anaphylatoxins (see text). Certain bacterial products, for example endotoxin, enhance the activity of the alternate pathway which acts as a positive feedback loop, providing additional C3 convertase and C5 convertase activity.

B, D and P are components of the alternate complement pathway.

Many of the reactions of the complement system are calcium- or magnesium-dependent.

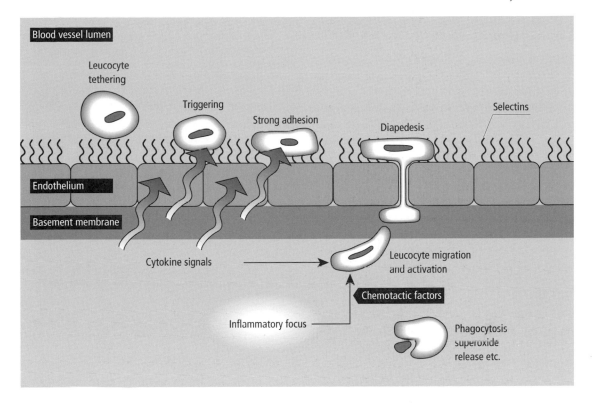

Fig. 4.5 Leucocytes migrate from the blood to sites of injury by a process involving adhesion and movement (diapedesis) through the capillary endothelium under the influence of chemotactic factors released from damaged tissues and bacterial cells.

Summary

It is clear from this chapter that inflammation is a process which involves integration of a number of body systems. These include components of the immune system, including various immune cells and their products (cytokines) and complement, together with components of the coagulation and fibrinolytic systems. An understanding of the complex interactions between these various systems is central to an understanding of the process of inflammation.

Key points

1 Inflammation is the body's response to injury.

2 In acute inflammation there is tissue oedema (increase in intercellular fluid) and the accumulation of neutrophils.

3 In chronic inflammation lymphocytes and macrophages are the predominant cell type. Chronic inflammation often follows unresolved acute inflammation. Alternatively, it may result from exposure to insoluble agents, foreign bodies or some intracellular parasites (e.g. *Mycobacterium tuberculosis*).

4 Tuberculosis represents an unusual form of chronic inflammation in which there is development of granulomas. Granulomas are collections of macrophages surrounded by a cuff of lymphocytes. Some of the macrophages may fuse together to form giant cells.

5 One outcome of inflammation is tissue repair. Where full regeneration is not possible the functional tissue is replaced by collagen fibres (scar tissue).

Further reading

Adams D.H. & Shaw S. (1994) Leucocyte/endothelial interactions and regulation of leucocyte migration. *Lancet*. **343**, 831–836.

Gallin J.I., Goldstein I.M. & Snyderman R. (1992) *Inflammation: Basic Principles and Clinical Correlates*. Raven Press, New York.

Meager A. (1990) *Cytokines*. Open University Press, Buckingham U.K.

The Immune System

Introduction

The immune system functions as a network of cellular interactions which take place in a wide range of different micro-environments throughout the body. These interactions are facilitated by receptor molecules on the outer surface of cells which bind to molecules in the micro-environment, often on the surface of other cells. This can initiate biochemical changes within the cells, leading in turn to changes in gene expression and consequently in cell function. In this respect, the immune system is just a subset of the cellular interactions which take place within the body and determine its physiology. An understanding of the way in which cells of the immune system are influenced by, and interact with, other subsets (e.g. those which characterize the neuro-endocrine or gastrointestinal systems) is only just beginning to emerge.

Lymphocytes and their receptors

The focus of attention for immunologists is on understanding the formation and function of cell surface receptors which recognize specific 'foreign' molecules, and as a result generate an immune response. There are two different types of receptor. The surface receptor of the *B lymphocytes* is a membrane bound form of the glycoprotein *immunoglobulin* (Ig). The counterpart on *T lymphocytes* is less imaginatively referred to as the *T cell receptor*. These receptors recognize a diverse range of foreign molecules including the components or products of micro-organisms such as viruses, bacteria, and fungi, other parasites such as helminth worms, and cells from unrelated human donors, as well as commonplace sub-stances such as pollen or animal hair. Collectively these are referred to as *antigens* (Ag).

The B and T cells are central to *acquired* or *adaptive* immune responses, which in more highly evolved organisms complement and enhance *natural* or *innate immunity*. The latter consists of a variety of mechanisms to counteract infectious agents which include physical and chemical barriers to infection, or the synthesis of antimicrobial agents which interact in a non-specific way with infectious agents and their products, and often promote their lysis by cytotoxic cells, or their uptake and degradation by phagocytic cells. Some of these aspects of natural immunity are dealt with in more detail in Chapter 4.

Acquired immunity

Acquired or adaptive immunity has certain characteristics which are outlined in the sections below.

Specificity

The antigen receptors on the surface of any individual B or T cell are specific for a single molecular cluster or arrangement within the structure of an antigen. This molecular cluster or arrangement is referred to as an *antigenic determinant* or *epitope*.

Diversity

The body is able to mount responses against a wide range of antigenic determinants. Although each B or T cell has surface receptors with a single specificity, collectively these cells have a wide range of specificities facilitating the recognition of a similarly wide range of epitopes. This diversity is generated during B and T cell development, by random rearrangement of the genetic information encoding the polypeptides that make up the receptor molecules and is independent of the presence of antigen. The range of receptors (or *immunological repertoire*) produced will be unique to the individual, may alter with time, and will contain receptors specific to epitopes that exist at present or which may by generated in the future as a consequence of evolutionary changes occurring in infectious organisms.

Memory

Once the immune system has encountered a particular antigen, it is able to make a quicker, more vigorous, and more effective response to the same antigen on subsequent re-exposure, so the B and T cells have 'memory'. This is probably the most widely known property of the immune system — every parent knows that an infant contracting measles in childhood is protected from the disease in later life. It is the basis of vaccination, the first demonstration of which by E. Jenner in 1796 really marked the foundation of immunology as a discipline. Despite this, immunological memory is still relatively poorly understood at the molecular level.

Self — non-self discrimination

Under normal circumstances the immune system is able to mount an effective response against 'foreign' antigens, but does not attack other components of the body (i.e. self). In part, this is due to the removal or deletion of cells that carry receptors specific for 'self', before they become fully able to respond to antigen (i.e. before they become *immunocompetent*). Cells with self-reactive receptors are present however, and mechanisms exist which either prevent their activation (*clonal anergy*), or actively suppress their function (*suppression*).

Generation of diversity in the immunological repertoire

Like other cells of the blood, B and T cells both originate from stem cells that are formed at first in the yolk sac, then in the fetal liver or spleen, and later in adult bone marrow. B cells complete their development in the bone marrow, but T cell precursors migrate from the bone marrow to the thymus where they mature. The bone marrow and the thymus are responsible for the production of the repertoires of immunocompetent B and T cells respectively, and are the *primary lymphoid organs* of humans.

The B and T cell receptors are both made up of two distinct types of polypeptide chain. These are the heavy and light chains of Igs on B cells, and the α and β chains in the most common form of the T cell receptor (Fig. 5.1). In both cases, the polypeptides have *a non-polymorphic* or *constant* region, and a *polymorphic* or *variable* region which forms the antigen recognition site. Hypervariable amino acid residues within this region are involved in antigen recognition and binding.

In each individual, within each haploid set of chromosomes, there are a number of different versions of the gene segments (variable, joining and diversity gene segments) which carry the information for the synthesis of the polymorphic regions of the receptors, but usually only single versions of the gene segments which encode the constant regions. Rearrangement of the gene segments occurs to produce functional coding information for the diverse repertoire of B and T cell receptors (Fig. 5.2). The mechanisms by which this occurs show the same essential features in both B and T cells. The main features of this process are outlined below.

1 The gene segments for a particular polypeptide are contained on a single chromosome. Although the gene segments can recombine in a large number of ways, a given chromosome in a particular cell can only make one rearrangement to produce a functional coding sequence. This is because the segments are brought together to form a functional sequence by looping out of DNA, and

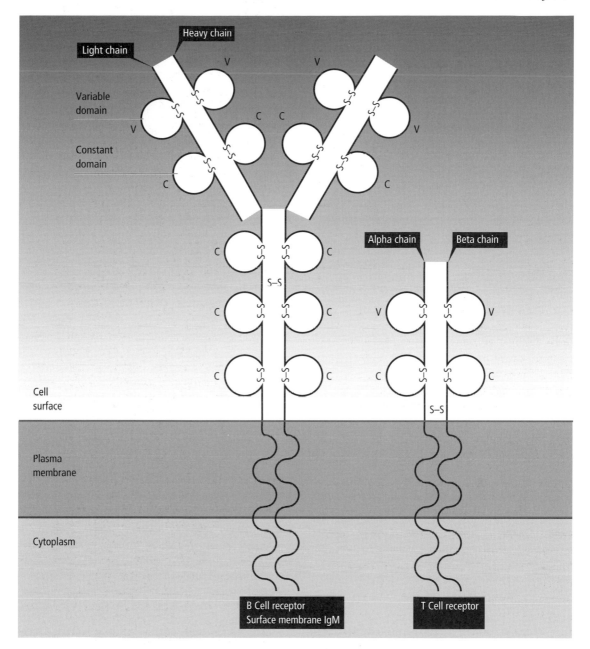

Fig. 5.1 Surface receptors of B and T lymphocytes. The specific antigen receptors of both B and T cells are composed of variable and constant region domains. These domains have a similar basic structure and are also found in a variety of other molecules which have an immunological function. They are members of the immunoglobulin (Ig) supergene family. Activated B cells can produce Igs with the same specificity, but with different heavy chain constant region domains. This allows them to be secreted from the cell as antibody molecules. Different heavy chain constant region domains also confer different effector functions on the antibody molecules. The subclasses of antibody IgM, IgD, IgG, IgA and IgE have μ, δ, γ, α, and ε heavy chains respectively.

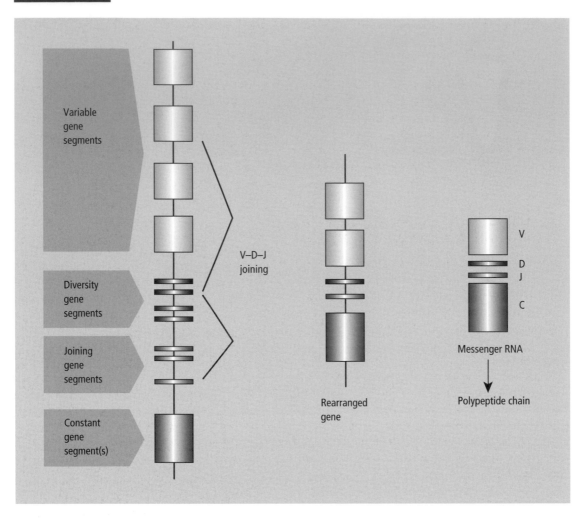

Variable
gene
segments

Diversity
gene
segments

Joining
gene
segments

Constant
gene
segment(s)

V–D–J
joining

Rearranged
gene

Messenger RNA

↓

Polypeptide chain

V
D
J
C

Fig. 5.2 Generation of diversity in the immunological repertoire. Each of the polypeptides making up the B and T cell receptors is encoded by a number of clusters of gene segments. There are a number of different versions of each of the gene segments in the variable, diversity (where present), and joining gene segment clusters. Functional genes are produced by rearrangements which bring together a gene segment from each of these clusters, with a constant region gene segment. The larger the number of gene segments in each of the clusters, the greater the number of functional gene combinations that can be produced by rearrangement. Additional variability is introduced through the random addition of nucleotides at the junctions between gene segments, and through flexibility in the precise point of joining.

the breakage and rejoining of the chromosome, which is an irreversible process. Even though the cells are diploid, and therefore contain two sets of gene segments on homologous chromosomes, successful rearrangement on one chromosome prevents rearrangement of the other. This is termed *allellic exclusion*. It ensures that each cell has only a single receptor specificity.

2 Gene rearrangement does not depend on the presence of antigen.

3 Rearrangements occur at random, so that different precursor cells can rearrange in different ways to produce functional genes that encode receptors with different specificities.

4 A functional gene is assembled from a single variable, joining, diversity (in some cases), and constant region segment. The more versions of the gene segments there are on the chromosome, the greater the number of possible combinations (combinatorial joining).

5 When a junction between segments is formed, there is some variation in the precise point of joining (*junctional flexibility*), and extra coding information can be added at the junctions (*random nucleotide addition*).

6 Functional receptors are formed by the pairing of the polypeptide products of two different types of rearranged gene (*heterodimer formation*). The number of possible receptor structures is therefore the product of the number of possible structures for each polypeptide.

Lymphocyte recirculation

Immunocompetent lymphocytes pass from the bone marrow or thymus into the lymphocyte circulation. They are transported around the body in the blood and the lymphatic system and reach the *lymph nodes* in arterial capillaries or *afferent lymphatics* (Fig. 5.3). They pass through the cuboidal endothelial cells of the venules (*high endothelial venules*) into the cortical tissues of the node. From here they are collected by *efferent lymphatics* draining the lymph nodes, and returned to the blood system via the thoracic ducts. Foreign antigens within the peripheral tissues are collected with other extracellular fluids, and drained to the nearest lymph node.

The lymph nodes, along with the other *secondary lymphoid organs* (the spleen and the mucosal-associated lymphoid tissues) provide a micro-environment which facilitates interaction between the lymphocyte surface receptors and foreign antigens. The secondary lymphoid organs are the location at which an immune response is initiated.

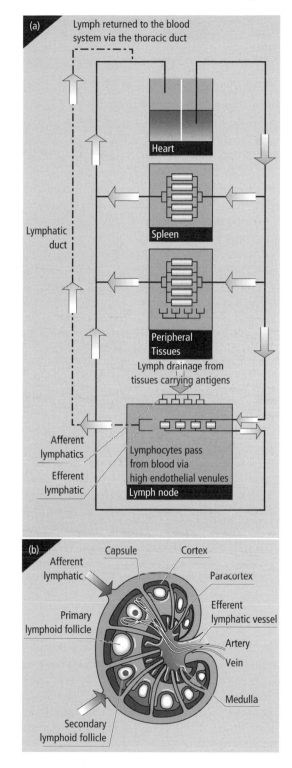

Fig. 5.3 (a) The routes of lymphocyte recirculation. Lymphocytes reach the lymph nodes in arterial capillaries or from afferent lymphatics draining the tissues. (b) The lymph node. This provides a site for the interaction between antigen and B cells carrying the appropriate surface receptor. B cell stimulation occurs in primary follicles, leading to proliferation and differentiation, to form memory cells and antibody-secreting plasma cells in the secondary follicles.

Lymphocyte activation

The immunological repertoire contains an enormous number of lymphocytes with receptors for different antigens. There is no reliable way to determine the size of the repertoire, but estimates suggest something like 10^{10} different B cell receptors and rather more, maybe as many as $10^{15}\alpha\beta$ T cell receptors. There are likely to be only a few cells with receptors of the same specificity. How then is the immune system able to effectively counteract a particular infection? This is explained by the *clonal selection theory*, which is the central concept of immunology (Fig. 5.4).

When a B or T cell encounters an epitope for which its surface receptor is specific, it is in effect *selected*. Binding of epitope to the receptor triggers biochemical changes inside the cell which lead ultimately to proliferation and the production of a clone of cells all with the same receptor specificity. The antigen is therefore responsible for *clonal selection*, and receptor binding results in *clonal expansion*. Changes occur within the cells as they differentiate to form either *effector cells* or *memory cells*. The same process occurs in both B and T lymphocytes, but the details of receptor interaction are very different, as are the effector functions and the characteristics of the memory cells.

The role of the major histocompatibility complex

B cell receptors are able to recognize epitopes on the surface of complex antigens (e.g. components of the surface coat of bacteria). They recognize a particular three-dimensional arrangement of molecules on the antigen which interact with key amino acid residues in the receptor-binding site. These amino acids are the hypervariable residues, often described as *complementarity-determining regions*. The B cell receptor therefore recognizes what is often described as a *conformational epitope*.

The situation in T cells is more complex. The T cell receptor can only recognize short peptides displayed on the surface of cells by glycoproteins which are encoded by genes of the *major histocompatibility complex* (MHC; Fig. 5.5 and Table 5.1). These genes were first identified in the context of transplantation. A graft between genetically identical animals is usually successful, but if there are genetic differences between donor and recipient, the graft is rejected. The genes which are most important in this context are those of the MHC. In humans this gene region is referred to as the *human leucocyte antigen (HLA)* region. There are two sets of genes which produce two different types of protein (see Table 5.1): the MHC Class I genes (HLA-A, -B and -C in humans), and the MHC Class II genes (HLA-DP, -DQ, and -DR in humans).

In the population there are many different alleles for each of these genes, although more have been identified for some than for others. So there is a high level of polymorphism at the population level. Each individual carries only two alleles (one from each parent) for each of the three Class I genes, and the same number for each of the Class II genes. It is the nature of these alleles which characterizes a tissue type, a vitally important feature when considering the suitability of donors for transplantation.

Different alleles encode MHC molecules which have the same overall structure, but which differ in the structure of their peptide-binding sites, and are therefore specific for peptides with different structural motifs. Effective peptide binding is essential for effective presentation of antigens to T cells. The MHC therefore exerts a genetic influence on the ability to respond to particular antigens — it regulates *immune responsiveness*.

Antigen processing and presentation

As T cells can only recognize peptides presented by MHC molecules, there must be mechanisms by which antigens can be processed to produce peptides which are bound to MHC molecules and presented at the cell surface. There are separate mechanisms for MHC Class I and MHC Class II molecules.

MHC Class I molecules are present on the surface

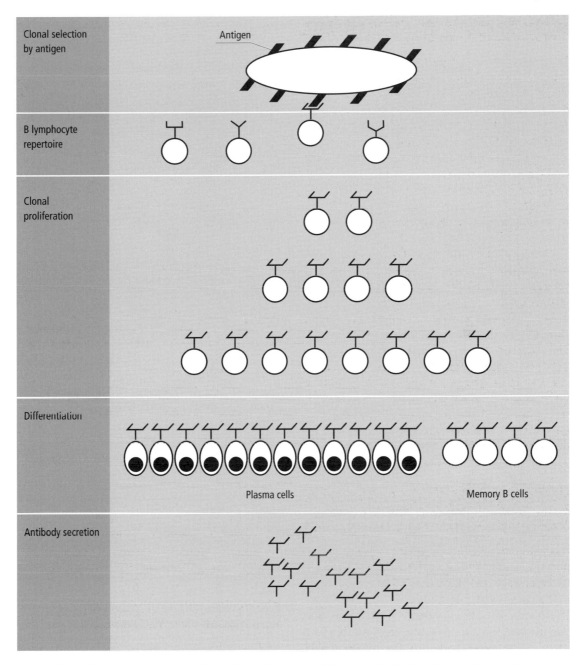

Fig. 5.4 Clonal selection. Lymphocytes from the B cell repertoire, with surface receptors that can bind to surface epitopes on the antigen, are selected and triggered to proliferate and differentiate, forming plasma cells and memory cells. The plasma cells secrete antibody molecules of the same specificity, which are able to interact with the antigen to bring about its elimination. A similar process of clonal selection and proliferation operates on the T cell repertoire, although the initial interaction between T cell and antigen is more complex.

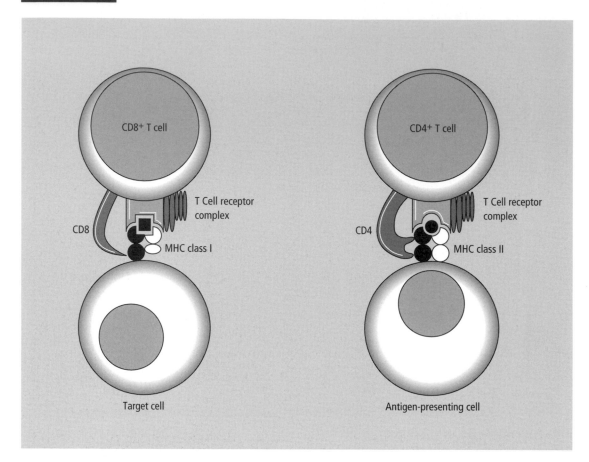

Fig. 5.5 Antigen recognition by T lymphocytes. T cell receptors can only recognize short peptides, derived from antigens, and displayed on the surface of cells by the major histocompatibility complex (MHC) glycoproteins. There are two types of MHC molecule, MHC Class I and MHC Class II. They have different patterns of expression, bind peptides from different locations derived from separate pathways of antigen-processing, and present peptides to different subclasses of T cell.

of virtually all cells. They are produced in the endoplasmic reticulum and depend on peptide binding at this site for their assembly and transport to the cell surface (Fig. 5.6). They provide a mechanism for sampling the peptides available in the cytoplasm and endoplasmic reticulum.

Transporter proteins in the membrane of the endoplasmic reticulum bring about the import of peptides from the cytoplasm. In most cases the peptides presented will be derived from 'self'

Table 5.1 Genes of the major histocompatibility complex (MHC)

MHC Class I	MHC Class II
Presents peptides to CD8 +ve T cells (usually cytotoxic)	Presents peptides to CD4 +ve T cells (usually helper)
Encoded by HLA-A, -B and -C genes	Encoded by HLA-DP, -DQ, and -DR genes
Expressed on the surface of virtually all cells	Expressed on the surface of antigen presenting cells e.g. B cells, dendritic cells, macrophages
Presents cytoplasmic peptides e.g. from viruses or tumour antigens	Presents peptides from extracellular antigens e.g. bacteria
Peptides complex with MHC by endogenous-processing pathway	Peptides complex with MHC by exogenous processing pathway

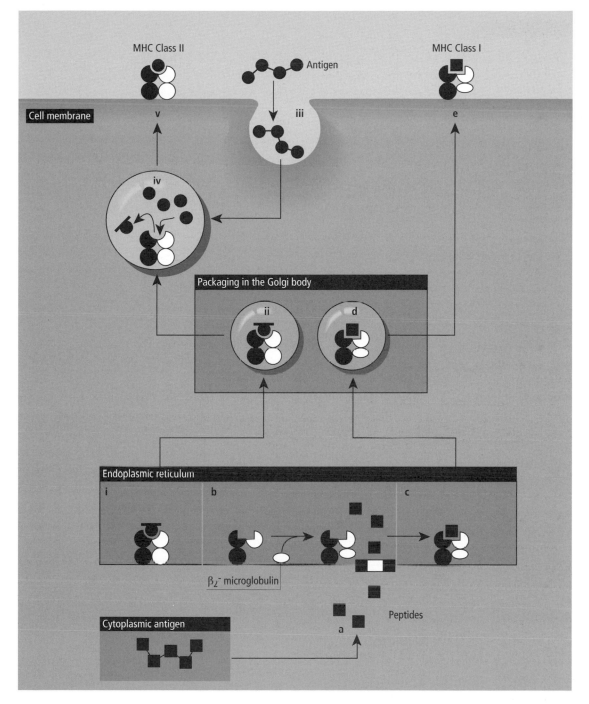

Fig. 5.6 Antigen processing and presentation. T cells only recognize peptides presented on the surface of cells by major histocompatibility complex (MHC) molecules. There are two discrete pathways of antigen processing by which peptides are produced and complexed with MHC molecules. Presentation by MHC Class I: endogenous pathway. (a) Peptides generated from cytoplasmic antigens are transported into the endoplasmic reticulum by a peptide transporter. (b) MHC Class I molecules are assembled in the endoplasmic reticulum and (c) bind peptides with appropriate structural characteristics. (d) Peptide binding facilitates the transport of the complex to the Golgi body and onwards to the cell surface. (e) Peptides are presented at the cell surface, to CD8 +ve T cells. Presentation by MHC Class II: exogenous pathway. (i) MHC Class II molecules are synthesized in the endoplasmic reticulum but in the presence of 'invariant chain', peptide binding is blocked. (ii) The molecules are transported to the Golgi body and on towards the cell surface. (iii) Extracellular antigen is taken into the cell by endocytosis in vesicles. (iv) In the endosomes, antigen is digested to produce peptides which may combine with MHC Class II after the dissociation of invariant chain. (v) Peptides are presented at the cell surface, to CD4 +ve T cells.

proteins. As T cells specific for 'self' are deleted in the thymus, this would not normally be expected to generate an immune response. However, if a cell is infected by a virus it may produce viral proteins which will be processed and presented at the cell surface where they will generate an immune response (see Chapter 8). In a similar way, tumour cells may produce antigens which are seen as 'non-self' (see Chapter 28). Peptides presented by MHC Class I are only recognized by a subset of T cells which carry the surface glycoprotein CD8. The majority of these cells have a *cytotoxic* function which brings about lysis of the target cell.

MHC Class II molecules are restricted to the surface of particular cells, often referred to as antigen-presenting cells, which are associated with the immune system (e.g. dendritic cells, B lymphocytes and macrophages). Like MHC Class I molecules they are produced in the endoplasmic reticulum, but are prevented from binding peptides at this site by the action of an additional polypeptide, referred to as the *invariant chain*. The molecules are eventually transported to the endosomal compartment where they are dissociated from the invariant chain and able to bind available peptides. These peptides are derived from proteins that have been taken up by endocytosis of exogenous antigens from the cell surface. MHC Class II therefore samples and presents antigens from the extracellular compartment. In this case, the presented peptides are recognized by a subset of T cells which are defined by the presence of the glycoprotein CD4 on their surface. The majority of these CD4+ve T cells have a *helper* function.

Effector functions

The role of lymphokines

The activation of helper T cells leads to the production and secretion of growth factors which are referred to as cytokines, or more specifically *lymphokines*. These interact with specific receptors on the surface of other cells and lead to changes in the cells which are associated with the processes of development, differentiation or activation (Fig. 5.7). The lymphokines usually act in a *paracrine* (on nearby cells) or *autocrine* (on the producing cell) manner, and are *pleiotropic* (i.e. they produce different effects in different cells).

Helper T cells have a central function in the immune response as the lymphokines that they produce have a role in the differentiation of other lymphocytes, and also play an important part in the activation of both B and T cells. They also link the acquired immune system to the innate immune system by activating non-specific effector cells such as macrophages and natural killer (NK) cells.

It now seems that there may be different subsets of helper T cells which produce different lymphokines. It may well be that different types of antigen activate different subsets of helper T cells which produce different 'cocktails' of lymphokines. Two subsets have been well characterized in mice. Helper T1 cells secrete interleukin-2, interferon-γ and tumour necrosis factor-β, in contrast to helper T2 cells which secrete interleukins (IL) -4, -5 and -10. Different lymphokine secretions lead to the activation of different cellular components of the immune system, giving a bias to the response based on the nature of the antigen by which it was induced.

B – T cell interactions and antibody production

B cells display MHC Class II molecules as well as specific antigen receptors on their surface. They are therefore able to recognize antigens, take them

---

Fig. 5.7 The key role of helper T cells. Helper T cells have a central role in the regulation of the immune response. The lymphokines which they secrete on activation can provide 'help' in the activation, proliferation or differentiation of other cells. For example, lymphokines provide essential 'help' for the clonal proliferation and differentiation of B cells in the presence of antigen. The plasma cells produced secrete antibody which can stimulate additional components of the immune system such as complement activation or antibody-dependent cell-mediated cytotoxicity.

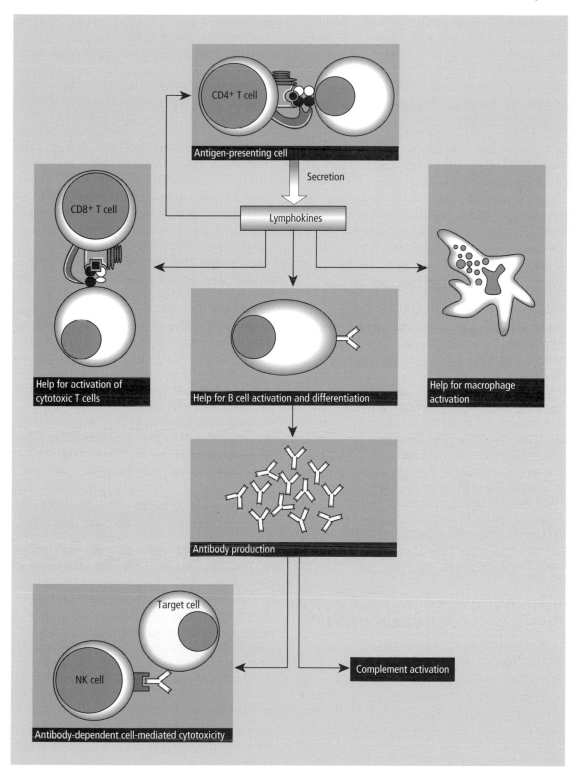

into the cell by endocytosis, and process them to produce peptides which can be combined with MHC Class II molecules and presented on the surface. Helper T cells recognizing the presented peptide may be activated and produce lymphokines which provide 'help' to the B cell. B cells that have never been exposed to a particular antigen before are called *naive* B cells. On activation, they proliferate and differentiate to produce plasma cells which secrete antibody. Other cells will differentiate to form memory cells. This is a *primary response*. Memory cells live longer, and on exposure to the same antigen on subsequent occasions, respond more rapidly and more vigorously to produce higher titres of antibody. This is referred to as a *secondary response*.

There are two further qualitative differences between primary and secondary responses. The antibody molecules produced in a primary response are usually IgM. Their heavy chains have a constant region encoded by the μ-gene segment. In the secondary response, antibody molecules are often produced from rearranged genes in which the information encoding the variable portion of the heavy chain is recombined with a different constant gene segment. The specificity of the antibody remains the same, but the portion of the molecule which is responsible for its effector function may be changed. This process is known as *class switching* and is regulated by lymphokines.

The antibodies generated in a secondary response also show an accumulation of changes in the amino acid residues which make up the antigen-binding site. These changes arise as a result of somatic mutation within B lymphocytes, and appear to be selected as they make the binding site of the antibody a better fit for its epitope. This increases the affinity of antibody for antigen and is called *affinity maturation*. Affinity maturation of B lymphocytes occurs within secondary lymphoid follicles (see Fig. 5.3).

Links with components of the innate immune system

There are many ways in which the antigen specific cells of the acquired immune system interact with components of the innate immune system (see Fig. 5.7) some of which are detailed below.

1 A subset of CD4+ve helper T cells produces lymphokines including IL-2, interferon (IFN)-γ, and tumour necrosis factor (TNF)-β which attract and activate macrophages and lead to localized tissue destruction.

2 Exposure to an antigen can generate plasma cells which secrete antibodies of the IgE subclass. These are able to bind to receptors on the surface of mast cells and basophils and sensitize them. Subsequent exposure of the cells to the same antigen results in degranulation of the sensitized cells, releasing chemicals which mediate a variety of physiological effects (see also Chapter 12).

3 Antibody molecules complexed to antigen can initiate a cascade of reactions – the classical complement pathway – which generates biologically active molecules that can act as anaphylatoxins, promote phagocytosis or bring about cell lysis through the formation of a membrane attack complex (see Chapter 4).

4 Antibody molecules binding cell surface antigens can attract cells such as NK cells which have receptors for the effector portion of the antibody molecule. The antibody thus forms a bridge between the two cells and facilitates the lytic killing of the target cell by the NK cell. This is *antibody-dependent cell-mediated cytotoxicity*.

Summary

This chapter has described the important features of acquired or adaptive immunity and how this relates to aspects of innate immunity. The importance of the immune system in the maintenance of health is well illustrated by the disorders of immunity. These may be grouped under three general headings: (a) hypersensitivity, characterized by abnormal or inappropriate responses to antigens; (b) autoimmunity, in which immune responses are directed against self antigens; (c) immunodeficiency, in which there is a deficiency in one or more components of the immune system. These disorders are the subject of Chapters 12–14.

Key points

1 Two forms of immunity may be recognized. Acquired or adaptive immunity and innate or natural immunity.

2 Acquired immunity has specificity, diversity and memory, and is able to discriminate between self and non-self.

3 Lymphocytes are of prime importance in acquired immunity. Lymphocytes have antigen receptors. The enormous repertoire of antigen receptor specificity is produced by rearrangement of the genes that encode the receptor proteins.

4 B lymphocytes have antigen receptors which are membrane-bound forms of the glycoprotein, immunoglobulin. Binding of antigen to the B cell receptor leads to clonal expansion of B lymphocytes and the secretion of antibody by mature B lymphocytes, known as plasma cells.

5 T lymphocytes also have surface receptors for antigen. Unlike B lymphocytes, these receptors can only recognize processed antigen (usually in the form of short peptides) displayed on the surface of cells in association with MHC molecules. MHC Class 1 molecules present intracellular antigens (e.g. virus proteins) to CD8 +ve T cells, whereas MHC Class II molecules present extracellularly derived antigens to CD4 +ve T cells.

6 CD4 +ve cells have a 'helper' function and secrete lymphokines necessary for the activation and function of other effector cells (e.g. B lymphocytes). CD4 +ve T lymphocytes have a central role in the generation of effective immune responses.

Further reading

Austyn J.M. & Wood K.J. (1993) *Principles of Cellular and Molecular Immunology*. Oxford University Press, Oxford.

Kuby J. (1993) *Immunology*, 2nd edn. Freeman, New York.

Nossal G.J.V. (1993) Life, death and the immune system. *Sci. Am.* **269**, 21.

Roitt I., Brostoff J. & Male D. (1993) *Immunology*. Mosby.

Roitt I. (1994) *Essential Immunology*. Blackwell Science, Oxford.

Staines N., Brostoff J. & James K. (1993) *Introducing Immunology*. Mosby, London.

Part 3
Infection

General Principles of Infection

Introduction

Despite significant advances in the treatment and control of infectious diseases, they remain a major cause of morbidity and mortality in the modern world. The worldwide epidemic of AIDS and the re-emergence of serious diseases such as tuberculosis, caused by drug resistant forms of mycobacteria, have highlighted the need for extensive research effort in order to understand the nature of these important diseases and improve strategies for their control.

This chapter considers the delicate nature of the host–parasite relationship in infectious disease. Definitions and basic concepts are considered and features of the parasite and the host that are important in the establishment of disease are outlined.

The relationship between humans and their microbes

Humans are hosts to a variety of micro-organisms and animals, not all of which cause disease. All associations in which one species lives in or on another are grouped under the general heading of symbiosis, which literally means 'living together'. A *parasite* may be defined as an organism which lives on or in another organism (the *host*), obtains nutrients directly from it, provides no benefit to the host and may also be harmful.

Humans support a wide range of micro-organisms, mostly bacteria living on the skin, in the mouth and in the gastrointestinal tract. These are often referred to as *commensals* or 'normal flora' and are generally harmless. Commensals may also provide some benefit to the host, for example,

the presence of gut commensals can prevent colonization from other, potentially harmful, organisms. However, if the host becomes immunosuppressed or if commensals colonize inappropriate sites then disease may result.

Parasites and pathogens

Some parasites are entirely dependent on the host for their reproduction and are therefore incapable of independent existence. These are termed *obligate parasites*. Viruses are examples of obligate parasites.

Those organisms that are capable of existing outside the host are called *facultative parasites*. Most bacterial parasites belong to this latter group.

Intracellular parasites (e.g. *Mycobacterium tuberculosis*, viruses), are adapted for life within cells whereas those that exist outside cells are *extracellular* parasites (e.g. *Streptococcus viridans*).

Parasites are aerobic if they have a strict requirement for oxygen (e.g. *Pseudomonas aeruginosa*) or anaerobic where oxygen is not required and for some organisms may be toxic (e.g. *Clostridium tetani*). *Facultative anaerobes* are micro-organisms that can survive whether oxygen is present or not (e.g. *Escherichia coli*).

A parasite growing in or on a host can cause an infection but when the infection leads to a disease state the parasite is referred to as a *pathogen*. Pathogenicity, therefore, is defined as the ability to cause disease. Many different types of organisms can cause disease. The most important groups are *bacteria, viruses, fungi, protozoa* and higher *eukaryotic* organisms such as *helminths*. In addition, very simple agents such as *prions* (*proteinaceous infective particles*) can cause important diseases such as scrapie in sheep but are yet to be fully characterized.

While infectious diseases are responsible for significant morbidity and mortality, in biological terms it is not in the best interests of the parasite to kill the host. Survival of the host enables the maintenance of a reservoir of potentially infectious organisms which may be transmitted to other susceptible hosts. Highly pathogenic organisms may therefore be regarded as poorly adapted symbionts.

Koch's postulates

The 19th century microbiologist, Robert Koch, devised a set of postulates that have to be satisfied before a particular organism can be named as the aetiological agent for a given disease. These are outlined below.

1 The pathogen must always be present when there is disease and absent when there is no disease.

2 The pathogen must be isolated from an infected host and grown in pure culture.

3 Disease must result from reintroduction of the pathogen into a healthy host.

4 Subsequently, the same pathogen must be isolated from the second host.

These postulates are not always easily satisfied. For example, the presence of specific antibodies to a given micro-organism is often the only indicator that infection has occurred. In addition, for pathogens which only infect human hosts, postulates **3** and **4** cannot be satisfied for ethical reasons.

Types of infectious disease

Infectious diseases are *acute* when they are of short duration. The signs and symptoms of acute infections are often severe and usually appear suddenly. In contrast, a *chronic* infection usually develops slowly and is long-lasting. There may also be periods of *latency* when overt symptoms are absent. This is often the case with viral infections, particularly of the *herpesvirus* family (see

Chapter 8). *Systemic* infections involve the whole body, whereas *localized* infections are restricted to a particular body site. *Opportunistic* infections are those caused by organisms that are non-pathogenic under normal circumstances. However, they can cause disease when there is impaired immunity or loss of normal flora.

Transmission of infectious disease

In order to produce infectious disease pathogens must be transmitted to the host. The following are several ways in which transmission can take place.

1 Transmission through air: pathogens can be transmitted in droplets or droplet nuclei in air to susceptible hosts (e.g. *Mycobacterium tuberculosis*).

2 Transmission by water and food: ingestion of contaminated water or food can lead to infection. Examples of organisms transmitted in this way include *Vibrio cholerae* and *Salmonella typhi*.

3 Transmission by contact: pathogens can be passed on by direct contact, for instance through sexual contact (e.g. *Treponema pallidum*, HIV), or be inoculated through the skin by animal (e.g. rabies virus) or insect bites (e.g. *Plasmodium falciparum*). Some infections can be transmitted by *fomites*, (that is inanimate objects or materials on which pathogens may be conveyed) such as dust particles (e.g. *M. tuberculosis*).

Factors contributing to the establishment of an infectious disease

Features of the pathogen

1 *Virulence* is the degree of pathogenicity and refers to the ability of the pathogen to invade and multiply within the host and cause damage, for instance by the production of toxins. Pathogens have many different types of virulence factors or *determinants* and these are dealt with in more detail in Chapters 7–10.

2 *Evasion of host immunity*. Some pathogens have

developed ways of evading the host's immune system. For example, African trypanosomes (see Chapter 10) can rapidly change their surface antigens thereby evading attack by specific antibodies and T cells. Other pathogens have devised mechanisms that allow intracellular survival. An example here is the survival of *M. tuberculosis* within phagocytic cells.

3 *The number of infectious organisms* to which an individual is exposed is important in determining whether or not disease will result. In general, the larger the infective dose, the greater the probability of disease. The *minimum infective dose* refers to the minimum number of organisms required for infection and varies for different pathogens. In this context, the ID 50 (*infective dose 50*) and the LD 50 (*lethal dose 50*) are important laboratory measures of the virulence of a pathogen. They refer to the numbers of organisms required to cause an infection in (ID 50), or kill (LD 50) 50 per cent of test host animals within a specified time period.

Features of the host

Host factors, such as age, nutritional status and genetic constitution are important in determining whether infection will occur following exposure to a potential pathogen. The very young and the very old are more susceptible to infection—a reflection of developing and gradually failing immune systems, respectively. Malnutrition also increases disease susceptibility. Some populations are more susceptible to certain types of infection as a result of genetic differences.

The status of the host's immune system is a crucial determinant. An alteration in any of the natural barriers to infection may enable entry of potential pathogens. For example, breaks in the integrity of the skin or decreased levels of mucosal antimicrobial proteins, such as immunoglobulin A (IgA), can predispose individuals to infection. Immunodeficiency, whether *inherited* (see Chapter 14) or *acquired* (e.g. by certain drug treatments or virus infections) can have devastating effects on the host, often allowing disease to occur as a result of opportunistic infection by those organisms not normally regarded as pathogenic.

Summary

Infectious diseases are caused by pathogens— parasitic organisms that are capable of causing disease. Subsequent chapters in this section of the book consider the diverse range of pathogens and the infinite variety of strategies that enable them to survive in or on the human host. An understanding of the mechanisms by which infectious agents cause disease should enable the development of more rational approaches to the treatment and prevention of infectious disease.

Key points

1 Pathogens are parasites that are capable of causing disease.
2 In general, Koch's postulates have to be satisfied before an organism can be identified as the aetiological agent for a given disease.
3 Parasite and host factors determine whether infectious disease will occur.
4 Parasite factors include the effect of virulence factors, the ability of the parasite to evade host immunity and the size of the infective dose.
5 Major host factors are age, nutritional status, genetic constitution and the integrity of the immune system.

Further reading

Mims C.A., Playfair J.H.L., Roitt I., Wakelin D., Williams R. & Anderson R.M. (1993) *Medical Microbiology*. Mosby.

Bacterial Infection

Introduction

Bacteria are amongst the most successful living organisms. Their ubiquity ensures that humans are obliged to live in constant and intimate contact with a wide variety of species and to encounter, if briefly, many more. Fortunately, relatively few species routinely cause disease (the so-called pathogenic bacteria) but many others have the potential to do so, given appropriate conditions.

Whether or not a bacterial encounter leads to disease is determined by the balance of two principal factors—host factors, including the state of the individual's immune system and features of the bacterium that enable it to cause disease. These bacterial features are often termed *virulence determinants*. Virulence determinants enable bacteria to: compete successfully with the normal microflora; survive in adverse conditions; adhere to or enter their targeted cells; and evade defence mechanisms.

This chapter examines some general characteristics of bacteria and considers in detail the structure of the cell wall of the major groups of bacteria. The classification of bacteria is briefly considered and routes of entry and modes of transmission are outlined. Finally, the important bacterial virulence factors are considered in detail.

General features of bacteria

Bacteria are *prokaryotes*, that is they lack an organized nucleus. Their genetic information is carried in a double-stranded, circular molecule of DNA which is often referred to as a chromosome although it differs from eukaryotic chromosomes in that no introns (non-coding sequences of DNA) are present.

Some bacteria possess small circular extra-chromosomal DNA fragments known as *plasmids* which replicate independently of the chromosomal DNA. Plasmids may contain important genes coding for virulence factors or antibiotic resistance and may be transferred from one bacterium to another. The cytoplasm of bacteria contains many ribosomes but no mitochondria or other organelles.

In all bacteria, the cell is surrounded by a complex cell wall. The nature of the cell wall is important in the classification of bacteria (see below) and in determining virulence.

The importance of the bacterial cell wall

In 1884, Christian Gram observed that the majority of bacteria could be classified into two broad groups, depending upon their ability to retain crystal violet dye after decolorization. Those retaining dye were termed Gram-positive and those failing to do so Gram-negative. This staining phenomenon, which is still of great importance in the initial laboratory identification of bacteria, results from fundamental differences in the cell walls of the two types of organism (Fig. 7.1).

All bacteria are bounded by a cytoplasmic membrane, composed of a typical phospholipid bilayer, the function of which is to supply the cell with energy via its associated enzyme systems and to regulate the passage of metabolites into and out of the cell.

Surrounding the cytoplasmic membrane is a layer of *peptidoglycan*, a complex polymer of polysaccharide chains linked by short peptides. This layer gives the cell its strength and shape and is much thicker in Gram-positive cells (accounting for more than 40 per cent of the dry

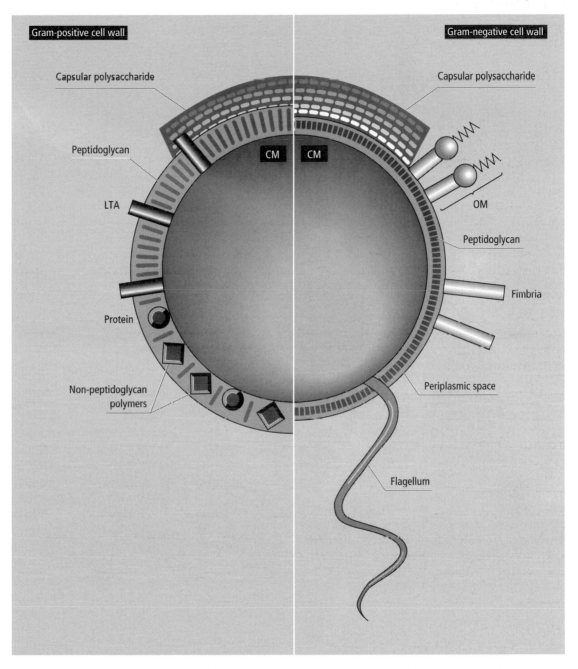

Gram-positive cell wall

Gram-negative cell wall

Capsular polysaccharide

Capsular polysaccharide

Peptidoglycan

CM   CM

LTA

OM

Peptidoglycan

Protein

Fimbria

Non-peptidoglycan
polymers

Periplasmic space

Flagellum

Fig. 7.1 Schematic illustration of the structure of the cell wall of
Gram-positive and Gram-negative bacteria. The cytoplasmic
membrane (CM) in both Gram-positive and Gram-negative
organisms is surrounded by a layer of peptidoglycan which is
much thicker in Gram-positive cells. In Gram-positive organisms
numerous surface proteins and polymers, including lipoteichoic
acid (LTA), are also present. Gram-negative organisms possess a
second outer membrane (OM) containing lipopolysaccharide and
protein. Flagella and fimbrae are also present in some Gram-
negative cells. An external layer of capsular polysaccharide is
common to both types.

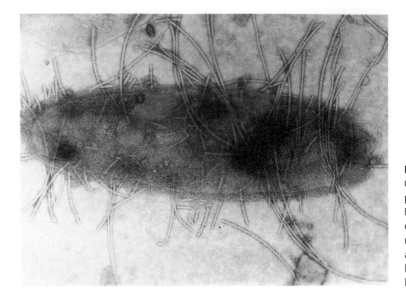

Fig. 7.2 Electron photomicrograph of a Gram-negative bacillus showing the presence of both fimbriae and flagella. Flagella are longer than fimbriae and enable the bacterium to move in a fluid medium. Fimbriae, on the other hand, are mainly involved in the adherence of bacterial cells to other bacteria and to host tissues.

weight of the cell wall) than in Gram-negative cells (where it accounts for around 10 per cent). In Gram-positive organisms, numerous surface proteins and polymeric molecules other than peptidoglycan are also found closely associated with the peptidoglycan layer. A second outer membrane is present in Gram-negative organisms which contains lipopolysaccharide and protein molecules.

Flagella and *fimbriae* are cell appendages, composed of tubular filaments of polymerized protein that project from the cell wall of some Gram-negative bacterial cells (Fig. 7.2). Flagella are much longer than most fimbriae and generate propulsive forces which enable the bacterium to move within a fluid medium. Fimbriae, often also referred to as *pili*, are mainly involved in the adherence of bacterial cells to other bacteria and to host tissues. The notable exceptions are the sex pili which are important in the transfer of bacterial DNA, usually plasmids, from one bacterium to another.

Finally, external to the cell wall, most pathogenic bacteria, whether Gram-positive or negative, are covered with a protective layer of carbohydrate known as *capsular polysaccharide*.

Classification of bacteria

It is beyond the scope of this book to consider in detail the classification systems in use for separating the major groups of bacteria. However, it is useful to acknowledge, in general terms, how this classification is achieved.

The simplest classification is based entirely on *staining characteristics* (e.g. Gram-positive or Gram-negative) and *morphology* (Fig. 7.3). However, this method alone will not differentiate significant pathogens from other organisms. Descriptions of the colony types produced when bacteria are grown on simple, artificial media, will improve differentiation considerably in experienced hands, but this is not reliable enough for routine, diagnostic use. For this reason, a range of biochemical properties, for example, the ability to ferment certain sugars, is normally examined; the wider the range, the more accurate the designation.

In practice, a combination of all these methods is used, thereby allowing bacteria to be characterized into families, genera, species and strains (Fig 7.4). For example, a Gram-negative *diplococcus* (spherical bacteria in pairs), which grows aerobically on serum-enriched media, and ferments

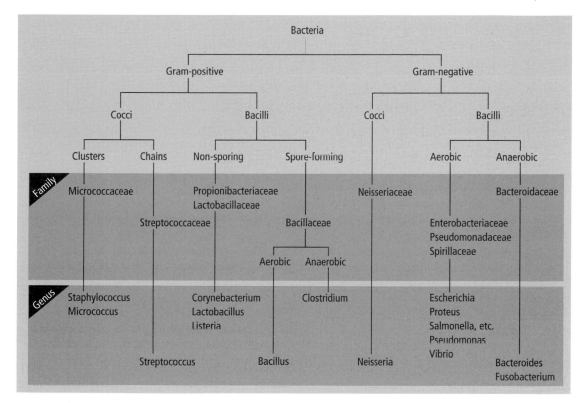

Fig. 7.3 Simple classification of Gram-stainable bacteria of clinical significance. A number of properties of bacterial cells may be exploited in order to classify bacteria into specific groups. Bacteria may be classified into broad groups depending upon their ability to retain crystal violet dye after decolorization. Those retaining dye are termed Gram-positive and those failing to do so, Gram-negative. Other characteristics including morphology (see also Fig 7.4) and biochemical properties may be used to further subdivide bacteria.

maltose and glucose, might be identified as *Neisseria* (genus) *meningitidis* (species) the causative agent of *meningococcal meningitis*.

Perhaps the most definitive method of classification is the examination of bacterial DNA sequence homology, although this is not a method which is routinely used in the laboratory identification of bacteria.

Routes of acquisition

Bacteria causing infection are acquired from two principal sources: either from amongst the patient's own normal flora (*endogenous infection*) or from external sources, for example from food (*exogenous infection*).

Exogenous infections may be acquired by one of the four principal routes detailed below.

1 *Ingestion* e.g. food poisoning associated with the consumption of foods contaminated with *Salmonella* species.

2 *Inhalation* e.g. inhalation of airborne droplets containing *Mycobacterium tuberculosis*, leading to pulmonary tuberculosis.

3 *Inoculation* e.g. rose-thorn punctures introducing *Clostridium tetani* and leading to clinical tetanus.

4 Direct contact e.g. *Neisseria gonorrhoeae*, acquired by intimate person to person contact.

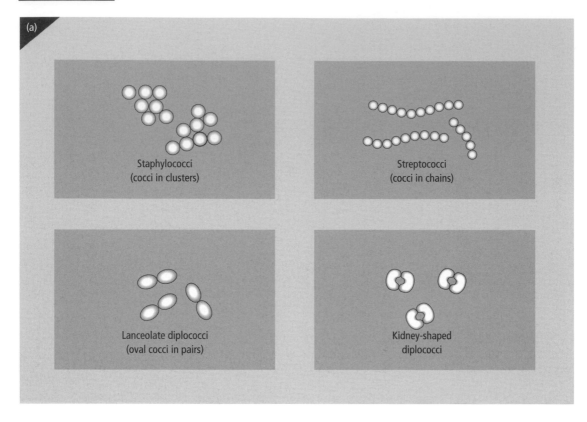

(a)

Staphylococci
(cocci in clusters)

Streptococci
(cocci in chains)

Lanceolate diplococci
(oval cocci in pairs)

Kidney-shaped
diplococci

Fig. 7.4 Basic bacterial forms. Microscopic examination of the morphology of bacteria in stained preparations is useful in classifying bacteria. Two major morphology types are recognized: cocci (a), which are roughly spherical in shape, and bacilli (b) which are rod-shaped. Within each major group certain variations exist, for example cocci are identified as streptococci if they are arranged in chains or diplococci if they are organized into pairs.

Transmission of infection

The transmission of a bacterial infection is dependent upon several factors including the characteristics of the 'host' population at risk, the bacterium concerned and the nature of the environment.

Important *host factors* include the degree of immunity to a particular pathogen within the population, the proximity of individuals to each other and the general state of health and hygiene. It is worth mentioning here that some individuals, while apparently healthy, may harbour and transmit pathogenic bacteria—these individuals are often referred to as *carriers*. For example, healthy individuals can excrete *Salmonella* species for prolonged periods, causing outbreaks of food poisoning if they are involved in the preparation of food.

Bacterial factors include: the general properties of the organism, in particular, its virulence; its ability to survive in the environment; the size of the infecting dose; and the route by which the bacterium is acquired.

Environmental factors affecting transmission include: climate (bacterial growth generally being favoured by warm humid conditions); the standard of sanitation; and the presence of non-human *'vectors'* for example ticks, which transmit bacteria whilst feeding on human or animal blood.

Bacteria can be transmitted between individuals of the same generation (horizontally e.g. *M. tuberculosis* spread by respiratory droplets) or

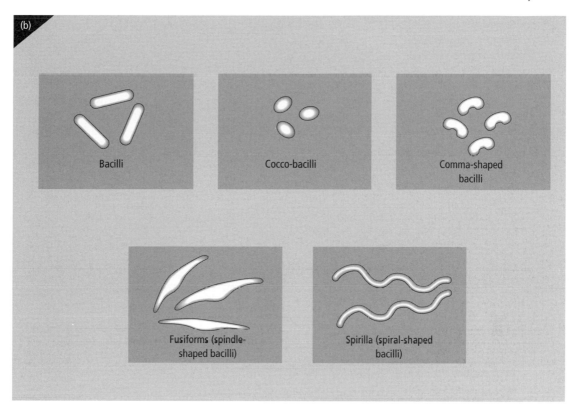

Labels within figure:
Bacilli

Cocco-bacilli

Comma-shaped bacilli

Fusiforms (spindle-shaped bacilli)

Spirilla (spiral-shaped bacilli)

Fig. 7.4 (Cont.)

from mother to baby (vertically). An example here is *Listeria monocytogenes*, which may be transmitted from mother to child *in utero* and cause generalized sepsis in the fetus or newborn child.

Virulence determinants

As alluded to earlier, pathogenic bacteria possess so called 'virulence determinants', which are responsible for their ability to cause disease. Many of these virulence determinants are cell wall constituents. An understanding of the nature and mode of action of virulence determinants is essential if we are to appreciate the mechanisms which underly the pathogenesis of bacterial diseases.

Virulence determinants specific to Gram-positive bacteria

Non-peptidoglycan polymers

These are a heterogeneous group of *teichoic acid-like polymers* containing sugar alcohols and phosphodiester linkages, which are found on the surface of Gram-positive cells, bound covalently to peptidoglycan. Their precise role in the pathogenesis of disease is unclear, but they are thought to be involved in the stimulation of the inflammatory response (see Chapter 4). They are strongly immunogenic and form the identifying group antigens of many species of streptococci.

Unlike these 'secondary' cell wall polymers, the closely related molecule, *lipoteichoic acid*, lies in contact with the cytoplasmic membrane and protrudes through the peptidoglycan layer. It is thought to be important in the adherence of bacteria to surfaces, in particular, the binding of decay-causing organisms, such as *Streptococcus mutans*, to tooth enamel.

Surface proteins

Many different cell surface proteins have been identified, the majority of which do not appear to be virulence factors. One notable exception, however, is the 'M' protein of group A beta-haemolytic streptococci (e.g. *Streptococcus pyogenes*). By binding to various serum proteins, bacteria expressing M proteins are able to avoid recognition and ingestion by phagocytic cells and inhibit neutrophil chemotaxis (see Chapter 4).

Virulence determinants specific to Gram-negative bacteria

Lipopolysaccharide

Lipopolysaccharide (LPS) is one of the most important bacterial virulence factors and is often referred to as *endotoxin*. It is an integral part of the outer surface of the outer membrane of Gram-negative cell walls and consists of an *inner glycolipid* (Lipid A) attached to a 'core' *oligosaccharide*, with or without a variable length, outer, 'O' *polysaccharide*.

Lipid A is a very potent toxin and is responsible for all the toxic properties attributed to endotoxin, although these are enhanced when the lipid molecule is associated with an O polysaccharide. Although incompletely understood, endotoxin exerts a profound effect when introduced into the host, producing widespread stimulation of the immune system and activation of the complement and the clotting cascades (see Chapter 4). This results in generalized damage to the host manifested in features collectively referred to as *endotoxic shock*, which may result in death.

The O polysaccharide chain of LPS additionally confers resistance to the bacteriolytic effects of serum and protects the bacterial cell from phagocytosis.

Outer membrane proteins

Numerous protein molecules can be found within the outer bacterial membrane. They are closely associated with LPS and often difficult to purify, but do appear to have functions in cell transport systems and ion binding. In some bacterial species, however, these proteins are also major virulence factors, enabling bacterial cells to adhere to their target tissues. Particular examples are found in enteropathogenic forms of *Escherichia coli* (EPEC) which cause diarrhoea in young children.

In other species, such as entero-invasive *E. coli* (EIEC) and *Shigella* species, which cause a dysentery-like illness, the outer membrane proteins not only help the bacteria to adhere to the gut epithelium, but also enable them to enter the host cell where they multiply and subsequently kill the cell. The precise mechanisms of this invasive process are not yet fully understood.

Flagella and fimbriae

Flagellar proteins are strong immunogens and represent the 'H' antigens used in typing many Gram-negative bacteria, notably the Salmonellae. However, apart from conferring active motility, which may be a useful attribute in certain circumstances, it is not thought that flagella are of major importance as far as virulence is concerned.

Fimbriae, on the other hand, are very significant virulence factors. Their presence is dependent upon the conditions under which the bacteria are growing but they are often present in the majority of Gram-negative bacteria. Traditionally, fimbriae have been divided into two groups, depending on whether or not their ability to agglutinate erythrocytes of several animal species can be blocked by the presence of D-mannose. The *mannose-sensitive* (MS) variants are commonly encountered and are referred to as '*common fimbriae*'. They facilitate binding to a number of cells and proteins, but their precise role remains unclear.

The role of *mannose-resistant* (MR) fimbriae,

however, is better understood, at least in certain species. The fimbriae of *N. gonorrhoeae*, for example, adhere to a number of host cell types. In addition, the fimbriae also prevent binding of the bacterium to leucocytes, thereby inhibiting phagocytosis. Certain strains of *E. coli* isolated from patients with infections of the kidney (*pyelonephritis*), possess specific fimbriae that bind to glycolipids present on the lining epithelium of the upper urinary tract. Bacteria possessing such fimbriae are less likely to be flushed away by the normal flow of urine and therefore more likely to produce clinical infection.

Another example of fimbrial adherence is seen in enterotoxin-producing *E. coli* which cause diarrhoeal disease, including the verotoxin-producing *E. coli* (VTEC) which can give rise to haemorrhagic colitis and renal failure. The fimbriae of these organisms adhere to the colonic epithelium allowing direct interaction between the potent toxins produced by the bacteria and the epithelial cells.

Virulence determinants common to Gram-negative and Gram-positive bacteria

Capsular polysaccharides

The polysaccharide matrix surrounding many bacteria is highly variable in structure and is often derived from either the non-peptidoglycan polymers in the case of Gram-positive organisms or the O polysaccharide chains of Gram-negative organisms, and is termed the 'K' antigen in enterobacteria.

Capsular polysaccharides enable the bacterium to adhere by forming a sticky layer on surfaces and are important in the formation of dental plaque and the colonization of implanted medical devices and intravenous cannulae. They also render the bacterial cell wall inaccessible to the action of complement and to phagocytosis. Some capsular polysaccharides have the added advantage of mimicking host tissue antigens and so are not recognized as foreign by the immune system. For example, certain strains of *E. coli* are able to

cause meningitis in newborn infants. These organisms possess the so-called K1 capsule, which is structurally similar to proteins found in the central nervous system of newborn infants. The immune system sees the K1 capsule as 'self' and the bacteria are therefore not destroyed.

Toxins and enzymes

Large numbers of toxins are known to be produced by bacteria. They are usually proteins of varying molecular weight and are traditionally referred to as *exotoxins* to differentiate them from the endotoxin of Gram-negative bacteria. They are numerous and wide-ranging in their effects and are conveniently grouped on the basis of the following three main characteristics.

1 *Site of action of the toxin.* Some exotoxins act only at the site at which they are released. For example, the enterotoxin of *Clostridium perfringens* acts locally on intestinal epithelial cells to cause diarrhoea. On the other hand, certain toxins may have more generalized systemic effects. Diphtheria toxin, for example, acts systemically, inhibiting host cell protein synthesis and resulting in damage to most major organs.

2 *Mode of action.* Exotoxins may either act directly to cause their effects or their effect may be mediated through other agents. Tetanus toxin, for example, acts directly by blocking the release of neurotransmitters, leading to paralysis, whereas *staphylococcal toxic shock syndrome toxin* causes the release of immune mediators from macrophages, resulting in widespread tissue damage.

3 *Structure of the toxin.* The toxin of *Streptococcus pyogenes*, streptolysin O, is a single molecule which binds to cell membranes causing lysis, whereas diphtheria toxin, after binding to a cell, requires cleavage by proteolytic enzymes before its active component can enter the cytoplasm.

Some toxins are enzymes but many other enzymes not regarded as toxins are produced by bacteria of all types. Their role as virulence factors is unclear, although some are able to lyse molecules of immunoglobulin A (IgA), which may enable them to become more easily established on mucous membranes, while others may assist in the local spread of bacteria once infection has occurred.

Other important enzymes, which cannot be classed as true virulence factors but are nevertheless important in human disease, are the enzymes produced by bacteria to counter the effects of antibiotics used to treat infections. Examples of this are the β-lactamase enzymes produced by bacteria that are capable of inactivating penicillin-like compounds.

Factors influencing bacterial virulence

Many bacteria do not have the potential to express virulence factors and are only able to do so if they acquire the necessary genetic material from plasmids or bacteriophages. Plasmid-mediated virulence factors are important in infections caused by several Gram-negative species. As transmissible units of genetic material, plasmids offer enormous potential for the exchange and recombination of gene sequences coding for virulence.

Bacteriophages are viruses capable of infecting bacterial cells and may also mediate the transfer of genetic material from one bacterial cell to another. The best example of bacteriophage-mediated virulence is *Corynebacterium diphtheriae* which requires the β-phage genome in order to produce its toxin. Environmental conditions (e.g. temperature, pH, available nutrients) also influence the expression of virulence factors, although this area is still incompletely understood.

Summary

There remains much to learn about the nature of bacterial pathogenicity, a task hindered by the diversity and adaptability of bacteria. By endeavouring to understand the basic mechanisms of bacterial infection it should be possible to devise new and more effective methods for their prevention and treatment.

Key points

1 Bacteria are prokaryotes that may be classified on the basis of staining properties, morphology and biochemical characteristics.
2 Bacterial infections may be acquired from two principal sources (a) from amongst the patients' own flora (endogenous infection) and (b) from external sources (exogenous infection).
3 Bacteria capable of causing disease (so-called 'pathogenic bacteria') possess virulence determinants that are responsible for their ability to cause disease.
4 Most virulence determinants are associated with the cell wall of pathogenic bacteria.

Further reading

Poxton I.R. & Arbuthnott J.P. (1990) Determinants of bacterial virulence. In Topley & Wilson, *Principles of Bacteriology, Virology and Immunity* (8th edn.), Vol. 1, pp. 331–353. Edward Arnold, London.

Kasper D.L. (1990) Bacterial Diseases. In Mandell G.L., Douglas R.G. & Bennett J.E. *Principles and Practice of Infectious Diseases* (3rd edn.), pp. 1484–1942. Churchill Livingstone, New York.

CHAPTER 8

Viral Infection

Introduction

Viruses are unaffected by antibiotics, are smaller than bacteria (30–200 nm) and are composed of a single type of nucleic acid (either DNA or RNA) surrounded by a protein coat (*capsid*) which may be further enclosed in an *envelope*. They are *obligate intracellular parasites*, that is, they can only replicate within a living host cell. During replication they utilize the protein and nucleic acid synthesis machinery of the cell to generate new virus particles or *virions*. The release of several hundred newly formed infectious virions invariably kills the host cell. Diseases caused by viral infection are therefore a direct result of this cell death, and/or the immune response to the virus. In some cases the immune system is itself a target for viral infection. This can lead to the destruction of important immune cells which in turn can lead to *immunosuppression*. An example of this is the immunosuppression which results from HIV infection of CD4 +ve T lymphocytes. In some cases viral infection may also contribute to the development of neoplasia.

In this chapter, virus structure and replication are briefly discussed. Modes of viral spread are then considered in relation to the important routes of transmission. The remainder of the chapter discusses in detail the effects of viral infection on the host, ranging from asymptomatic infection through to severe debilitating disease and death.

Virus structure and replication

Viruses are classified into a number of families based on differences in their structure and modes of replication. Table 8.1 summarizes the properties of some virus families and Fig. 8.1 shows a diagrammatic representation of four selected virus particles.

During replication, viruses undergo a series of steps which ultimately lead to the successful release of several hundred progeny virions.

In Step I (*attachment and penetration*) the virus attaches, via the viral capsid or envelope, to a specific receptor on the surface of a target cell, triggering off a series of events which allows the virus to penetrate the cell. It is this initial interaction which accounts for the predisposition of certain viruses to infect particular species or tissue types. For example, HIV attaches to the CD4 receptor found on certain cell types (T helper cells, see Chapter 5) via a 120 kDa envelope glycoprotein (gp120). The influenza virus attaches to sialic acid residues present on the epithelial cells of the respiratory tract. Following penetration of the cell the virus is uncoated, releasing the virus genome. In the case of many viruses, the genome migrates rapidly to the host cell nucleus where it may integrate within the host cell DNA or exist as a separate extrachromosomal entity (*episome*). In others the genome remains within the cytoplasm.

In Step II (*macromolecular synthesis*) viral nucleic acid is used for the synthesis of virus structural proteins (those proteins that will make up new virions) or non-structural proteins (that is, the virus enzymes required for the manufacture of the structural proteins). The nucleic acid also replicates to provide the genome for progeny virions. The complexity of the different mechanisms used by viruses to reproduce themselves is well illustrated by the RNA viruses. In the case of 'positive strand' RNA viruses, the viral RNA is the messenger RNA (mRNA) and is translated directly the virus enters the cell. The 'negative strand' RNA viruses firstly make mirror image copies of their genome which act as the mRNA. The retroviruses

Table 8.1 Taxonomic chart of selected virus families

Family	Characteristics	Typical members	Diseases caused
Poxviridae	Double-stranded DNA, 'brick'-shaped particles; largest virus	Vaccinia Variola	Laboratory virus Smallpox (now eradicated)
Herpesviridae	Double-stranded DNA, icosahedron capsid enclosed in an envelope, latency in host common	Herpes simplex Varicella-zoster Cytomegalovirus Epstein–Barr virus	'Cold' sores, genital infections Chicken pox, shingles Febrile illness or disseminated disease in immunosuppression Glandular fever. Virus is also associated with certain malignancies e.g. Burkitt's lymphoma
Adenoviridae	Double-stranded DNA, icosahedron with fibre structures, non-enveloped	Adenoviruses (many types)	Respiratory and eye infections, tumours in experimental animals
Papovaviridae	Double-stranded circular DNA, 72 capsomeres in capsid, non-enveloped	Human papilloma viruses	Warts, association with some cancers (e.g. cervical cancer)
Hepadnaviridae	One complete DNA minus strand with 5' terminal protein, DNA circularized by an incomplete plus strand, 42 nm enveloped particle	Hepatitis-B virus	Serum hepatitis, association with hepatocellular carcinoma
Paramyxoviridae	Single-stranded RNA, enveloped particles with 'spikes'	Parainfluenza virus Measles virus Respiratory syncytial virus	Respiratory tract infection ('croup') Measles Bronchiolitis
Orthomyxoviridae	8 segments of single-stranded RNA, enveloped particles with 'spikes', helical nucleocapsid	Influenza virus	Influenza
Reoviridae	10–12 segments of double-stranded RNA, icosahedron, non-enveloped	Rotavirus	Infantile diarrhoea
Picornaviridae	Single-stranded RNA, 22–30 nm particle of cubic symmetry, non-enveloped	Poliovirus Coxsackie virus Rhinovirus Hepatitis-A virus	Poliomyelitis Myocarditis Common cold Infectious hepatitis
Togaviridae	Single-stranded RNA, enveloped particles, icosahedron nucleocapsid	Rubella virus Arbovirus	German measles Yellow fever
Rhabdoviridae	Single-stranded RNA, bullet-shaped, enveloped particle	Rabies virus	Rabies
Retroviridae	Single-stranded RNA, enveloped particles with icosahedral nucleocapsid, employ reverse transcriptase enzyme to make DNA copy of genome on infection	Human T lymphotropic virus-1 Human immunodeficiency virus (HIV)	Adult T cell leukaemia and lymphoma Acquired immune deficiency syndrome (AIDS)

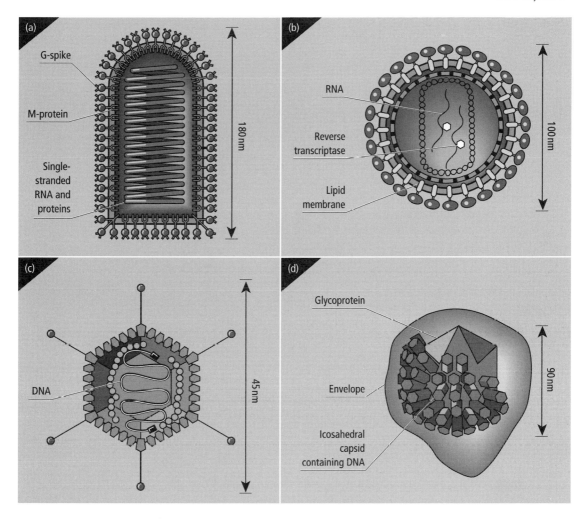

Fig. 8.1 Diagrammatic representation of the structure of four virus particles. Rabies virus (a) and HIV (b) have tight-fitting envelopes, herpes simplex (d) has a loose-fitting envelope, whereas adenovirus (c) is non-enveloped. The diagrams are based on electron microscopic observation and molecular configuration exercises.

have a more complex replication mechanism (Fig. 8.2) which involves the use of a viral *reverse transcriptase* enzyme which makes a DNA copy of the viral RNA. This DNA copy is integrated into the host cell DNA where it is referred to as a *provirus*. The provirus is then transcribed to generate the early viral proteins required for replication.

In Step III (*assembly*) the newly formed viral proteins enclose the viral nucleic acid to form mature virus particles.

In Step IV (*release*) these particles leave either by lysing the infected cell or by budding from the host cell plasma membrane. In some cases host-derived membrane proteins may form part of the virus envelope. Virus release often leads to cell death.

During infection, viral proteins are processed by the host cell into peptides and presented on the surface of the cell in association with MHC Class 1 molecules (see Chapter 5). Infected cells, therefore, can be recognized and destroyed by cytotoxic T lymphocytes carrying the CD8 surface receptor. Although an effective immune

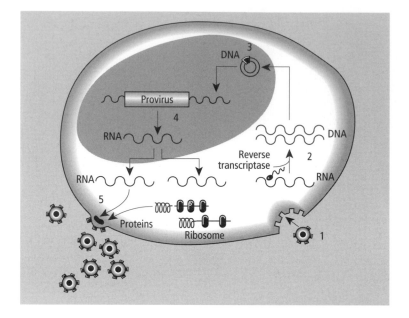

Fig. 8.2 Life cycle of a retrovirus: (1) retrovirus binds to a specific receptor on the cell surface and enters the cell; (2) the virus is uncoated and reverse transcriptase employed to make a double-stranded DNA copy of the RNA genome; (3) the DNA copy is transported to the nucleus and integrates into the cellular genome where it is known as a provirus; (4) viral DNA is transcribed to produce genomic RNA and mRNA for the synthesis of structural virus proteins and enzymes; (5) new virus particles are assembled and leave the cell by budding at the cell membrane.

response against a virus-infected cell often depends upon an efficient cytotoxic T cell response, other immune effector systems may also be important. The immune responses to virus infection are summarized in Fig. 8.3. It is important to emphasize that while replication of viruses can cause cell death and therefore tissue damage, in many cases this is further exacerbated by the immune response to the infection which will also lead to significant tissue destruction.

Viral spread

In order to persist and evolve in nature, viruses need a large population of susceptible hosts and an efficient means of spread between these hosts. The *respiratory route* is the most common pathway for virus entry and exit. Following inhalation, viruses often infect and replicate within epithelial cells of the upper or lower respiratory tract. Following release from these cells, progeny virions enter surrounding airways and exit via sneezing and coughing. Examples of viruses which are transmitted in this way include the influenza and parainfluenza viruses, the common cold viruses, adenoviruses and the respiratory syncytial virus (RSV).

Although the entry and exit of many viruses is via the respiratory tract, some viruses do not remain within the respiratory tract but may enter the bloodstream causing *viraemia* (defined as the presence of infectious virions in the bloodstream) and subsequent infection of other target organs. Examples of such viruses include: the varicella-zoster virus, which is responsible for chicken pox; the measles virus; and the rubella virus, the causative agent of German measles.

The *oral-gastrointestinal* route is used mainly by those viruses responsible for gut infections (rotavirus, Norwalk virus, and the enteroviruses, including, polio and coxsackie viruses). Again many of these viruses (e.g. polio and coxsackie viruses) leave the gastrointestinal tract and cause

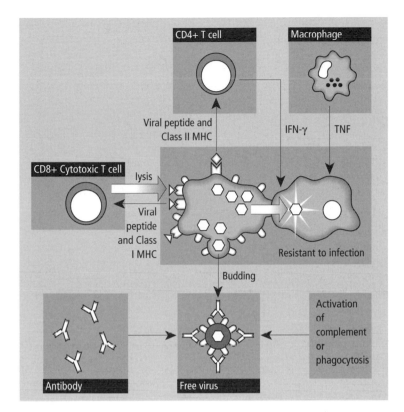

Fig. 8.3 Summary of immune responses to viral infection. A virus-infected cell is able to process viral peptides and present these on the surface of the cell in association with MHC Class I molecules. This complex is recognized by CD8 +ve T cells which are able to lyse the infected cell. CD4 +ve T cells recognize viral antigens associated with MHC Class II molecules and these cells, together with macrophages release cytokines that act on other cells, making them resistant to further viral infection. Free viruses released by infected cells may be bound by specific antibody. Subsequent activation of complement may lead to lysis of viral particles or promote their phagocytosis.

serious debilitating diseases elsewhere, in many cases within the central nervous system (CNS). Vast numbers of infectious virus particles can be excreted in faecal material (e.g., of the order of 10^{12} particles/gm) facilitating the easy spread of these viruses in conditions of poor sanitation. The drinking of faecally contaminated water, and consumption of contaminated shellfish or other food prepared by unhygienic food handlers are ways in which these viruses are spread between susceptible hosts. Infections caused by these viruses are widespread in 'developing' countries where poor sanitation is a particular problem.

Whilst the *skin* normally provides an impenetrable barrier to virus invasion, infectious viruses can enter following trauma to the skin. This may be a bite from an animal vector (e.g. transmission of the rabies virus from the bite of an infected canine), or an arthropod vector (e.g. the transmission of the yellow fever virus by mosquitoes). HIV or hepatitis-B virus may be transmitted by the injection of blood or blood products either in the form of a blood transfusion, a needle-stick injury, or by intravenous drug abuse.

Sexual transmission of viruses is an important route for the spread of herpes simplex virus (HSV) and the papilloma viruses. The advent of the acquired immune deficiency syndrome (AIDS) has highlighted the ease with which viruses, in this case HIV, can be transmitted during unprotected

63

sexual intercourse. Unprotected penetrative anal intercourse among homosexual men has been the main route by which HIV has been transmitted in the 'developed' world. In Sub-Saharan Africa and the Caribbean, where the virus is endemic in the heterosexual population, transmission during vaginal intercourse is the most important route for viral spread.

Viruses may also be transmitted *vertically* that is, from mother to offspring via the placenta, during childbirth, or in breast milk. For example, rubella virus and cytomegalovirus (CMV) infections acquired by the mother during pregnancy may be transmitted to the developing embryo and can lead to severe congenital abnormalities and/or spontaneous abortion. Some viral infections, for example HSV infections, if acquired *in utero* or during birth can present as an acute disease syndrome in a neonate. Alternatively, the child may be born without any overt signs of disease but may still carry the virus as an asymptomatic infection. The development of this 'carrier state' follows congenital infections with viruses like HIV or the hepatitis B virus. The developing fetus of an HIV-positive mother has an estimated 40–60 percent chance of becoming infected with HIV.

Some of the routes for virus spread within the host are summarized in Fig. 8.4.

The clinical results of viral infections

The outcome of a viral infection is dependent on several factors. These include various host-related factors, including age and immune status. Thus, HSV infection is usually fatal in a neonate but may cause inapparent infections or minor epithelial lesions (e.g. 'cold' sores) in older children and adults. Epstein–Barr virus (EBV) causes a very mild febrile illness in infants but infectious mononucleosis (glandular fever) in teenagers. The same virus in parts of tropical Africa and in China is believed to contribute to the development of Burkitt's lymphoma and nasopharyngeal carcinoma respectively (see Chapter 29). CMV in a healthy individual may cause a mild febrile illness, but in immunosuppressed individuals can

lead to fatal pneumonia. Measles rarely causes severe complications in healthy well nourished children, but kills around 900 000 children per year in 'developing' countries.

There are also many 'unknowns' in studies on viral infections. Why, for example, even in the absence of vaccination, do most people infected with polio virus show no signs of ill health, and in those with symptoms why do only about 10 percent suffer CNS damage? Likewise, why do a very small proportion of cold sore sufferers develop fatal HSV encephalitis?

For the purpose of the current discussion, the clinical outcome of a viral infection will be considered under seven general headings. It will be seen that the distinction between these clinical groups is not always clear cut and in some cases there may be considerable overlap between them.

Inapparent (asymptomatic) infection

Many virus infections are *sub-clinical*, there being no apparent outward symptoms of disease. This is virtually always true in the immune host, where recovery from a previous infection or vaccination protects the host from virus growth following reinfection by the wild-type virus. However, several viruses, including some respiratory viruses and enteroviruses, do not produce clinical symptoms even in non-immune individuals. Thus, the polio virus, in 80 percent of infected individuals, replicates in the epithelial cells of the gastrointestinal tract, is excreted in the faeces, but causes no symptoms. After a few days, the virus is eradicated and the host acquires life-long immunity.

Disease syndrome, virus eradication and recovery

The pattern we expect following most viral infections in otherwise healthy individuals, is that of clinical symptoms of varying degrees of severity (i.e. disease syndrome), followed by virus eradication by the immune system, recovery and often life-long immunity. This is true of most childhood viral infections, for example measles, mumps and

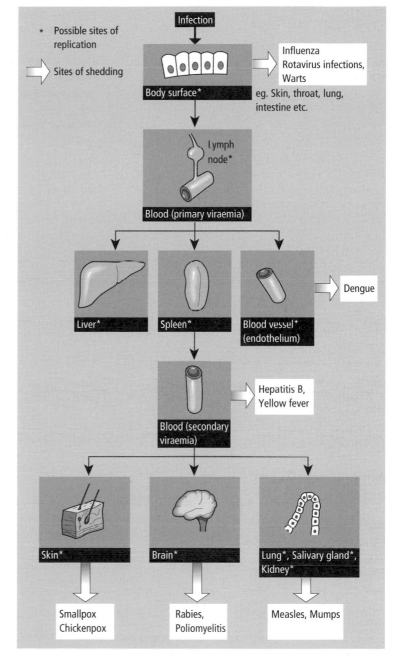

Fig. 8.4 Virus spread within the host. Different viruses have different modes of spread within the host. Some viruses remain localized at the site of entry, whereas others may spread to involve other tissues. Routes of infection are shown, together with examples of possible clinical outcomes (white boxes).

German measles, and most respiratory infections, for which there are a huge number of viruses responsible. A vast spectrum of other viral infections also follow this pattern, including those resulting from hepatitis-A virus (infectious hepatitis), rotavirus (gut infections) and coxsackie virus (myocarditis, pericarditis, conjunctivitis). The following section outlines the typical patterns of infection seen with both a local and a systemic virus infection.

65

Local virus infection

RSV infections are confined to the respiratory tract and are responsible for severe respiratory distress in children less than 12 months old. RSV infection causes necrosis of the bronchiolar epithelium which sloughs off, blocking the small airways. This in turn leads to obstruction of air flow and respiratory distress. Obstruction is compounded by the increased secretion of mucus and the presence of inflammatory exudates within the airways. The bronchiolar inflammation (bronchio-litis) may progress to pneumonia, when oedema and necrosis of the lung parenchyma result in the filling and collapse of the alveoli. Children recovering from acute RSV bronchiolitis are often left with a weakened and vulnerable respiratory system, predisposing them to a lifetime of chronic lung disease. Figure 8.5 illustrates the possible outcomes of respiratory invasion by viruses.

Systemic virus infection

Following respiratory infection with measles, the

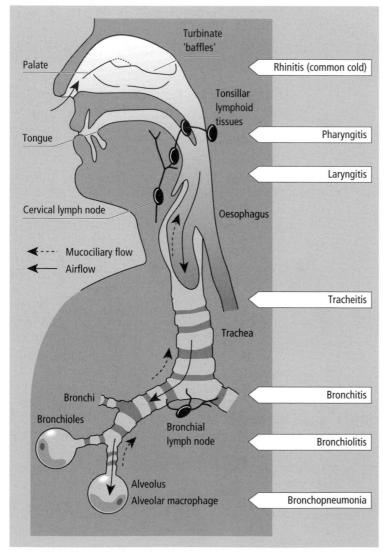

Fig. 8.5 Routes of infection in the respiratory tract. Virus infections can produce a variety of respiratory disorders depending on the area of the respiratory tract infected.

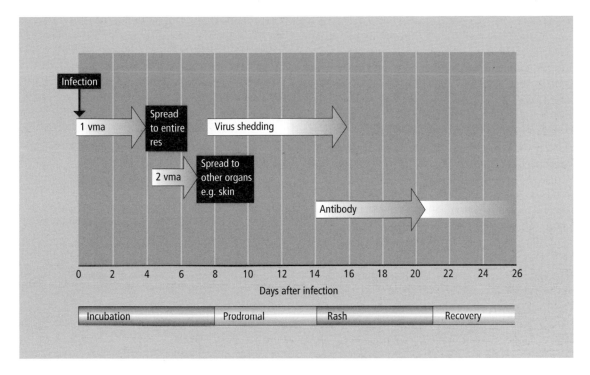

Fig. 8.6 The course of clinical measles. Measles is characterized by a primary viraemia (1 vma) followed by a secondary viraemia (2 vma). Virus shedding occurs, at which point the patient is highly infectious. A prodromal phase is followed by the typical symptoms and signs of measles, including a rash. The appearance of antibody is usually followed by complete recovery and life-long immunity. res, reticuloendothelial system.

virus replicates in the lymph nodes that drain from the infected tissue. The virus spreads to the rest of the lymphoid system and respiratory tract through the blood in a primary viraemia. Giant cells infected with the measles virus are formed in lymphoid tissues and on epithelial surfaces, these giving rise to free viruses which again enter the bloodstream in a secondary viraemia. Subsequently, this 'second wave' of viruses infect the skin and viscera, kidney and bladder. At this stage the patient is highly infectious and may present with fever, malaise, sneezing, rhinitis, respiratory congestion, conjunctivitis and a cough. The distinctive measles rash appears about 14 days post-infection. The rash is characterized by vascular congestion, oedema, and epithelial necrosis. The

primary events of a measles infection are summarized in Fig. 8.6.

Latency

A restricted range of viruses, most being in the herpesvirus family (HSV, varicella-zoster, EBV and CMV), are not eradicated from the body following recovery, but instead become *'latent'* within the host. Virus replication may be initiated some time later (*reactivation*) and cause clinical symptoms which are similar to those observed in primary infection.

HSV can reactivate many times during the life of an individual and produces the typical painful cold sore lesions on the mouth or genitals. Following primary infection, HSV travels via the nerve axon to the CNS where it lays dormant in the trigeminal or sacral ganglia. It may remain dormant for the lifetime of the patient, for several years, or occasionally only for a few months before reactivating. A variety of stimuli including menstruation, exposure to ultraviolet light and stress induce the virus to reactivate and travel back down the axon to the periphery, where it causes the characteristic lesions. HSV can spread by cell-to-cell fusion, thus protecting it from the high concentrations of HSV antibody found in the sera of infected patients. Cytotoxic T cells are eventually responsible for abrogating clinical infection.

Alternatively, a very different clinical syndrome may result following virus reactivation. Thus, primary infection with the varicella-zoster virus produces chickenpox, whereas reactivation is associated with the development of shingles. Shingles is characterized by a localized area of extremely painful vesicles from which the varicella-zoster virus can be isolated. The lesions may clear after 1–2 weeks but often result in an aftermath of severe neuralgia which may persist for months or years. However, it is unusual for patients to present with further attacks of shingles unless they are immunocompromised.

It is important to make the distinction here between clinical latency and microbiological latency. *Microbiological latency* defines a situation where the virus exists within a cell but does not replicate, usually producing only those virus proteins required to maintain the virus within the cell. *Microbiological latency* usually also results in *clinical latency*, there being no outward signs of infection. The difficulty in accurately defining latency is well illustrated in the case of EBV. Following primary infection, EBV persists within the host within B lymphocytes where the virus is latent. This latent state is characterized by the production of only those viral proteins required for the maintenance of the viral genome within the cell and there is no viral replication. However, free viruses can be isolated from the saliva of normal individuals during this clinically latent infection, implying that viruses are replicated at low levels in the oropharyngeal epithelial cells. Reactivation of EBV often occurs during immunosuppression and is characterized by the onset of the typical symptoms of infectious mononucleosis with or without the development of lymphoproliferative disease (see Case Study 31.2).

Carrier state

Although a rare event following viral infection, the virus carrier state is induced by hepatitis-B virus and HIV. Five to 10 percent of individuals infected with hepatitis-B virus will carry the infective particles in their blood for months or years. Estimates suggest that 200 million individuals worldwide carry the virus in their blood and body fluids. One reason for this is that, in addition to being transmitted horizontally, the virus is also passed from mother to offspring. Unfortunately, chronic hepatitis-B carriers also have a greatly increased risk of developing hepatocellular carcinoma (see Chapter 29).

Following exposure to HIV, the virus nucleic acid becomes integrated into the chromosome of host cells where it may remain for months or years before causing disease. The infected individual becomes antibody-positive, this positivity denoting the presence of free infectious virus or virus-infected cells within blood, semen, vaginal fluid and saliva. In 1994 there were estimated to be 14 million HIV-positive virus carriers in the world with predictions of 38−110 million by 2015AD.

Host immunosuppression

Mild immunosuppression can often result from viral infections such as measles and glandular fever. However, the advent of AIDS has highlighted the dramatic consequences of viral infection of the immune system.

HIV infects and grows best in cells which express the surface glycoprotein CD4 (i.e. T helper cells). The progression from HIV positivity to a pre-AIDS syndrome and ultimately to AIDS is usually best indicated by a dramatic drop in the CD4 +ve cell count, extremely low levels demonstrating the extent to which the patient may become immunosuppressed. This drop in CD4 +ve cells is brought about by activation of the virus, which lyses the cell in which it is harboured, releasing hundreds of progeny virions which infect and kill other CD4 +ve cells. The T helper cell is of central importance in the immune system (see Chapter 5) and depletion rapidly leads to invasion by opportunistic pathogens including HSV, CMV, *Pneumocystis carinii* and *Candida albicans* (see Case Study 11.2).

The appearance of widespread lesions of Kaposi's sarcoma is also typical of a person with AIDS. Some relief from these AIDS-associated conditions is possible with chemotherapy, but restoring the CD4 +ve cell count on a long-term basis is ineffective. Severe immunosuppression eventually leads to death, most often from an opportunistic infection.

Neoplastic growth

Introduction of genetic material and the re-arrangement or 'switching on' of cellular genes are events that can be mediated by viruses. In some situations this can contribute to the development of neoplasia. This is discussed in detail in Chapter 29.

Death

Whilst many viral infections are fatal in distinct circumstances and others in a percentage of victims, some are always fatal. Rabies, HIV infection leading to AIDS, and a range of neurological conditions resulting from viral infections, including sub-acute sclerosing panencephalitis (SSPE), are examples. SSPE is a very rare condition which occurs some months or years after a primary measles infection and is the result of the slow and persistent growth of the measles virus within brain cells.

Whilst the incubation period of rabies is 30–90 days, patients with initial symptoms of the disease die within 7–12 days. Following a bite, the virus may enter the peripheral nerves and moves to the spinal cord and brain where it replicates. The virus then leaves the CNS and spreads to virtually all tissues of the body, including the salivary glands where it is shed in saliva. The patient develops a variety of abnormalities including hydrophobia (aversion to water), rigidity, photophobia (aversion to light), fasciculations (muscle twitches) and paresis (motor weakness), cerebellar signs, cranial nerve palsies, hypo- or hyper-

reflexia, focal or generalized convulsions and a variety of autonomic disturbances. Development of a flaccid paralysis and onset of coma precede fatal complications.

Summary

Viral infections are responsible for more visits to family doctor surgeries than any other single disease condition and yet, to date, most remain untreatable. Whilst a handful of vaccines are available, for several the efficacy is poor and their cost is prohibitive to countries with poor economies. Viral infections will therefore continue to

Key points

1 Viruses are intracellular parasites that are composed of a single type of nucleic acid (either DNA or RNA) surrounded by a protein coat (capsid) and in some cases by an outer envelope.

2 Viruses can only survive and replicate inside host cells. Distinct stages in virus replication can be recognized. These are: (a) attachment and penetration; (b) macromolecular synthesis; (c) assembly; and (d) release, which often results in cell death.

3 The tissue damage caused by viral infections is the result of the direct cytopathic effects of the virus or the immune response to the virus, or a combination of both.

4 Viruses can gain access to the host through the skin and mucous membranes, via the respiratory or gastrointestinal tracts, or through sexual contact. Viruses may also be transmitted vertically from the mother to her offspring.

5 Infections caused by viruses are either localized at or near the site of virus entry, or systemic, where the virus spreads from its point of entry to involve one or more target organs.

6 In humans the outcome of a viral infection follows basic patterns. These include: (a) inapparent infection; (b) disease syndrome, virus eradication and recovery; (c) latency; (d) carrier state; (e) immunosuppression; (f) neoplasia; and (g) death.

cause severe morbidity and mortality until such a time as scientific know-how and a favourable economic climate allow the development of effective vaccines and chemotherapeutic agents.

Further reading

Collier L. & Oxford J. (1993) *Human Virology*. Oxford University Press, Oxford.

Mims C.A., Playfair J.H.L., Roitt I., Wakelin D., Williams R. & Anderson R.M. (1993) *Medical Microbiology*. Mosby, London.

Zuckerman A.J., Banatvala J.E. & Patterson J.R. (Eds) (1987) *Principles and Practice of Clinical Virology*. Wiley.

Fungal Infection

Introduction

Fungi are micro-organisms that obtain nutrients from the dead remains of animals or plants, or occur as parasites on living hosts. Of the thousands of species known, the vast majority do not cause disease in humans or other mammals. Those which do, commonly cause disease by invading the tissue or by eliciting an allergic response. Another type of disease (*toxicosis*) occurs when the metabolic products of fungi, present in spoiled food, cause poisoning on ingestion.

This chapter deals mainly with infection resulting from invasion of the tissues of the host. Selected examples of important pathogenic fungi are used to illustrate the essential features of fungal infection.

Classification of pathogenic fungi

The fungi responsible for human disease can be divided into two major groups, on the basis of either the type of infection they produce or their growth characteristics.

Type of infection

Two types of fungal infection (*mycoses*) are recognized (Table 9.1): (a) *superficial mycoses*, where fungus growth is confined to body surfaces, including skin, hair and nails; and (b) *deep mycoses*, when infection of internal organs occurs.

Growth characteristics

Pathogenic fungi may exist as *branched filamentous forms* or as *yeasts*. Some fungi show both growth forms depending on the environmental con-

ditions and are often referred to as *dimorphic fungi*. The filamentous forms (often referred to as *moulds*) produce branching *hyphae* (Fig. 9.1a) which extend as a result of transverse divisions forming a network of hyphae, or *mycelium*. Asexual reproduction results in the formation of spores known as *conidia*. Dispersal of the spores is the means by which the fungus is spread. Yeasts are single cells (Fig. 9.1b) that can reproduce by simple division. Budding of yeast cells may occur resulting in the formation of *pseudohyphae*.

Among fungi causing human infection, many are normally free-living saprophytes or plant parasites and infection follows their accidental introduction into the host tissues. Many of these species have an optimum growth temperature close to blood heat, resulting from saprophytic adaptation to other warm habitats such as self heating accumulations of decomposing vegetation. Such fungi, whilst they may cause devastating disease, are nevertheless poorly adapted mammalian pathogens and there is no spread to a second individual. This is in direct contrast to the infection of skin, nail and hair by the adapted parasitic fungi known as the *dermatophytes*, which depend upon contagious spread to new hosts for their survival.

Candidosis

Candida albicans is a commensal organism, found in the gut of many species of mammals and birds, particularly those which habitually have a diet high in sugar and other carbohydrates. Approximately 60–70 percent of healthy people carry the species in the intestine, and probably 40–50 percent also in the mouth. In addition, some 40 percent of women have *C. albicans* in the vaginal

Table 9.1 Selected examples of superficial and deep mycoses. Organisms that can produce deep mycoses may also cause infections which remain localized to the skin and mucous membranes (e.g. *Candida albicans*)

Superficial mycoses	Deep mycoses
Ringworm	Candidosis
	Aspergillosis
	Histoplasmosis
	Cryptococcosis

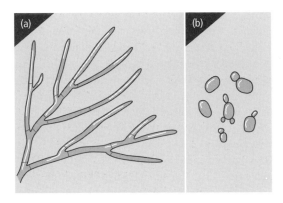

Fig. 9.1 Growth characteristics of fungi. Some fungi exist as filamentous forms, producing branched hyphae (a). Others exist as single cells and are known as yeasts (b). A third group, known as dimorphic fungi, can exist in both filamentous and yeast forms. Their transition from one form to another is dependent upon the prevailing environmental conditions.

mucosa. In most healthy people *C. albicans* is harmless. However, under certain circumstances, such as during immunosuppression, it may cause serious disease.

Infection by *C. albicans* (and, less commonly, by other species of *Candida* such as *C. tropicalis*, *C. krusei* and *C. parapsilosis*) can take many forms depending upon the part of the body involved. Symptoms range from fatal infection of deep organs to superficial skin rashes and diseases of mucous membranes of the alimentary and genito-urinary systems.

Deep infections

Serious, often fatal, deep infection occurs in two main groups of hospitalized patients. Firstly, among patients undergoing immunosuppressive therapy for malignancy or organ transplantation, *Candida* infections of deep organs such as liver, kidney, and brain represents a common cause of morbidity or mortality. A second major group of cases occurs among surgical patients, often without severe immunosuppression but in whom physical barriers to infection have been removed. A smaller third group is represented by intravenous drug abusers who may inject *Candida* organisms directly into the bloodstream.

Candida septicaemia (the presence of *Candida* organisms in the bloodstream) is a serious compli-

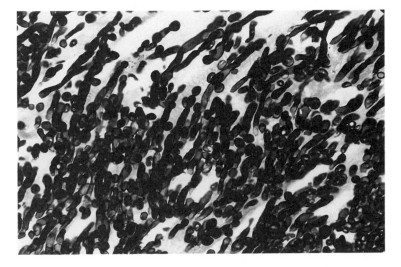

Fig. 9.2 Growth of *Candida albicans* in the tissue of a heart valve. (From a case of candida endocarditis.)

cation in immunosuppressed patients. Clinical indicators of systemically spread *Candida* are the development of discrete cutaneous lesions and *endophthalmitis* (infection within the eye). *Candida* septicaemia in immunocompetent individuals may result in colonization of the endocardium (Fig. 9.2) leading to endocarditis, particularly if there is already some abnormality of heart structure.

Superficial infections

Candida infection of the skin of the napkin area is a common problem in infants, producing *macular erythema* (discrete patches of redness) especially in the skin folds and inguinal fold. Smaller 'satellite' lesions also occur outside the main area of reddening. Similar changes are seen in adults, especially in diabetics who are particularly prone to skin infections.

Candida infection of the mouth and vagina (often referred to as 'thrush') represents another common form of superficial infection. White plaque-like lesions are produced on the epithelia which are seen to be reddened if the plaque is removed. The plaque consists of a mixture of keratinized epithelial cells and fungal hyphae and yeast cells.

Oral thrush is common in infants, in diabetic patients and under denture plates. It is also commonly encountered in patients with AIDS (see Case Study 11.2). Vaginal thrush causes itching and burning sensations and a discharge is common. Women with diabetes, and those in advanced pregnancy are particularly prone to vaginal thrush.

Chronic mucocutaneous candidosis is a special type of superficial infection that occurs in children, at least some of whom have been shown to have inherited defects of the immune system. It is characterized by the development of extensive and persistent skin infection and oral thrush at a very early age. As the child grows, the infection causes disfiguring scaly swellings.

Aspergillosis

Aspergillosis is the clinical term given to disease produced by members of the genus *Aspergillus*. These saprophytic filamentous fungi are ubiquitous in the environment where they are commonly isolated from decaying organic debris. *Aspergillus fumigatus* is the most common pathogen in this genus, although *A. flavus*, *A. terreus*, *A. nidulans* and *A. niger* may occasionally cause disease.

Asexual spores (conidia) are produced in vast numbers from the heads of maturing conidiophores (Fig. 9.3) from which they are liberated into the environment. Inhalation of these spores can lead to infection. Aspergillus species are opportunistic pathogens that are unable to invade or colonize healthy lungs but can cause devastating systemic infection in immunocompromised patients. The two most common forms of aspergillosis in non-compromised patients are allergic aspergillosis and aspergilloma; in neither of these is the fungus invasive.

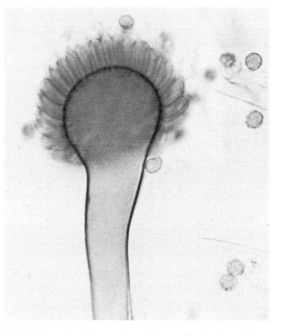

Fig. 9.3 Spore-producing structure of *Aspergillus fumigatus*, from *in vitro* culture.

Allergic aspergillosis

This is a localized reaction to inhaled spores and the mycelium produced by their subsequent germination in the bronchi. It is primarily a Type 1 (IgE-mediated) hypersensitivity response (see Chapter 12) and may be particularly severe in atopic individuals. In addition, the production of circulating aspergillus-specific IgG antibody results in the formation of antibody–antigen complexes leading to complement activation (Chapter 4) and localized tissue damage.

Aspergilloma

Aspergilloma is the name given to the fungus ball that can colonize old tuberculous or other preexisting lung cavities. The fungus grows as a compact mass of mycelium and normally does not invade adjacent tissue. This infection is only serious if the patient becomes immunosuppressed or if the fungus ball impinges on a blood vessel. Damage to the blood vessel can lead to bleeding in the lungs which is often clinically apparent as *haemoptysis* (the coughing up of blood).

Invasive aspergillosis

The most serious form of the disease is invasive aspergillosis. This is seen in immunocompromised patients, especially those with low neutrophil counts. In these patients, inhalation of spores may be followed by extensive growth of fungal forms within the lungs and frequent dissemination to other organs, especially the brain. Invasive aspergillosis is rapidly fatal and is often only diagnosed *post mortem.*

Histoplasmosis

This is one of several mycoses in which a normally saprophytic mould-like fungus changes to a unicellular, budding, growth form upon infection. Spores from the mycelium of *Histoplasma capsulatum* living in the soil are inhaled deep into the lungs where they are phagocytosed by macro-

phages. Instead of succumbing to the lytic enzymes of the macrophage, the conidia begin to reproduce as yeast cells. Eventually, the organisms burst from the host macrophages and are phagocytosed by other macrophages, thus spreading the infection (Fig. 9.4).

H. capsulatum is known to be restricted to certain soil types and geographical areas, notably guano-enriched soils in the Mississippi and Ohio river valleys of the USA, and in many tropical areas. In these regions, skin testing with a fungal extract (histoplasmin) has shown that almost all the human and mammalian population have been infected, probably experiencing a self-limiting sub-clinical or flu-like illness. In a small percentage of cases there will be a recurrence of symptoms and some of these patients will develop chronic disease of the lung. Occasionally, particularly in immunosuppressed patients, there is dissemination through the reticulo-endothelial system to cause fatal infection of many organs.

As with other deep mycoses, the fungus does not normally spread to other hosts, although pseudo-epidemics can occur where a group of cases can be traced to inhalation of conidia from a common source.

Cryptococcosis

This is caused by the yeast *Cryptococcus neoformans,* a saprophyte which exists in dried accumulations of the droppings of pigeons and other birds. The disease is rare but it is probable that sub-clinical infection of the lungs is common. The most common form of cryptococcosis involves infection of the central nervous system, which is often manifested as meningitis, although infection can occur in any deep organ or in the skin.

As with other opportunistic fungal infections, cryptococcosis is commonly seen in immuno-suppressive states, including AIDS. The yeast cells of this fungus secrete a mucilaginous capsule which is thought to protect the fungus from phagocytosis by host cells.

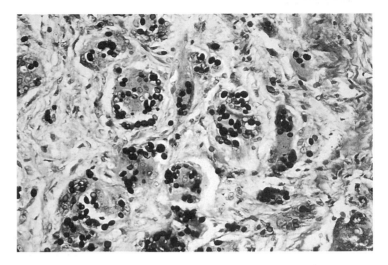

Fig. 9.4 Lung infection with *Histoplasma capsulatum*. The organisms are present within macrophages.

Dermatophytosis (ringworm)

Ringworm is caused by a group of fungi known as dermatophytes. These fungi live on the keratinized tissue of skin, hair and nails and although closely related to certain soil fungi, many have become adapted to a purely parasitic existence.

Human infections can be caused by *anthropophilic*, *zoophilic* or *geophilic* species. Anthropophilic dermatophytes are entirely dependent on passage from one human host to another and infections can occur in any body site. They are passed on to susceptible hosts by direct contact or contact with shed infected skin cells in which the fungus can lie dormant for several years.

Zoophilic species have become adapted to life on animal hosts; when passed to humans, infection most often occurs in the exposed sites of the head, neck, trunk and limbs.

Infections with geophilic species are rare. These dermatophytes are more suited to a saprophytic existence in the soil but can cause infection following contact with contaminated soil.

There are three main genera of dermatophyte fungi: *Trichophyton*, *Microsporum* and *Epidermophyton*. The three genera are indistinguishable in tissue. In culture, all three genera produce distinctive multicellular macroconidia or large spores. In addition, *Trichophyton* and *Microsporum*

species produce unicellular microconidia. Hair infections are characterized by the production of large numbers of arthroconidia (spores formed from fragmentation of hyphae). These may be *ectothrix*, forming a sheath around the hair, or, *endothrix* in which hair penetration is followed by spore production within the hair shaft.

Probably the most common and therefore the best known anthropophilic dermatophytosis is athlete's foot or *tinea pedis*, caused most often by *Trichophyton rubrum* or *T. interdigitale*. Athlete's foot is common in affluent countries where there is ready access to swimming baths and sports facilities where use of communal changing rooms facilitates transfer from host to host. Occlusive footwear also provides the warm, moist conditions in which the fungus thrives. Athlete's foot is characterized by itching, skin peeling, maceration and fissuring of the toe webs often with concomitant nail infection in which the nails may become discoloured and crumbly. Lesions on smooth skin are itchy, *erythematous* (red) and flaky and may take on the circular appearance from which the term 'ringworm' was derived.

Infections with zoophilic species often induces a more marked inflammatory response. Occasionally, suppurating, highly inflammatory lesions known as *kerions* may be produced. Scalp infections in children in the UK are now most often caused by zoophilic species acquired from animals. Scalp infections with the anthropophilic species *Microsporum audouinii* are still common in 'developing' countries but are now rare in the UK.

Mycetoma

This exemplifies a range of mycoses which are mainly subcutaneous in nature, resulting from traumatic inoculation of a saprophytic fungus through the skin. Many fungal species and aerobic actinomycetes (bacteria capable of forming hyphal forms) are able to cause mycetoma and whilst they show minor differences in histological appearance there are several unifying features. The inoculated fungus grows slowly in the presence of a massive and intense host inflammatory response. The resulting mycelial microcolonies appear as tightly packed 'grains' just visible to the naked eye. These microcolonies break apart and re-form, enabling a slowly progressive, localized infection to develop. There is often massive swelling of the affected area, which may penetrate and erode underlying bone. Sinus tracts filled with pus develop around the grains and these may drain out onto the surface of the skin. Left untreated, many mycetomas will continue an inexorable spread further and further from the original site and cause death if vital viscera become involved. Initial infections most often occur on the feet and render amputation a possible form of treatment.

Summary

Many of the fungi that cause human infection are normally free-living saprophytes or plant para-

sites and infection often occurs following their accidental introduction into host tissues. The establishment of an infection by these organisms often occurs in the absence of a competent immune system. This is in contrast to the dermatophytes that infect skin, hair and nails. These organisms are the only fungi that are adapted to contagious spread between individuals.

Key points

1 Fungi can cause disease in humans by invasion of tissue, by eliciting an allergic reaction or by toxicosis.
2 Dermatophytosis or ringworm of skin, nails and hair is the only truly contagious fungal infection.
3 *Candida albicans* and related yeasts living harmlessly in the body can cause serious infection in people with lowered immunity.
4 *Aspergillus fumigatus* and *Cryptococcus neoformans* are examples of free-living fungi capable of causing serious deep infection following inhalation of airborne spores. These infections are common in immunosuppressed individuals.
5 Many serious deep fungal infections such as histoplasmosis and mycetoma are encountered in tropical regions and in North America.

Further reading

Evans E.G.V. & Gentles J.C. (1985) *Essentials of Medical Mycology*. Churchill Livingstone, Edinburgh.
Kwon-Chung K.J. & Bennett J.E. (1991) *Medical Mycology*. Lea & Febiger, Philadelphia.
Warnock D.W. & Richardson M.D. (eds.) (1991) *Fungal Infection in the Compromised Patient* (2nd edn.) Wiley, Chichester.

Parasitic Infection

Introduction

In Chapter 6, a parasite was defined as an organism (plant or animal) which lives on or in another organism (the host), takes nutriment directly from it and which, under certain circumstances, may be harmful. However, in the study of microbiology, the term 'parasite' is often used to designate protozoa and members of the animal kingdom that infect and cause disease in other animals including humans. This chapter describes the general features of parasitic infection. Selected examples of important parasitic infections are summarized.

Classification of parasites

Three groups of parasites are recognized. These are *protozoa, helminths* and *arthropods*.

Protozoa

Protozoa are single-celled organisms that are larger than bacteria and whose DNA is organized in a nucleus. Protozoa are further subdivided into *amoebae, flagellates, ciliates* and *sporozoa* (Table 10.1).

Helminths

These are the parasitic worms. They are large multicellular organisms and are divided into three groups: the tapeworms (Cestoda), flukes (Trematoda) and roundworms (Nematoda). Examples of important disease-causing helminths are given in Table 10.2.

Arthropods

Most arthropods which attack humans are bloodfeeders (e.g. mosquitoes, ticks and fleas) and reside only briefly on the host. Many of these arthropods are vectors for the transmission of other infectious agents (Table 10.3).

Some arthropods, notably the louse, *Pediculus humanus,* and the crab louse, *Phthirus pubis*, can reproduce on humans and produce inflammatory reactions following penetration of the skin during feeding. The scabies mite, *Sarcoptes scabei*, lives permanently on humans, burrowing into the skin to feed and lay eggs.

General features of parasitic infection

Some parasites (*ectoparasites*) live on the surface of the host and others (*endoparasites*) live inside the host. Some ectoparasites are important as disease agents in their own right (e.g. scabies mites) or as vectors of infection (e.g. fleas transmitting the plague bacillus, *Yersinia pestis*). However, in general, endoparasites are potentially much more important as causes of disease, due to the much greater degree of intimate contact between parasite and host. (An extreme example is the malaria parasite which for part of its cycle lives inside the erythrocytes of humans.)

Where and in which groups of people parasitic infection is more likely to occur is determined to a large extent by environmental conditions (housing, water supply and sanitation) and climate (particularly rainfall and temperature). Even where infection is common, individuals differ in the degree to which they are exposed to infection, such factors as personal protection or

Table 10.1 Important classes of pathogenic protozoa

Group	Features	Example	Disease produced
Amoebae	Move by extending pseudopodia	*Entamoeba histolytica*	Amoebiasis
Flagellates	Move by beating of one or more flagella	*Trypanosoma spp.*	Trypanosomiasis
		T. cruzi	Chagas' disease
		T. brucei gambiense, *T. brucei rhodesiense*	African trypanosomiasis or sleeping sickness
		Giardia lamblia	Giardiasis
Ciliates	Move by beating of cilia	*Balantidium coli*	Balantidiasis
Sporozoa	All are intracellular parasites	*Plasmodium spp.* *P. falciparum, P. vivax,* *P. ovale, P. malariae*	Malaria

personal hygiene being particularly important.

Although parasitic infections are most common in the 'developing' communities of the tropics and subtropics, they can occur wherever conditions are suitable. Furthermore, individuals may be infected with more than one parasite at any one time and this is particularly likely where a number of parasites are transmitted by a common route (e.g. the faecal–oral route).

Factors affecting the shift from parasitic infection towards disease

In the individual, the balance between parasitic infection and disease can be affected by a number of factors acting either independently or in concert. The inter-relationships between host and parasite are complex and are grouped under three broad headings: *host-related*; *parasite-related*; and *immunological*.

Host-related factors

Age

Children up to about 6 months old are rarely susceptible to parasitic infection because of the protection afforded by maternal antibodies and also because of a significantly lower risk of exposure to infection. After about 6 months, a child is exposed to a wide variety of infectious agents and the prevalence and severity of infections rise dramati-

cally, reaching a peak in the age group 6 months to 5 years. While older people may continue to be at risk of infection, the degree of exposure, the intensity of infection and the occurrence of disease are often lower.

Nutrition

Malnourishment is important in shifting the balance from infection towards disease, a malnourished person being much less able to withstand the adverse effects of disease. This is a particular problem in the 'developing' world where malnutrition is common.

Parasite-related factors

Parasite-related factors include the physical size and/or number of parasites, their site of occurrence, their rate of multiplication, their metabolism, and differences in pathogenicity shown by different parasite strains.

Size

Parasites which grow to a large *physical size* or multiply rapidly have a much greater potential for causing disease than those which are small or multiply slowly. Many protozoan parasites, such as *Plasmodium* spp. (malarial parasites), and those which live in the intestine, are capable of very rapid asexual multiplication so that they make up in numbers what they may lack in individual size.

Table 10.2 Examples of medically important helminths

Group	Examples	Comments
Tapeworms	Human tapeworms (e.g. *Taenia solium* and *T. saginata*)	Human infection follows ingestion of larvae in pork (*T. solium*) or beef (*T. saginata*). Adult tapeworms found in gut of humans but larvae may develop in other tissues of pig and occasionally humans (*T. solium*) and cattle (*T. Saginata*)
	Dog tapeworm (*Echinococcus granulosus*)	Hydatid disease is acquired by ingestion of eggs from faeces of infected canines. Embryos migrate through gut to form hydatid cysts, especially in the liver of sheep, other herbivores and occasionally of humans
Flukes	*Schistosoma haematobium* *S. japonicum S. mansoni*	Larvae released by aquatic snails penetrate human skin and pass through blood to liver where they mature to form adults. Adults migrate to final site (*S. haematobium* to veins surrounding bladder, *S. japonicum* and *S. mansoni* to veins around the small intestine)
	Human liver fluke (*Clonorchis sinensis*)	Organism acquired by ingestion of fish containing larval stages. Young flukes released in the intestine move up the bile duct and attach to bile duct epithelium
	Common liver fluke of sheep (*Fasciola hepatica*)	Infection follows ingestion of vegetation contaminated by larvae.
	Oriental lung fluke (*Paragonimus westermanii*)	Human infection acquired by ingestion of crustacea containing larvae. Larvae migrate from the intestine across the diaphragm and penetrate the lungs. Normally, the adult flukes develop within fibrous cysts that connect with the airways allowing an exit route for the eggs produced by these organisms
Nematodes	*Ascaris lumbricoides*	Human infection acquired by ingestion of eggs. Larvae hatch in intestine, penetrate bowel wall and migrate to lungs. From the lungs the worms are swallowed once again reaching the intestine. Adult worms live freely in gut lumen. Female worm lays eggs which are passed in faeces
	Hookworms (e.g. *Ancylostoma duodenale*)	Human infection acquired when larvae present in faeces penetrate the skin and migrate to the lungs and bronchi where they are swallowed. Adult worms live in gut and attach to the intestinal mucosa using their specialized mouth parts. Female hookworms lay eggs that hatch in the faeces shortly after defaecation
	Filaria (e.g. *Wuchereria bancrofti*)	Larvae are introduced through the skin by mosquitoes and develop slowly into long, thin, adult worms located in lymphoid tissues and lymphatic vessels. Blockage of lymphatic vessels can lead to gross enlargement of affected tissues ('elephantiasis')
	Toxocara canis	Eggs from dog are ingested and hatch in the intestine. Larvae migrate from the gut to many tissues including lung, liver, eyes and CNS

Thus, it is perhaps more meaningful to consider *biomass* rather than physical size as the important factor.

Multiplication rates

Inherent differences in the rate of multiplication between closely related parasites are also important. *P. falciparum* has a considerably faster rate of

Table 10.3 Examples of vector-borne disease transmitted by arthropods

Infectious agent	Disease	Arthropod vector
Arboviruses	Dengue fever	Mosquitoes
	Yellow fever	Mosquitoes
Bacteria		
Yersinia pestis	Plague	Fleas
Borrelia burgdorferi	Lyme disease	Ticks
Protozoa		
Trypanosoma cruzi	Chagas' disease	Reduviid bugs
T. brucei gambiense,	Sleeping sickness	Tsetse flies
T. brucei rhodesiense		
Plasmodium spp.	Malaria	Mosquitoes
Helminths		
Wuchereria bancrofti	Filariasis	Mosquitoes

multiplication than the other three species of malarial parasite affecting humans and this contributes substantially to the greater severity of the disease it causes.

Dose size

Another factor related to the rate of multiplication is the size of the infective dose necessary to establish an infection. The minimum infective dose for *Giardia lamblia* may be as low as 10 cysts whereas that for *Entamoeba histolytica* may be in the region of several thousand cysts.

Site of occurrence

Site of occurrence is particularly important in determining whether infection shifts towards disease. For example, parasites in the intestine of an otherwise healthy individual generally cause little or no disease unless they become invasive (such as some strains of *Entamoeba histolytica*), multiply rapidly (such as *Giardia lamblia*) or migrate to inappropriate sites (such as adult *Ascaris lumbricoides* in the bile or pancreatic duct).

Parasites which have stages in the tissues or which become tissue invaders are generally more pathogenic than those which live in the intestine. This is because parasites in the tissues have more intimate contact with the body than those in the intestine, where parasites and their products (including metabolic products and eggs) are carried away in the gut contents and faeces.

While most parasites have a 'normal' site of occurrence in the body where they may or may not cause disease, some parasites may occasionally be found in inappropriate sites where their effects can be much more serious. For instance, during its development, the human lung fluke, *Paragonimus westermanii*, migrates from the intestine through the diaphragm to the lungs where it produces eggs. Normally, these eggs pass harmlessly out of the body in sputum, causing no ill effects to the host. However, occasionally some immature worms migrate to other body sites where they lay eggs. These eggs are unable to escape and a granuloma (see Chapter 4) develops round them. If this occurs in the central nervous system, the consequences for the patient are quite different from the more typical lung infection.

Parasite metabolism

By definition, the parasite depends on the host for its nutrition and therefore the host is deprived (to a greater or lesser extent) of material which it could otherwise use for its own metabolic purposes. Severe infection with some intestinal parasites (such as hookworm) can exacerbate an already poor nutritional state, even to the point where it becomes life-threatening. A second aspect is the effect that some parasite metabolites have on the host. The intra-erythrocytic stages of the malarial parasite metabolize haemoglobin in the infected red cell. When the red cell bursts, the products of this metabolism are released into the general circulation and provoke the characteristic malaria fever. The fever is itself an important part of the chain of events leading to severe illness or death in the untreated patient.

Strain differences

It is well known that some strains of parasite are potentially more pathogenic than others. Infection with *Entamoeba histolytica* acquired in the tropics is much more likely to cause disease than infections acquired elsewhere.

Immunological factors

Although parasitic infections may stimulate the production of antibodies, in most cases these antibodies are not protective although they may be useful as indicators of existing, or of relatively recent, infection. Most antiparasite antibodies persist for some time after successful treatment and, in general, antibody tests are of little value as tests of cure. A marked feature of the immune reaction to helminthic infections is the high level of immunoglobulin E (IgE) antibody produced. Various roles are attributed to IgE in protective responses to parasitic infections including release of mast cell secretory products. The effectiveness of an individual's immune response to a parasitic infection may be affected by a number of factors, including those outlined below.

1 Other infections (such as measles, which is particularly common in 'developing' countries) can lower the host's resistance to, or tolerance of, parasitic infection and permit opportunist infections to develop.

2 Pregnancy lowers the mother's general resistance to infection and a parasitic infection which has been in a state of equilibrium may become life-threatening during pregnancy.

3 Inherited or acquired immunodeficiency may substantially lower an individual's immunity to a parasitic infection. This is well illustrated in the case of HIV infection and AIDS (see Chapter 8 and Case Study 11.2) where affected individuals are more prone to a range of infections including those caused by parasites.

4 Immunosuppressant drugs may have a similarly dramatic effect on an existing (and perhaps unsuspected) parasitic infection.

There are two other aspects of the immunological relationship between the parasite and the host that are important. These are the host's response to antigens of the parasite and the parasite's response to host immunity.

Much of the pathology caused by heavy infec-

tion with schistosome parasites results from the host's reaction to metabolites produced by the small proportion of eggs laid by the female worms which become trapped in the tissues (around 95 percent of eggs pass out in the urine or faeces). The host response is initially in the form of a giant cell reaction followed by progressive fibrosis, the formation of a granuloma round each egg (the final lesion being several times the volume of the egg that provoked it) and the replacement of normal tissue by these granulomas. The fibrous reaction associated with heavy infection of *Schistosoma mansoni* can cause constriction of the hepatic portal circulation leading to enlargement

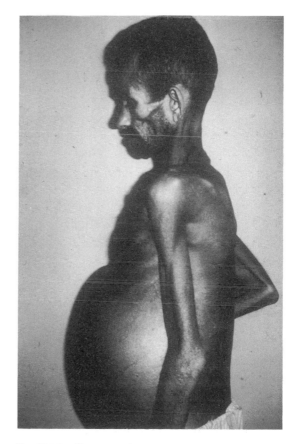

Fig. 10.1 Brazilian man with acute hepato-splenomegaly resulting from heavy *Schistosoma mansoni* infection. In cases as severe as this, the hepatic portal blood system becomes constricted as a result of a fibrous reaction to the trapped eggs.

of the liver and spleen (hepato-splenomegaly, Fig. 10.1).

Some species of parasite are able to avoid or to counteract the effects of host immunity. Some parasites are able to survive within macrophages and so are sheltered from any immune response. To do this they must block the normal microbiocidal mechanisms of the macrophage. *Toxoplasma gondii*, for example, inhibits phagosome–lysosome fusion, whereas *Leishmania* spp. are surrounded by a dense coat which can protect them from the oxidative burst (see Chapter 4).

During the early stages of their migration through the host, schistosome parasites incorporate host material into their outermost layers, effectively camouflaging their identity and preventing the host immune system from recognizing and destroying them. On the other hand, trypanosomes causing African sleeping sickness provoke an immunological response by the host which is potentially fatal to the parasites. However, these organisms are able to evade this immune response by producing broods of antigenically different parasites in quick succession. The host's immune response never quite catches up with these frequent changes in antigenicity and the parasites are able to survive.

Examples of parasitic infection

The following examples are intended to illustrate some of the general principles of parasitic infection discussed above. It is beyond the scope of this chapter to consider in detail all important parasitic infections. The interested reader is referred to the further reading list.

Amoebiasis

Entamoeba histolytica infections occur throughout the world and account for the third most common cause of death from parasitic disease. Infection is particularly common in warm, moist environments and where sanitation is poor. Transmission is faecal–oral and the parasites are normally found in the lumen of the large intestine feeding on food particles. The parasites become invasive in less than 20 percent of infections, lesions usually starting in the large intestine as small discrete, button-like ulcers. The advancing ulcer becomes flask-shaped, eventually extending through all layers of the gut wall. Amoebae may be carried in the blood to other parts of the body where an abscess may develop. The liver (particularly the right lobe) is most frequently affected. The liver abscess is usually single but may be multiple, does not have a well defined wall and is usually bacteriologically sterile.

Liver abscess is about 10 times more frequent in adults than in children and about five times more common in males than in females, but the degree to which differences in exposure are responsible for these variations is not clear. Malnourishment may increase the severity of infection and immunodeficiency may elicit or worsen the clinical effects of infection. Asymptomatic female carriers may develop severe amoebiasis during pregnancy and the puerperium.

Malaria

The four species of malarial parasites which infect humans are *P. falciparum*, *P. vivax*, *P. ovale* and *P. malariae*. The infective stages (*sporozoites*) are inoculated by an infected female mosquito during a blood meal and subsequently invade and develop inside hepatocytes. Each parasite multiplies asexually as a liver *schizont*, producing (according to species) between 10–40 000 *merozoites*. When the mature liver schizont bursts, the merozoites are released. They invade the erythrocytes, mature to *trophozoites* (ring forms) and then begin another cycle of asexual multiplication as erythrocytic schizonts. Each erythrocytic schizont contains, at maturity, between about eight and 24 merozoites. When mature, the erythrocytic schizont bursts, releasing the merozoites which invade other erythrocytes, develop into schizonts and so on, the cycle repeating itself every 36–72 hours according to the species.

The four species differ in their degree of pathogenicity. *P. falciparum* is the most pathogenic because it produces more merozoites in both liver and erythrocytic schizont stages, invades red cells of all ages, and has the shortest schizogany cycle in the blood. Numbers of *P. falciparum* organisms in the blood can rapidly reach life-threatening levels (see Fig. 10.2). Although the other three species can cause severe disease, their parasitaemias are rarely life-threatening.

The disease process in malaria is complex (Fig. 10.3). The liver stages have no effect on the individual but illness results directly or indirectly from the destruction of erythrocytes, the number destroyed increasing progressively with each schizogany cycle. The regular destruction of red cells results in increasing anaemia, while the release of parasite metabolites causes fever which can itself have serious consequences if severe (when the erythrocytic schizogany cycle is well synchronized, the fever pattern may become sufficiently regular to be characteristic of the species). Blockage of the capillaries by the erythrocytic schizonts (especially those of *P. falciparum*) leads to tissue anoxia and cell death (see Fig. 10.4). The kidneys, digestive and respiratory systems can all be affected, with accompanying renal failure,

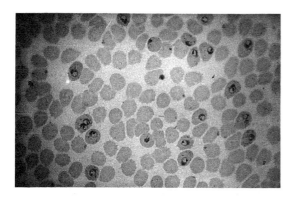

Fig. 10.2 A blood film from a patient with malaria, showing trophozoites of *Plasmodium falciparum* within red blood cells. The slide shows a heavy parasitaemia (approximately 10 percent of cells are infected). The trophozoites show the characteristic 'signet ring' appearance. Some infected cells contain more than one parasite, some also show characteristic stippling (Maurer's clefts) and some have peripheral parasites (accolé forms). Infected cells are not enlarged when compared with uninfected cells. Taken together these features identify the parasite as *P. falciparum*. © J.M. Jewsbury.

vomiting and diarrhoea. When capillary blockage occurs in the brain, cerebral malaria, coma and death result, unless treatment is initiated as an emergency.

Hydatid disease

The adult tapeworms, *Echinococcus granulosus*, live in the intestine of dogs and other carnivores. Eggs are passed in the faeces of the dog and the larval stages form so-called 'hydatid cysts' (cysts of varying sizes composed of developing larvae) in infected sheep and other herbivores (Fig. 10.5). Dogs become infected when they eat carcasses or offal containing the hydatid cysts. Human infection occurs in areas where there is a close association between sheep, sheep dogs and humans and results from the accidental ingestion of *Echinococcus* eggs (see Fig. 10.6). The eggs hatch in the intestine and the larvae bore their way into the gut wall and are carried around the body in the bloodstream before developing into the hydatid cyst. The usual site is the liver but they can lodge in other parts of the body such as the bone marrow or brain. As the hydatid cyst can grow to 100 mm or more in diameter its physical size can have serious effects on the organ in which it occurs. The fluid in the centre of the cyst is also highly allergenic and if the cyst bursts (or is ruptured during surgical removal) the patient may well suffer a severe and possibly fatal anaphylactic reaction (see Chapter 12).

Ascariasis

Although all age groups are susceptible to infection by *Ascaris lumbricoides*, children between the ages of about 1 and 5 years have the highest prevalence and intensity of infection (children living in poor environmental conditions may harbour more than 100 worms). Adult worms are large (females measure up to about 35 cm in length and males up to about 20 cm), physically strong and normally live in the lumen of the small intestine. Provided the worms remain in the lumen of the intestine, light infections in a well nourished person cause little or no

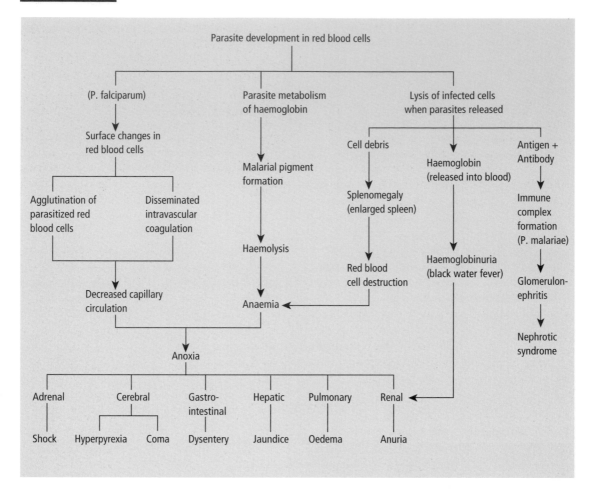

Fig. 10.3 Pathological effects of malaria. The chain of events following malarial infection is complex and can affect many parts of the body. The central feature is the destruction of red cells, the consequent reduction of the capacity for oxygen transport, tissue anoxia and the disruption of many metabolic processes throughout the body resulting in a wide variety of signs and symptoms. Following the treatment of some cases of *P. falciparum* malaria massive haemolysis occurs, releasing large amounts of haemoglobin into the circulation. This haemoglobin appears in the urine (haemoglobinuria) causing renal failure. After Garcia and Bruckner (1993).

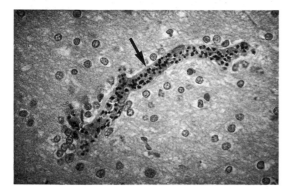

Fig. 10.4 Section of brain tissue from a fatal case of cerebral malaria showing a capillary (arrowed) within which are schizonts of *Plasmodium falciparum*. Schizonts of *P. falciparum* sequester in the capillaries of the deep circulation and are usually only seen in blood films in heavy infections. Blockage of the capillaries is one of the effects of *P. falciparum* infection and contributes substantially to tissue anoxia–this affects many organs and when it occurs in the brain is the cause of cerebral malaria. © J.M. Jewsbury.

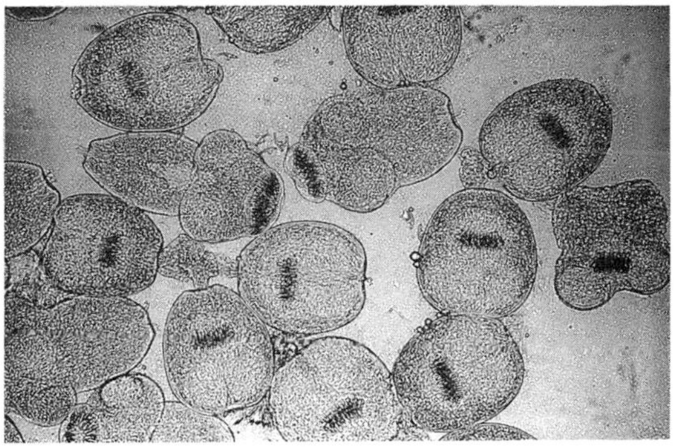

Fig. 10.5 The contents of a hydatid cyst consisting of scolices of *Echinococcus granulosus* plus hooks and calcereous corpuscles from disintegrated scolices. Each scolex is capable of developing into an adult tapeworm if ingested by a dog (or, less commonly, another carnivore). The hydatid fluid itself can cause an anaphylactic shock in a sensitized host if it leaks from a ruptured hydatid cyst. © J.M. Jewsbury.

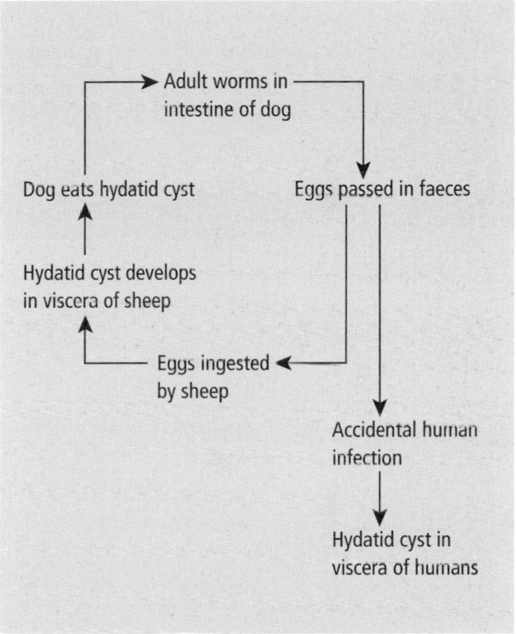

Fig. 10.6 Life cycle of *Echinococcus granulosus*. The adult worms of the dog tapeworm, *Echinococcus granulosus*, live in the intestine of dogs. Eggs are passed in the faeces and may be ingested by sheep or humans, whereupon the eggs hatch in the intestine. Subsequently, the larvae bore through the wall of the small intestine and are carried in the hepatic portal circulation from which a few pass to other organs including the lung, bone marrow or brain. Large hydatid cysts containing the larvae of *Echinococcus* may develop at these sites where they may damage the organ involved or lead to fatal anaphylaxis (see Chapter 12) if the cyst ruptures. Dogs are infected when they eat sheep carcasses or offal containing the hydatid cysts.

problem. About 85 percent of infections are asymptomatic.

Obstruction of the intestine occurs more frequently in heavy infections and can be a surgical emergency—in some parts of the world more than 50 percent of children admitted to hospital with acute abdominal conditions suffer from ascariasis. Single worms occasionally migrate into and obstruct the bile or pancreatic duct, and the passage of relatively large numbers of larvae through the lungs at any one time causes a pneumonitis (lung inflammation) lasting a few days.

Summary

Parasitic infections are still an important cause of mortality and morbidity throughout the world, particularly where poor environmental conditions, malnourishment and lack of appropriate preventive measures greatly increase the risk of infection. Diseases such as malaria and amoebiasis are, in principle preventable diseases given the implementation of appropriate strategies.

Key points

1 In a broad sense, any organism that derives benefit from the host and has the potential to cause it harm may be defined as a parasite. In microbiology the term 'parasite' is often used to denote protozoa and members of the animal kingdom that infect and cause disease in other animals including humans.

2 The main groups of medically important parasites are the protozoa, helminths and arthropods.

3 The balance between infection and disease is a delicate one and is the net result of host-related, parasite-related and immunological factors.

4 Host-related factors include age and nutrition. Parasitic infections are more common in the very young and in the malnourished.

5 Parasite-related factors include the number and size of the infecting species, their relative pathogenicities and the site at which infection occurs.

6 The risk of parasite-induced disease is greater in individuals with lowered immunity.

7 Certain parasites have evolved strategies for evading the immune system.

8 Disease caused by parasites may be the result of direct damage to tissues (e.g. intestinal amoebic ulcer and amoebic liver abscess caused by *Entamoeba histolytica*), the result of an inflammatory response to the parasite (e.g. schistosomiasis), or the induction of an allergic reaction (e.g. bursting of a hydatid cyst).

Further reading

Crewe W. & Haddock D.R.W. (1985) *Parasites and Human Disease*. Edward Arnold, London.

Garcia L.S. & Bruckner D.A. (1993) *Diagnostic Medical Parasitology*, 2nd edn. American Society for Microbiology, Washington.

Muller R. & Baker J.R. (1990) *Medical Parasitology*. Lippincott, Philadelphia & Gower Medical, London.

Case Studies

11.1 Fever, vomiting and neck stiffness in a child

Clinical features

A 10-month-old boy presented with a short history of fever, persistent vomiting and marked drowsiness. On examination he was febrile (temperature: 38.5°C), with photophobia and neck stiffness. Kernig's sign (see below) was positive.

Investigations

A specimen of cerebrospinal fluid (CSF) was taken by lumbar puncture and the investigations shown in Table 11.1.1 were performed.

A Gram stain was performed on the CSF and showed the presence of Gram-positive diplococci. Culture of the CSF revealed the presence of *Neisseria meningitidis* organisms which were sensitive to penicillin.

Diagnosis

The cardinal clinical features of bacterial meningitis are fever, depression or disturbance of the level of consciousness, and vomiting. Other features which are more specific but appear later include photophobia (aversion to light), and neck stiffness. A specific clinical test for meningitis is Kernig's sign. This is elicited by attempting to straighten the knee while the hip is held flexed. This manoeuvre pulls the spinal nerves where they penetrate the meninges, and therefore stretches the meninges themselves. Because the meninges are inflamed in meningitis this is exquisitely painful and the muscles go into spasm to prevent it from happening.

Diagnosis: bacterial meningitis

Discussion

Meningitis is inflammation of the meninges (the membranes around the brain). It can be caused by infections with bacteria, viruses, protozoa or fungal organisms. Viral meningitis is not usually serious, unless the brain itself is also affected (viral encephalitis) when brain damage can ensue. Fungal and protozoal meningitis are essentially confined to those individuals who are immunosuppressed or immunodeficient.

Seventy percent of cases of bacterial meningitis occur in childhood. Three organisms— *Haemophilus influenzae*, *Neisseria meningitidis* and *Streptococcus pneumoniae*—are responsible for the majority of cases. All of these organisms have a carbohydrate (polysaccharide) capsule that is essential for virulence (see Chapter 7). The ability to mount an immune response to this capsule is an important protective mechanism. Antibodies to carbohydrate antigens, unlike antibodies directed to many protein antigens, are thymus-independent (that is they do not require T cell help, see Chapter 5) and do not show 'memory' from previous exposure to antigen. More importantly, the immune responses to carbohydrate antigens mature relatively late in development. Therefore, children under 2 years of age are particularly susceptible to infection with the organisms listed above.

The low level of glucose in the CSF is characteristic of bacterial meningitis. This was originally

Table 11.1.1 Investigations performed

Analyte	Value	Reference range
CSF		
White cell count	$4600 \times 10^9/l$, 90% of which were neutrophils	Less than $5 \times 10^9/l$, no neutrophils
Glucose	0.7 mmol/l (blood glucose was 2.6 mmol/l)	CSF glucose levels are normally greater than two-thirds of blood glucose levels

explained by bacterial metabolism of the CSF glucose. However, probably more important is the finding that neurones and glial cells switch from aerobic to anaerobic metabolism. The inflammatory response produced by infection leads to the local accumulation of fluid (oedema) and compression of blood vessels with subsequent impairment of blood supply. This is compounded by blood clotting in the local microcirculation. Under conditions of reduced oxygen the cells switch from aerobic to anaerobic metabolism, with increased consumption of glucose and the production of lactate. It is not surprising, therefore, that the lower the CSF glucose and the higher the CSF lactate, the poorer the prognosis in bacterial meningitis.

Much of the tissue damage in bacterial meningitis is the result of the inflammatory response rather than a direct effect of the organism. Lipopolysaccharide (LPS, endotoxin) is a structural component of the cell wall of Gram-negative bacteria and is a potent stimulator of the inflammatory response. Gram-positive organisms have a similar component known as lipoteichoic acid. These cell wall molecules stimulate host cells (particularly macrophages) to secrete cytokines, including tumour necrosis factor-alpha (TNFα) and interleukin-1 (IL-1). These cytokines act on a wide variety of cells to initiate inflammation (see Chapter 4), leading to increased capillary permeability (with associated local oedema), an ingress of neutrophils and stimulation of the complement and coagulation cascades. Cerebral oedema in turn can lead to an increase in intracranial pressure and impairment of cerebral blood flow.

Treatment and prognosis

Antibiotics are the cornerstone of management of bacterial meningitis. They need to be given intravenously, at least during the acute stages of the illness, since vomiting, impaired consciousness, and possible shock make oral administration impossible. In addition, many antibiotics do not cross the blood–brain barrier effectively, and thus have very poor penetration into CSF. Currently, third generation cephalosporins are drugs of choice, but as more organisms are detected with resistance to these antibiotics, others are replacing them. In some areas of the world, antibiotic resistance in meningitis is a serious problem.

Over the last few years, the addition of dexamethasone (a corticosteroid) has become widespread as adjunct treatment. If given early, that is, at the same time as the initial dose of antibiotic, dexamethasone can reduce the release of pro-inflammatory cytokines and limit the inappropriately severe host inflammatory response. There is clinical and laboratory evidence that this improves the long-term prognosis.

Despite modern antibiotic therapy, the overall mortality remains around 10 percent in bacterial meningitis. Of the survivors, 10 percent will be deaf due to direct cochlear damage. There is a small canal (the cochlear aqueduct) connecting the cochlea directly with CSF, and bacteria can thus pass directly to the inner ear and damage it, even in the early stages of the disease. Other complications include epilepsy and other neurological damage, and up to 30 percent of survivors of meningitis are left with long-term sequelae.

Questions

1 In some cases of bacterial meningitis there is marked clinical deterioration within hours of starting appropriate antibiotic therapy. Can you suggest why this is?

Answer: antibiotics destroy bacteria, resulting in the release of cell wall components (see above). This leads to the release of large amounts of pro-inflammatory cytokines and a particularly marked and potentially harmful inflammatory response.

2 Despite the inability of infants to mount an antibody response to carbohydrate antigens, they can still be successfully immunized against *Haemophilus influenzae* capsular material. Do you know how this is achieved?

Answer: haemophilus vaccine is produced by conjugating the carbohydrate component of the bacterial cell wall to a protein 'carrier'. The infant's immune system sees the whole molecule as protein and produces antibodies to a variety of epitopes on it, including the carbohydrate portion. Similar vaccines are in preparation against the carbohydrate antigens of other clinically important bacteria.

11.2 Shortness of breath and vaginal discharge

Clinical features

A 28-year-old woman presented with a 3-day history of fever, shortness of breath on exertion and a dry cough. She denied chills, night sweats, nausea, vomiting, diarrhoea or abdominal pain. She had no headache, change in vision, muscle weakness, or change in sensation. She had lost 10 pounds in the last 3 months despite eating what she described as a 'healthy' diet. She had noted a new vaginal discharge accompanied by itching, as well as some burning in her mouth when she drank coffee.

She was not on any medication. She had no history of contact with homosexual or bisexual men, but had used intravenous drugs during a period from 1983 to 1989 and had traded sex for drugs during this period. In the last 2 years, she had had one steady male partner with whom she continued to have a sexual relationship. There was no other significant past medical history, no allergies, and all members of her family were in good health.

Investigations

On physical examination the patient was thin, in moderate respiratory distress and febrile (temperature: 39.4°C). Blood pressure was 100/60. Pulse was regular at 100 beats/minute. Respiratory rate was 24/minute.

Examination of the oral cavity revealed three discrete white patches on the hard palate, but was otherwise normal. There was no apparent lymphadenopathy (enlargement of lymph nodes). Pulmonary examination revealed bilateral, diffuse end-inspiratory rales (see below), but no rhonchi (wheezes) and no sign of consolidation or pleural effusion (fluid in the pleural cavity.) Cardiovascular examination was normal. Abdominal examination showed no hepatomegaly (enlargement of the liver) or splenomegaly (enlargement of the spleen), and no masses or tenderness. Neurological examination revealed normal mental status, no muscle-wasting and no focal weakness or sensory abnormalities. On pelvic examination a thick white vaginal discharge was noted. There was no cervical tenderness and no cervical discharge. A cervical smear was performed.

Laboratory investigations yielded the results shown in Table 11.2.1.

Table 11.2.1 Investigations performed

Analyte	Value	Reference range
Blood		
Haemoglobin	9.8 g/dl	11.5–15.5
White blood cell count	1.2×10^9/l	4.0–11.0
Urea	5.2 mmol/l	2.5–6.7
Creatinine	120 μmol/l	70–150
Sodium	140 mmol/l	136–145
Potassium	4.8 mmol/l	3.4–5.2

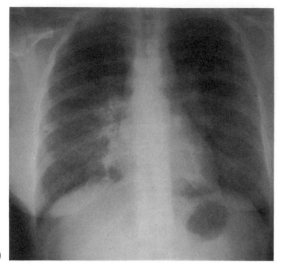

(a)

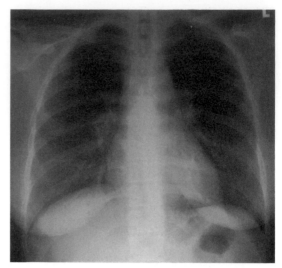

(b)

Fig. 11.2.1 Clinical features of *Pneumocystis carinii* pneumonia (a) Chest radiograph from the case patient showing bilateral interstitial lung disease, which is worse in the right lung. These features are characteristic of *P. carinii* pneumonia (PCP). (b) Chest radiograph from the same patient taken 6 weeks later showing clearing of the disease after therapy.

Initial laboratory work-up included an enzyme-linked immunosorbent-assay (ELISA) test for the presence of antibodies to HIV which was positive. This was confirmed by Western blot analysis. A CD4 +ve cell count revealed 150 cells/mm³ (reference range, 800–1200 cells/mm³). CD8 +ve cell count was 300 cells/mm³ (reference range, 400–600 cells/mm³). Microbiological cultures of blood were negative.

A chest radiograph (Fig. 11.2.1) showed bilateral interstitial infiltrates, no cavities, consolidation or pleural effusion.

No sputum was available for analysis and so sputum induction was performed. Microscopic examination of the specimen obtained revealed the presence of *Pneumocystis carinii* organisms. Microscopic examination of swabs taken from the oral cavity lesions and the vagina revealed the presence of fungal forms consistent with *Candida albicans*. The cervical smear showed a grade 3 cervical intra-epithelial neoplasia (CIN 3) reflecting infection with the human papilloma virus (HPV).

Diagnosis

The patient has *P. carinii* pneumonia and *C. albicans* infection of the vaginal and oral cavities. An HIV antibody test was positive. Center for Disease Control (CDC) classification was used as a reference for clinical categorization of HIV/AIDS (Table 11.2.2).

Diagnosis: acquired immune deficiency syndrome (AIDS).

Discussion

HIV infection is currently the most common cause of immunodeficiency. The risk factors associated with acquisition of the virus in the case of this patient include multiple sexual partners and the use of intravenous drugs. Although HIV can infect a wide variety of cell types it most efficiently binds the CD4 receptor and enters CD4 +ve helper T cells. Destruction of the CD4 +ve helper T cell results in an extensive cascade of immunological abnormalities since this cell is central to almost every function of the immune system (see Chapter 5).

During the early stages of HIV infection much of the virus load is concentrated within the

Table 11.2.2 1993 revised classification system for HIV infection and AIDS (Center for Disease Control, USA) in adolescents (aged 13 and above) and adults. Persons with AIDS indicator conditions (i.e. categories C1–C3) as well as those with CD4 + ve T lymphocyte counts less than 200/μl (i.e. categories A3 and B3) are reportable as AIDS cases

	Clinical categories		
CD4 + ve T cell count	(A) Asymptomatic, acute HIV infection or PGL	(B) Symptomatic but not (A) or (C) conditions	(C) AIDS indicator conditions
Greater than 500/μl	A1	B1	C1
200–499/μl	A2	B2	C2
Less than 200/μl	A3	B3	C3

The clinical categories are defined in the following sections.

Category A consists of one or more of the conditions listed below with documented HIV infection. Conditions listed in Category B or C must not have occurred.

- Asymptomatic HIV infection.
- PGL – Persistent generalized lymphadenopathy (lymph node enlargement).
- Acute (primary) HIV infection with accompanying illness or history of acute HIV infection.

Category B consists of symptomatic conditions in HIV infection that are not included in Category C and that meet at least one of the following criteria:

(i) the conditions are attributable to HIV infection or are indicative of defective cell-mediated immunity

(ii) the conditions are considered to have a clinical course or require management that is complicated by HIV infection.

Examples of conditions in clinical **Category B** include:

- oral Candidosis.
- constitutional symptoms, such as fever (>38.5°C) or diarrhoea lasting for more than one month.
- cervical intra-epithelial neoplasia (CIN).
- herpes zoster (shingles) involving at least two distinct episodes or more than one site.

Category B conditions take precedence over those in Category A (for example, a patient who is now asymptomatic but has previously had a condition listed under Category B should be classified under category B.

Category C conditions are AIDS indicator conditions. Examples of conditions in this category are:

- oesophageal candidosis
- invasive cervical cancer (see text)
- Kaposi's sarcoma
- lymphoma, Burkitt's
- lymphoma, immunoblastic
- lymphoma, primary of brain
- *Mycobacterium avium* complex or *M. kansasii*, disseminated or extrapulmonary
- *M. tuberculosis*, any site
- *Pneumocystis carinii* pneumonia
- toxoplasmosis of brain.

lymphoid system, including the spleen. With time there is a steady decline in the CD4 +ve helper T cell population and with increasing destruction of this population, as well as other components of the immune system, opportunistic infections may occur. An opportunistic infection is infection by an organism which is ubiquitous in the environ-ment and which rarely establishes an infection in an immunocompetent host.

P. carinii infection of the lungs is one of the most common opportunistic infections seen during HIV infection and may rapidly progress to pneumonia. The clinical features of *P. carinii* pneumonia (PCP) include fever, a dry cough and progressive dyspnoea (breathlessness). On examination the lungs often sound normal or end-inspiratory rales may be heard. Rales or 'crackles' are short explosive sounds that are thought to represent the equalization of pressure within collapsed small airways as they open during inspiration. Rales heard at the end of inspiration suggest fibrosis or the accumulation of fluid (oedema) within the lungs. Untreated patients with PCP become incapacitated from dyspnoea and eventually die of hypoxaemia (reduced blood oxygen levels). Vaginal and oral infections with the fungal organism *C. albicans* (see Chapter 9) are also common in the immunocompromised host.

The decline in the CD4 +ve cell count is a useful indicator of the severity of immune dysfunction and is measured frequently in HIV-positive individuals. Clinically the decline in immune function can be charted through a number of distinct stages, these are summarized in Table 11.2.2. The increased frequency of cervical intra-epithelial neoplasia (CIN) lesions in HIV-positive females is becoming increasingly well recognized. CIN refers to premalignant transformation of the squamous epithelium of the uterine cervix. In CIN, the transformed cells are retained within the epithelium by the underlying basement membrane. CIN 3 is at the most severe end of the spectrum of these disorders and, if left untreated, frequently progresses to invasive squamous carcinoma of the cervix. In invasive squamous carcinoma, the cells comprising the CIN lesion breach the basement membrane and spread into surrounding connective tissues causing local tissue destruction. Extensive spread throughout the connective tissues and lymphatics has serious consequences for the patient and can lead to the blockage of vital pelvic organs.

The severity of CIN in immunosuppressed females may be explained in part by the association of HPV with CIN (see Chapter 29). Certain subtypes of HPV (particularly subtypes 16 and 18) are believed to contribute to the development of CIN. Immunosuppression might allow outgrowth of HPV-infected tumour cells whose proliferation might otherwise be efficiently controlled by a competent immune system.

Treatment and prognosis

Unfortunately no cure exists for AIDS or HIV infection. Patients are encouraged to lead a normal healthy life and have all associated infections treated promptly. The antiviral compound zidovudine (AZT, Retrovir) has been shown to prolong survival in some patients and acts by inhibiting the HIV reverse transcriptase (see Chapter 8). However, the compound is highly toxic to bone marrow cells resulting in pancytopenia (see Chapter 20). Blood transfusions may therefore be required during therapy.

When treated early, PCP responds well to therapy with trimethoprim and sulphamethoxazole. These agents may also provide effective prophylaxis for HIV-positive individuals who have not yet developed PCP.

Locally active agents such as nystatin and amphotericin-B may be used to treat *C. albicans* infections. Treatment is also available for many other opportunistic infections such as cerebral abscesses due to *Toxoplasma gondii* and meningitis due to *Cryptococcus neoformans*. Patients who complete treatment for an opportunistic infection frequently remain on the same medication at a lower dose for the rest of their lives as prophylaxis.

There is no specific treatment for HPV. Rather, the infected cervical tissue must be removed through any number of approaches, including freezing the tissues, electrocautery or surgical removal.

Questions

1 This patient presented with CIN 3 which is regarded as a precursor to invasive carcinoma of the cervix. Is the incidence of other types of tumour increased in HIV-positive individuals?

Answer: HIV infection is associated with a progressive increase in the frequency of certain tumours, including aggressive lymphomas of B lymphocytes, anal cancer (in HIV-positive homosexual men) and Kaposi's sarcoma. This suggests that the immune system may be important in preventing the development of some of these tumours in immunocompetent individuals (see also Chapter 28) Many tumours arising during immunosuppression are associated with viruses, for example, lymphomas (EBV), Kaposi's sarcoma (human herpesvirus-8) and more recently CIN (HPV).

2 AIDS-associated tumours are often treated less aggressively than are the same tumours arising in immunocompetent individuals. Why do you think this is?

Answer: patients with AIDS-associated tumours present a therapeutic dilemma because of the risk of further bone marrow suppression and hence immunosuppression that results from treatment with cytotoxic drugs (see Chapter 30).

Part 4
Immunological Disorders

Hypersensitivity

Introduction

Hypersensitivity defines situations where the immune system reacts inappropriately or excessively to antigens which often appear to be harmless. These responses are classified into four different types based on their different underlying immunological mechanisms and clinical manifestations. The term 'hypersensitivity' is often used interchangeably with *allergy* which literally means 'altered reactivity'.

Substances which induce an immune response are usually foreign to the individual and are termed *antigens*, those which elicit a hypersensitive response may also be described as *allergens*. Hypersensitive reactions may also be directed against 'self-antigens' in the context of auto-immune diseases (see Chapter 13), as well as to foreign antigens.

Multiple factors determine whether a hypersensitive rather than a normal immunological response occurs, including the genetic make-up of the individual, the physical and chemical properties of the agent, and its mode of delivery into the patient.

An individual disease may involve more than one hypersensitivity mechanism, and an understanding of the four types of hypersensitivity helps to explain the immunopathogenesis of many conditions.

Type 1 hypersensitivity

In humans there are five classes of immunoglobulin: *IgG, IgM, IgA, IgD* and *IgE* which differ in their structure and function. Type 1 hypersensitivity reactions appear within minutes of exposure to allergen, and involve the inter-

action of *allergen, allergen-specific IgE* and tissue *mast cells*. IgE is normally present in very low concentrations in the serum. However, IgE levels are increased in patients with parasitic infections, and in most atopic patients, as well as in many apparently healthy individuals. The physiological role of IgE is thought to be the eradication of parasitic infections. Type 1 hypersensitivity appears to be a particular problem in areas of the world where these infections are no longer endemic.

In order to mount a Type 1 response, an individual's immune system must previously have encountered the antigen and stimulated B cells to produce antigen/allergen-specific IgE. Mast cells, found in the mucosae of the airways and gut as well as in connective tissues, bind this IgE via specialized surface receptors for the Fc portion of IgE molecules (Fig. 12.1). On re-exposure to allergen, the IgE molecules on the surface of the mast cell bind allergen via their available antigen-binding (Fab) portion and become cross-linked. This initiates a series of biochemical signals which results in the release of the mast cells' cytosolic granular contents into the surrounding micro-environment. These consist of a series of pre-formed mediators including histamine, heparin, lysosomal enzymes and proteases, neutrophil chemotactic factor (NCF) and eosinophil chemotactic factor (ECF). This release of mediators, and their effect on surrounding blood vessels, smooth muscle, and in attracting certain types of white blood cells to the area, is responsible for the early clinical manifestations of Type 1 hypersensitivity.

In addition to this *immediate response*, allergen exposure activates the metabolism of arachidonic acid within the mast cell via the lipo-oxygenase and cyclo-oxygenase pathways (see Chapter 4).

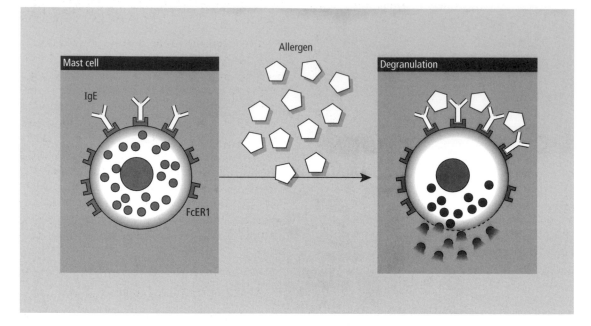

These pathways result in the synthesis of leukotrienes, prostaglandins, thromboxanes and chemotactic and activating factors (the slow-reactive substance of anaphylaxis, SRS-A, is a mixture of leukotrienes LTC4 and LTD4). This second group of mediators, which are released late (usually 4–6 hours after allergen exposure) have important clinical consequences in exacerbating disease. The physiological effects of early and late phase mediators are summarized in Table 12.1.

The clinical manifestations of Type 1 hypersensitivity include allergic rhinitis, asthma, eczema and urticaria. Individuals predisposed to this group of conditions are referred to as 'atopic', and an atopic tendency can often be traced back through families. The effects of the mediators described (see Table 12.1) directly accounts for the clinical features of these conditions.

Allergic rhinitis is characterized by facial flushing, itching of the nose, mouth and eyes and watery nasal discharge (rhinorrhoea), following exposure to allergens such as pollens (hay fever) or dust mite (perennial rhinitis). The flushing and rhinorrhoea are caused by vasodilatation and transudation of vascular fluid. The intense itching is a result of local histamine release.

Fig. 12.1 Type 1 (immediate) hypersensitivity involves the interaction of allergen specific IgE, mast cells bearing receptors for the Fc portion of IgE (FcER1), and allergen. Release of preformed mediators shown here is followed 4–6 hours later by release of newly formed mediators.

Table 12.1 The physiological effects of early and late phase mediators in Type 1 hypersensitivity reactions

Mediators	Effect
Preformed (early)	
Histamine	Vasodilatation, increased vascular permeability, bronchoconstriction
Heparin	Anticoagulation
Lysosomal enzymes	Proteolysis
Neutrophil chemotactic factor	Chemotaxis of neutrophils
Eosinophil chemotactic factor	Chemotaxis of eosinophils
Newly synthesized (late)	
Leukotrienes (LTC4, LTD4, LTB4)	Vasodilatation, Bronchoconstriction, Chemotaxis
Prostaglandins, thromboxanes	Vasodilatation, platelet activation, bronchoconstriction
Platelet-activating factor	Platelet activation

Allergens which penetrate further into the respiratory tree and lodge in the bronchi cause the features of *asthma* (see Case Study 15.2), with narrowing of the airways being caused both by constriction of smooth muscle and accumulation of fluid within the mucosa.

The most severe form of Type 1 hypersensitivity is termed *systemic anaphylaxis* and is a life-threatening condition. The patient collapses due to acute loss of blood pressure caused by the generalized vasodilatation, and is also likely to have breathing difficulty (due to broncho-constriction), skin rash, abdominal pain and vomiting or diarrhoea. The features result from the widespread activation of mast cells and circulating basophils. Basophils are a small subset of polymorphonuclear granulocytes which, like mast cells, bind IgE molecules and when these are cross-linked, release their mediators into the systemic circulation. This may occur in particularly sensitive individuals in response to any allergen, but usually occurs in response to parenterally administered protein antigens such as insect (e.g. bee/wasp) venom, or drugs (e.g. penicillin allergy).

The most important part of the management of any patient with Type 1 hypersensitivity is the identification of the likely precipitating allergen from the history and its careful avoidance where possible. An understanding of the underlying mechanisms of the condition have led to rational approaches to drug therapy both in the acute stage and in long-term prevention.

Disodium cromoglycate is a mast cell stabilizer which prevents degranulation and release of mediators. Its use is confined to the prevention of attacks and in order to be effective, it must be taken on a daily basis whether or not the patient is symptomatic.

Corticosteroid preparations are useful in long-term management and may also be given during the acute attack to prevent the occurrence of late-phase manifestations.

Type 2 hypersensitivity

Type 2 hypersensitivity reactions are also mediated by antibody, but in contrast to Type 1 reactions the antibodies involved are either of the IgG or IgM class. A characteristic of Type 2 reactions is that the antibody response is directed against antigens that are expressed on cell surfaces and therefore the damage that results from these responses tends to be limited to a particular organ or cell type. The pathogenic antibodies in this situation bind to cells via their Fab portion.

There are several possible consequences of antibody binding to cell surface antigens (Fig. 12.2). These are explained in detail in the sections below.

Activation of complement system

Activation of the complement cascade at the surface of the cell leads to the production of the anaphylatoxins C3a and C5a, with recruitment of inflammatory cells to the area (see Chapter 4). Ultimately, pores will be formed in the cell wall by the assembly of the terminal complement pathway components C5–C9 into the membrane attack complex (MAC). Cellular damage is enhanced via the deposition of C3b on the cell wall (opsonization) which allows phagocytes to bind and release their lysosomal enzymes.

Antibody-dependent cell-mediated cytotoxicity

The direct interaction of the Fc portion of the bound antibody with Fc receptor-bearing cells (NK cells, platelets, phagocytes) allows these cells to engage the target tissues, focusing their damaging effects onto the antigen-expressing cellular membrane. This is antibody-dependent cell-mediated cytotoxicity (ADCC, see also Chapter 5).

These two mechanisms, complement activation and ADCC, are part of the immune system's normal armamentarium for fighting infection. A normal response causes damage to cells bearing foreign (e.g. microbial or tumour) antigens. These

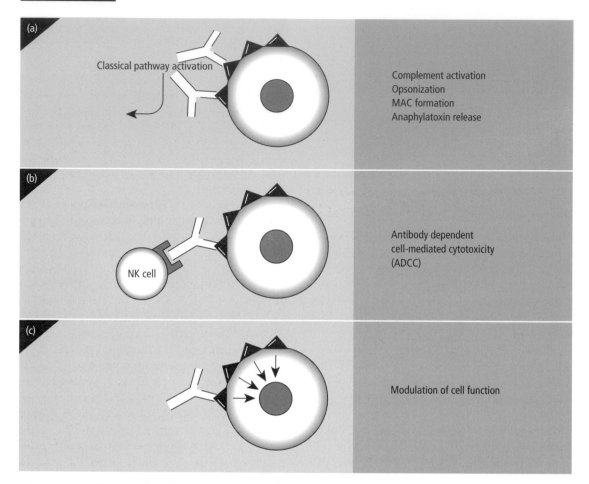

responses may be considered to be hypersensitive when they are directed against an individual's own cellular antigens, or when the scale of the response to a foreign antigen is such that it causes damage to the individual's own cells disproportionately to the potential hazard of the antigen(s) concerned.

Typical examples of Type 2 hypersensitivity include transfusion reactions, autoimmune haemolytic anaemias, hyperacute graft rejection, Goodpasture's syndrome, and Grave's disease. Transfusion reactions and hyperacute graft rejection involve the recognition of truly foreign antigens and ought to be preventable conditions with adequate blood-grouping, tissue-typing and cross-matching. In autoimmune haemolytic anaemias, the antibody is directed against 'self' blood group antigens, for example

Fig. 12.2 Type 2 hypersensitivity involves the interaction of antibody with cell bound antigen. This may have several consequences including (a) activation of the complement cascade; (b) recruitment of cytotoxic cells or (c) modulation of cellular function.

the Rhesus system (see also Chapter 20).

Goodpasture's syndrome is characterized by autoantibodies to glomerular basement membrane (GBM) which can cause acute renal failure but also react with pulmonary basement membranes causing severe pulmonary haemorrhage (see Case Study 15.1).

Antibody-mediated modulation of cellular function

Graves' disease is a good illustration of how antibody recognition of a cell-surface antigen may result in modulation of the cell's function. The autoantibodies in this case are directed against the thyroid stimulating hormone (TSH) receptor. The result is that the antibody mimics the effect of TSH and causes the gland to secrete an excess of thyroxine, causing clinical hyperthyroidism. Therapy in this condition is directed towards reducing thyroid response with drugs or by surgical resection.

Type 3 hypersensitivity

Type 3 reactions are also antibody-mediated. In contrast to Type 2 reactions, the antigenic targets of Type 3 reactions are soluble and not cell membrane bound. The combination of soluble antigen and specific antibody, of IgG or IgM class, results in the formation of circulating *immune complexes* (ICs). As a consequence, the damage caused is not limited to one particular cell type or organ, but may occur at remote sites throughout the body.

ICs are formed during normal antibody responses as a means of assisting antigen disposal, but are quickly cleared by the monocyte/macrophage system, in particular by the phagocytes of the liver, the Kupffer cells. When ICs are allowed to persist, either in the circulation or as deposits within tissues, they activate a number of inflammatory pathways and the response becomes hypersensitive. Antigens which cause IC formation may be either *exogenous* (infection or environmental agents) or *endogenous* (e.g. in autoimmune responses). Two classic examples of Type 3 reactions demonstrate the effector mechanisms involved.

The *Arthus reaction* occurs in animals that have been repeatedly immunized with antigen, resulting in high levels of antigen-specific IgG. An intradermal injection of antigen causes the rapid local accumulation of ICs and a reaction which peaks approximately 6–24 hours later. The ICs cause local complement activation, with recruitment of polymorphonuclear phagocytes to the perivascular area. The release of lysosomal enzymes causes vascular damage resulting in oedema and haemorrhage seen as raised, reddened areas on the skin.

Serum sickness is a condition which was seen in the pre-antibiotic era when patients were treated with large doses of antibody made in other species, for example horses. It was characterized by urticaria, arthralgia (joint pain) and glomerulonephritis (inflammation of the renal glomeruli) and the reaction is reproduced by the injection of foreign antigen into experimental animals. Approximately 1 week after injection, antibody is formed which reacts with the persisting antigen to form ICs in the circulation (Fig. 12.3); this causes complement activation and the appearance of clinical features. Immunofluorescent examination demonstrates deposition of ICs and complement components within glomeruli and small blood vessels, and symptoms persist as long as ICs are detectable in the circulation. Repeated injections of antigen cause persistence of the ICs and the serum sickness syndrome.

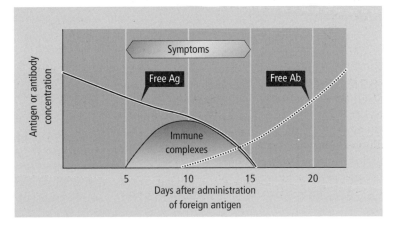

Fig. 12.3 Experimental serum sickness illustrates the formation of immune complexes typical of Type 3 reactions. Ag, antigen; Ab, antibody.

A number of factors including complex size, duration of antigen exposure, host response and local tissue factors, determine when immune complexes persist and cause hypersensitive reactions.

Complex size

Large ICs generally activate complement efficiently and become coated with complement fragments (e.g. C3b). This enables blood cells which bear the CR1 receptor to bind the ICs via C3b and transport them to the liver for degradation by Kupffer cells. Small ICs are also cleared by the reticuloendothelial system, whereas intermediate-sized ICs are less efficiently dealt with by this pathway. Therefore, intermediate-sized ICs are most likely to persist and cause hypersensitivity.

Duration of antigen exposure

Chronic antigen exposure allows continuous IC formation, analogous to the serum sickness model using repeated injections of antigen. Clinical examples of conditions in which chronic antigen exposure is believed to be important in generating a Type 3 response include infections (e.g. hepatitis-B virus infection, bacterial endocarditis), or autoimmune conditions (e.g. systemic lupus erythematosus).

Host response

Host responses are considered important in both the production of ICs and in the failure to remove them from the circulation. Individuals who preferentially produce low affinity antibody favour the production of small/intermediate ICs which are difficult to clear. In addition, individuals deficient in the early components of the classical pathway, C2 and C4, have an increased incidence of immune complex-mediated diseases (see Chapter 14). This is due to their reduced ability to cleave C3 via the classical pathway and therefore their diminished ability to effectively coat circulating ICs with C3b and so facilitate their disposal.

Local tissue factors

Local tissue factors are also important in determining where ICs are deposited and hence where inflammation is focused. Haemodynamic factors such as *blood pressure, turbulence* and *filtration* affect IC deposition. High blood pressure and increased filtration rate contribute to IC accumulation in the renal glomerulus. Turbulence occurs particularly at sites of vessel bifurcation and increases IC deposition at these sites. Furthermore, physicochemical properties of the antigen or IC, including particle size, electrostatic charge and degree of glycosylation of complexes, will also influence their ultimate tissue destination.

Classical examples of human disease involving Type 3 hypersensitivity are immune complex-mediated glomerulonephritis, systemic lupus erythematosus (SLE) and extrinsic allergic alveolitis. In immune complex-mediated glomerulonephritis (see also Case Study 24.2) the nature of the glomerular damage is greatly influenced by the type of IC involved and its rate of deposition. With rapidly deposited ICs, a proliferative response is likely (e.g. post-streptococcal glomerulonephritis), whereas with slower deposition, membranous glomerulonephritis occurs.

In extrinsic allergic alveolitis (e.g. allergic aspergillosis, see Chapter 9), the patient has preformed IgG antibody to inhaled allergen and develops an Arthus-type reaction in the alveoli upon exposure. The clinical features of acute alveolitis usually occur about 6 hours after exposure, corresponding to immune complex formation and recruitment of the damaging effector mechanisms, including complement and polymorphonuclear phagocytes.

Type 4 hypersensitivity

Type 4 hypersensitivity reactions are cell-mediated and differ from Types 1–3 in that they cannot be transmitted from animal to animal by injection of serum. Type 4 responses are also referred to as 'delayed-type hypersensitivity' as the reactions occur 12 hours or more following expo-

Table 12.2 Peak response times for the three forms of Type 4 hypersensitivity reactions

Type 4 reaction	Peak response
Contact	48–72 hours
Tuberculin	48–72 hours
Granulomatous	21–28 days

sure to allergen. They are further classified into three sub-types based on the time of peak response, their clinical manifestations, and the cell types and sites involved (Table 12.2). The common feature is the involvement of T lymphocytes (particularly the CD4 + ve T helper subset), and antigen-presenting cells (APCs).

Contact hypersensitivity

This is caused by low molecular weight antigens which alone are incapable of eliciting an antibody response. They act as *haptens* by binding to normal body proteins and in this form are capable of stimulating the immune system. The most common example is nickel hypersensitivity where affected individuals develop a hyper-reactivity to nickel (which may be contained in costume jewellery, watches, trouser buttons etc.). The rash that appears is red and itchy, eczematous and is usually limited to areas which have been directly exposed.

The mechanism of the reaction is well defined and is divided into *sensitization* and *elicitation* phases. Nickel (or another low molecular weight hapten) is absorbed directly through the skin and is taken up in the epidermis by *Langerhan's cells*. These are related to interdigitating dendritic cells and are APCs. They migrate from the skin to the paracortical regions of local lymph nodes where the antigen is presented to T cells, stimulating the development of memory T cells. This results in the sensitization of the individual to the allergen. In the elicitation phase, cutaneously absorbed antigen is presented to the memory T cells in the dermis causing the secretion of cytokines such as interferon gamma (IFN-γ) and tumour necrosis factor alpha (TNF-α). These soluble mediators

cause keratinocytes to express MHC Class II molecules and the adhesion molecule ICAM-1 which is also expressed on dermal endothelial cells. These two factors contribute to the recruitment of further lymphocytes and macrophages to the inflamed area and within 24 hours lymphocytes are entering the epidermis. By 48 hours, the epidermis contains lymphocytes, macrophages and is oedematous, causing the clinical appearance of an eczematous rash. This sequence of events explains the mechanism of the 'patch test' used in the clinical diagnosis of contact hypersensitivity.

Tuberculin hypersensitivity

In contrast to contact hypersensitivity, tuberculin hypersensitivity is a phenomenon chiefly involving the dermis (Fig. 12.4). Koch observed that when patients suffering from tuberculosis were administered an intradermal injection of tuberculin (an antigen derived from *Mycobacterium tuberculosis*) they suffered both a local and a systemic reaction. The local skin reaction is characterized by an area of induration and swelling and is now recognized as being mediated by sensitized lymphocytes.

This Type 4 reaction is used clinically as a means of determining the sensitization status of individuals in tests for tuberculosis and leprosy. The *Mantoux test* and *Lepromin test* involve the intradermal injection of *M. tuberculosis* and *M. leprae* extracts, respectively. Following the intradermal injection of antigen, lymphocytes begin to accumulate around blood vessels at about 12 hours and peak at approximately 48 hours. There is a predominance of CD4 + ve cells, with a CD4 + ve:CD8 + ve ratio of 2:1. Macrophages accumulate in the dermis simultaneously with lymphocytes and there is migration of some Langerhan's cells from the epidermis. These cells are focused at the site of foreign antigen in the dermis and the response is usually self-limiting as the antigen is removed by the immune system. Both contact sensitivity and tuberculous reactions may be contrasted with a Type 3 Arthus reaction in that they do not involve antibody, complement

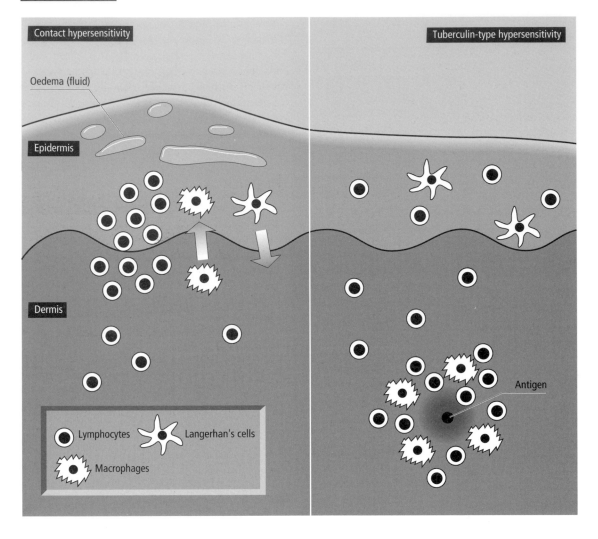

Fig. 12.4 The anatomical sites of contact (epidermal) and tuberculin-type (dermal) hypersensitivity (see text).

activation or recruitment of neutrophils and other polymorphonuclear cells.

Granulomatous hypersensitivity

Where antigen persists, however, the initial tuberculin response may develop into a granulomatous hypersensitivity which is the most severe form of Type 4 hypersensitivity and clinically the most important. Granulomas are collections of macrophages, some of which coalesce to form giant cells, surrounded by a cuff of small lymphocytes (see Chapter 4). The macrophages often have the appearance of epithelial cells, and are known as *epithelioid* cells. Granulomas are formed when the immune system fails to remove foreign antigen which is then allowed to persist, usually within macrophages. Granuloma formation is not confined to skin reactions but occurs in many organs.

Study of experimental models of granulomatous conditions has recently focused attention on the factors involved in initiation and persistence of Type 4 lesions. Antigen presentation is associated with production of the cytokine interleukin-1 (IL-1) by APC, causing the activation of T cells which in turn produce interleukin-2 (IL-2) and express the IL-2 receptor on their cell membrane. These events contribute to the proliferation of T cells and induction of the cellular response. High levels of IL-1 have been demonstrated in early experimental lesions, suggesting that macrophage production of this cytokine is an important early event in recruitment of cells for granuloma formation.

The activated T cells are predominantly of the T helper 1 phenotype, i.e. they preferentially produce IFN-γ and IL-2. They are therefore potent activators of monocytes/macrophages and of other T cells and hence contribute to the accumulation of the cells necessary for granuloma formation. In the later stages of experimental lesions, TNF-α production appears to predominate over IL-1 suggesting that there is an initial cellular recruitment phase and a longer-term maintenance phase in immunological granuloma formation which may be defined in terms of the local production of different cytokines. Clinical conditions associated with significant immunological granuloma formation include *tuberculosis, leprosy, schistosomiasis* (see Chapter 10), *leishmaniasis* and *sarcoidosis*.

In pulmonary tuberculosis, much of the lung damage is due to granuloma formation. Reactivation of the disease, which is often seen in later life, is associated with an age-related reduction in memory T cell function, allowing mycobacterial growth.

Leprosy is an excellent example of how the immune status of an individual determines the clinical manifestation of disease. There are two forms of leprosy, *tuberculoid* and *lepromatous leprosy*. Tuberculoid disease is largely asymptomatic and is characterized by a few hypopigmented (pale) areas of the skin which histologically show typical granulomatous features but few mycobacteria. These patients have potent Type 4 hypersensitivity responses to *M. leprae*, the CD4+ve T cell population being predominantly of the T helper 1 phenotype. In lepromatous leprosy, there are widespread skin lesions containing numerous bacilli but few lymphocytes

These patients have a predominant T helper 2 phenotypic response to the organism (T helper 2 cells secrete IL-4, IL-5 and IL-10) and no clear granuloma formation. Consequently *M. leprae* are able to proliferate and disseminate more freely in lepromatous leprosy and the patient suffers the systemic effects of the infection. Host response in the form of hypersensitivity may therefore be advantageous under certain circumstances.

Key points

1 Hypersensitivity defines situations where the immune system responds inappropriately or excessively to antigens which often appear harmless. The term hypersensitivity is often used interchangeably with allergy, which literally means 'altered reactivity'.

2 Hypersensitivity responses are classified into four types, based upon their different underlying mechanisms and clinical manifestations.

3 Type 1 hypersensitivity reactions are immediate and involve allergen, allergen-specific IgE and mast cells. In its most severe form, a Type 1 hypersensitivity reaction leads to the development of systemic anaphylaxis which is a life-threatening condition.

4 Type 2 hypersensitivity reactions are also antibody-mediated, but in contrast to Type 1 reactions, the antibodies involved are either IgG or IgM. Type 2 reactions are directed against antigens expressed on the surface of cells.

5 Type 3 hypersensitivity reactions are also antibody-mediated but the antigenic targets of Type 3 reactions are soluble and not cell membrane bound. The combination of soluble antigen and specific antibody results in the formation of circulating immune complexes.

6 In contrast to Types 1–3, Type 4 hypersensitivity reactions are cell-mediated, commonly involving the participation of T lymphocytes and antigen-presenting cells.

Summary

A knowledge of the mechanisms of hypersensitivity reactions is essential to the understanding of many disease processes. Different hypersensitivity responses may occur in a single disease process and they are best understood as physiological responses which happen either out of context or to an abnormally severe degree, resulting in deleterious effects to the host.

As our understanding of hypersensitivity increases at the cellular and molecular level, new therapeutic strategies will undoubtedly evolve.

Further reading

Chapel H. & Haeney M. (1993) *Essentials of Clinical Immunology* 3rd edn. Blackwell Scientific Publications, Oxford.

Reeves G. & Todd I. (1990) *Lecture Notes in Immunology* 2nd edn. Blackwell Scientific Publications, Oxford.

Roitt I., Brostoff J. & Male D. (1993) *Immunology* 3rd edn. Mosby-Year Book Europe Ltd., London.

Autoimmunity

Introduction

The role of the immune system is to protect the host against invading pathogens and to mount responses to them leading to their elimination. The immune response involves complex interactions between a variety of cell types. These include T lymphocytes, whose role is recognition of a pathogen and control of the immune response to it; B lymphocytes, which produce specific antibodies capable of recognizing and binding to the pathogen; and phagocytic and cytotoxic cells which destroy the pathogen.

The immune system is highly specific in the recognition of antigens and a critical feature is its ability to discriminate between self and foreign antigens. Self-reactivity is prevented by a number of processes which occur early during lymphocyte development. Under certain circumstances, these mechanisms break down and the body reacts against itself. This concept is known as *autoimmunity* and was first proposed by Paul Ehrlich in 1899 who gave it the name 'horror autotoxicus'. The earliest evidence for the existence of *autoimmune disease* was the identification of *autoantibodies* to red blood cells in a haematological complication of syphilis. It is now recognized that almost every organ and system of the body can be affected by autoimmune disease.

This chapter introduces the concept of *self-tolerance* and examines how its breakdown leads to the development of autoimmunity both at the cellular and humoral level. The spectrum of autoimmune diseases is described and factors predisposing individuals to autoimmune disease are discussed. Current and potential treatments for autoimmune conditions are considered.

Immunological tolerance

Immunological self-tolerance is the failure to respond to self-antigens. Tolerance occurs predominantly at the T cell level and the thymus gland plays a critical role in 'educating' T cells to discriminate between self and non-self. Immature T cells arise in the bone marrow and migrate to the thymus for further development. T cells possess surface receptors which enable them to recognize antigens and an early event in T cell maturation in the thymus is the rearrangement of the genes which code for these receptors (see Chapter 5). This gives rise to a vast repertoire of receptors able to bind to a wide range of antigens. Inevitably, some of these receptors will recognize self-antigens and the T cells which bear them are eliminated by a process called *apoptosis* in which the cells degrade their own DNA (see Chapter 3).

Some T cells which are reactive against self-antigens escape elimination in the thymus and are released into the general circulation. In this situation *peripheral tolerance* plays a role in protecting against self-reactivity, in which T cells are 'switched off' when they interact with antigen in the absence of other signals necessary for activation. Also, other regulatory T cells may suppress self-reactive T cells.

Autoimmune B cells can exist in the general circulation but they are prevented from mounting an antibody response by lack of appropriate T cell help. Some B cells need to be tolerized directly and these are either deleted in the bone marrow or are rendered unresponsive.

As discussed later in this chapter, breakdown in tolerance is central to the development of autoimmunity. However it should be emphasized that although many individuals mount autoreactive responses, only a few develop autoimmune diseases. This is probably because normal individuals can control the activity of autoreactive cells.

The spectrum of autoimmune diseases

Autoimmune diseases may be classified as either *organ-specific* where the autoantigen is localized in one organ only (e.g. thyroid peroxidase and thyroglobulin in Hashimoto's thyroiditis) or *systemic* where the autoantigen is widespread (e.g. components of the cell nucleus in systemic lupus erythematosus.) The more common autoimmune diseases together with their target antigens are shown in Table 13.1.

There is considerable overlap between the autoimmune diseases at either end of the spectrum. For example, patients with systemic lupus erythematosus (SLE) may have the clinical features of scleroderma and rheumatoid arthritis (RA), and patients with autoimmune thyroid disease quite often have gastric autoimmune disease.

Such patients are said to have 'overlap syndrome'. However there is usually little overlap between organ-specific and systemic diseases.

Different autoimmune processes may occur in the same tissue, leading to different clinical outcomes. For example, Hashimoto's thyroiditis involves the destruction of the thyroid cells resulting in hypothyroidism and is associated with immune recognition of thyroid peroxidase and thyroglobulin. Graves' disease involves the opposite effect of hyperthyroidism due to autoantibodies triggering the thyroid stimulating hormone receptor. Conversely, different autoimmune processes affecting the same tissues may have similar clinical effects. Thus, Goodpasture's syndrome and SLE can both cause glomerulonephritis, but through Type II and Type III hypersensitivity mechanisms, respectively (see Chapter 12).

Much of what we know about autoimmune diseases comes from studies of animal models. Such models are disease-specific and exhibit some clinical and immunological features with similarities to the human conditions. Some disease

Table 13.1 Autoimmune diseases, target autoantigens and HLA associations

Diseases	Autoantigen	HLA type
Organ-specific		
Hashimoto's thyroiditis	Thyroid peroxidase and thyroglobulin	DR3, B8
Graves' disease	Thyroid-stimulating hormone receptor	DR3, B8
Pernicious anaemia	Intrinsic factor	DR4, DR2 DR3
Addison's disease	Secretory cells of adrenal cortex	DR3, B8
Insulin dependent (Type 1) diabetes mellitus (IDDM)	Pancreatic islet cells	DR3, DR4 B8, B15
Goodpasture's syndrome	Glomerular and alveolar basement membrane	DR2, B7
Myasthenia gravis	Acetylcholine receptor	DR3, A1, B8
Pemphigus vulgaris	Intercellular component of epidermis	DR4, DR6
Bullous pemphigoid	Epidermal basement membrane	No known associations
Primary biliary cirrhosis	Bile ducts of liver	DR3, B8
Systemic		
Autoimmune haemolytic anaemia	Red blood cells, rhesus antigen	B8
Sjögrens syndrome	Extractable nuclear antigens	DR3, DR4, DR1, A1, B8
Rheumatoid arthritis	IgG rheumatoid factor	B44, B15
Dermatomyositis	Soluble nuclear proteins	DR3, B8, B14
Scleroderma	Nucleoli	DR5, B8
Mixed connective tissue disease	Ribonucleoprotein	DR4
Systemic lupus erythematosus	Double-stranded DNA	DR3 DR2 B5 B8

models may occur spontaneously. For example, the BB rat and NOD mouse are models of insulin-dependent diabetes mellitus (IDDM, also often referred to as Type-1 diabetes mellitus) and spontaneously develop diabetes. The islets of Langerhan in the pancreas become infiltrated with lymphocytes and complete loss of the insulin-producing beta cells follows. Onset of the disease is associated with the presence of autoantibodies reacting with islet cell components. These features are similar to events occurring in the pancreas of diabetic human patients.

Another spontaneous model is the obese strain (OS) chicken which develops thyroiditis and autoantibodies to thyroid components. Neonatal bursectomy (surgical resection of the bursa of fabricus to remove maturing B cells) dramatically reduces thyroiditis which suggests an important role for antibodies in the pathogenesis. Other animal models for autoimmunity can be induced experimentally. For example, injection of thyroglobulin produces thyroiditis in some susceptible mouse strains.

T Lymphocytes and cytokines in autoimmunity

T helper (Th) cells are central to the generation of an immune response to both foreign and self-antigens. They recognize antigens on the surface of antigen-presenting cells (APC) in association with Class II HLA molecules, and are thus activated to produce a cascade of cytokines which control the immune response at various levels. Th cells can be classified according to the profile of cytokines they secrete. Th1 cells produce primarily interleukin-2 (IL-2) and interferon-gamma (IFN-γ) and are associated predominantly with cell-mediated immunity whereas Th2 cells produce IL-4, IL-5 and Il-10 and are implicated mainly in the control of antibody responses.

Th1 cytokines, although beneficial in the clearance of some pathogens, also produce deleterious effects in a number of models of autoimmunity. For example, mice manipulated experimentally to express IFN-γ in the islets of Langerhan sponta-

neously develop IDDM. In contrast, the systemic administration of IL-4 and IL-10 inhibits the onset of diabetes in the NOD mouse model. This would suggest a role for Th2 cells in the prevention of diabetes and a role for Th1 cells in disease pathogenesis.

A wide range of cytokines have been isolated from the joints of patients with RA. These include IL-1α, IL-1β, IL-6, tumor necrosis factor-alpha (TNF-α), IL-8 and transforming growth factor (TGF). TNF is central to the production of other cytokines and in RA the cytokine network operates in series with TNF, promoting the secretion of IL-1 followed by IL-6. Blocking TNF action suppresses the production of most of the other pro-inflammatory cytokines, these effects being more profound than just blocking IL-1 alone.

Cytokines play an important role in regulating the expression of Class II HLA molecules, which in turn may contribute to autoimmune pathogenesis. The aberrant expression of Class II molecules by target epithelial cells was first reported in autoimmune thyroiditis but there is now a growing list of autoimmune diseases where abnormal epithelial expression has been observed (Table 13.2). It has been hypothesized that expression of Class II on these cells enables them to present their own surface molecules to activated autoreactive T cells, thus bypassing the need for conventional antigen-presenting cells. IFN-γ is a strong inducer of Class II expression. In autoimmune thyroiditis, for example, it has been

Table 13.2 Examples of aberrant HLA Class II expression by epithelial cells in autoimmune diseases

Disease	Cells expressing Class II
Autoimmune thyroid diseases	Thyroid epithelium
Insulin-dependent (Type 1) diabetes mellitus	Pancreatic beta cells
Inflammatory bowel disease	Gut epithelium
Autoimmune protracted diarrhoea of infancy	Immature jejunal enterocytes
Alopecia areata	Hair follicular cells
Primary biliary cirrhosis	Bile duct epithelium
Sjögrens syndrome	Salivary ducts

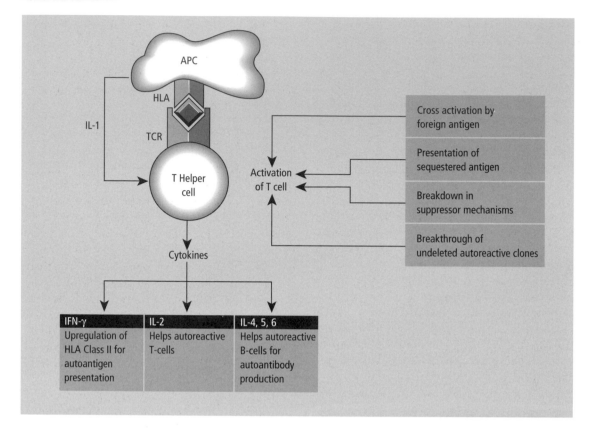

Fig. 13.1 Activation of autoreactive cells and the role of cytokines in autoimmunity.

suggested that autoreactive T cells infiltrating the thyroid gland produce IFN-γ which causes the spread of Class II expression through the gland, thus potentiating the autoimmune process. Figure 13.1 summarizes the role of activated Th cells and cytokines in the induction of autoimmunity.

Autoreactive T cytotoxic (Tc) cells are likely to contribute significantly to the tissue damage in some autoimmune diseases, for example IDDM and autoimmune thyroiditis.

B Lymphocytes and antibodies in autoimmunity

B lymphocytes capable of producing autoantibodies are present in the normal human B cell repertoire. Normal human serum contains natural autoantibodies of the IgM and IgG classes that can recognize a wide range of self-antigens including nuclear antigens and membrane components. These natural autoantibodies are produced by a subset of B lymphocytes expressing a molecule called CD5, and are usually *polyreactive*, that is, they recognize bacterial antigens and also show cross reactivity with self components. However, in normal individuals these antibodies are thought not to be auto-aggressive and may be beneficial in providing an early form of natural immunity to bacterial infections. Furthermore natural autoantibodies may actually prevent pathological autoimmunity by binding to microbial epitopes that are similar or identical to epitopes of self-antigens.

The production of autoantibodies by B cells is normally only possible when T lymphocytes recognize the self antigen and produce the appropriate cytokines necessary for B cell triggering.

However the CD5 +ve B cells do not require T cell help and these cells are found in increased numbers in SLE, multiple sclerosis, Hashimoto's thyroiditis and RA.

In contrast to natural polyreactive autoantibodies, specific disease-associated autoantibodies in the serum are helpful markers for diagnostic purposes and may be particularly useful for predicting disease onset. For example, autoantibodies to islet cell components are found several years prior to the onset of Type I diabetes. Studies of first degree relatives of IDDM patients have established that there is an increased risk for disease development in individuals who have antibodies to islet cell antigens, especially if the titre of the antibodies is high. Autoantibodies that are associated with the disease may, or may not, be directly pathogenic. The autoantibodies to cytoplasmic islet cell antigens are probably produced as a consequence of islet cell destruction and may not cause islet damage themselves. By contrast, other autoantibodies are directly involved in producing clinical disease, for example, antibodies to the thyroid-stimulating hormone receptor in Graves' disease and antibodies to the glomerular and alveolar basement membrane in Goodpasture's syndrome (see Case Study 15.1).

Contributory factors in the aetiology of the autoimmune diseases

Genetics

Family studies

Much evidence for the role of genetic factors in autoimmune diseases has come from family studies. Familial tendencies have been seen in IDDM, autoimmune thyroid disease and RA. For example, relatives of patients with IDDM have a greater chance of developing the disease than age-matched controls.

Studies with identical and non-identical twins are useful for identifying genetic susceptibility. The disease concordance rate is higher in identical twins. For example, in IDDM disease concordance is 50 percent in identical twins compared to five percent in non-identical twins. However, the disease concordance rate in identical twins is never 100 percent which would suggest that environmental factors are also important in triggering the development of autoimmunity.

HLA Associations

The genes of the human leucocyte antigen (HLA) system have been associated with susceptibility to autoimmune disease. These genes code for cell surface molecules which serve as identity markers and play a major role in antigen recognition. The HLA system is the human equivalent of the major histocompatibility complex (MHC) and comprises a set of tightly linked genes located on chromosome number 6. Three classes of HLA have been identified and autoimmune diseases are usually associated with the HLA Class II alleles DP, DQ and DR. For example, 80–90 percent of patients with RA carry either the DR1 haplotype or one of three variants of the DR4 haplotype (Dw4, Dw14 or Dw15). Similarly, for IDDM, DR3 and DR4 lead to increased susceptibility, compared to DR2 and DR5 which are protective. Further details of HLA associations are given in Table 13.1.

Hormone effects

The sex hormones have a major effect on the functioning of the immune system. Generally autoimmune diseases are more common in females and this has been demonstrated in animal models of SLE where the female sex hormones accelerate the disease process. Oestrogens can increase the level of antibody production by inhibiting suppressor T cell activity.

Environmental factors

Infectious agents

Autoimmune diseases can occur following chronic infection. An example is the development of rheumatic heart disease following infections

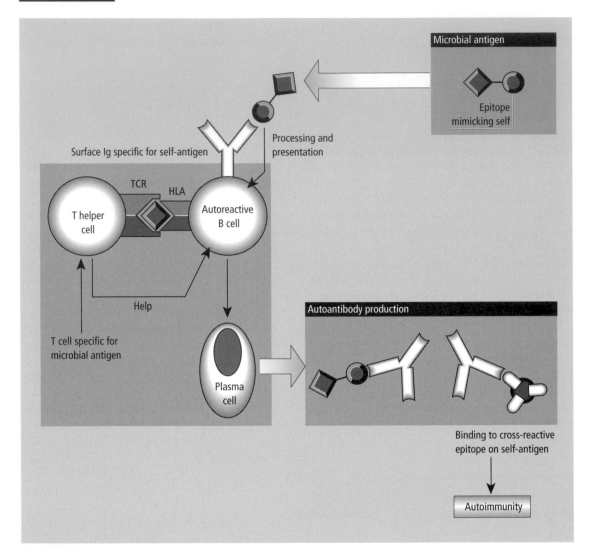

Fig. 13.2(a) Autoreactive B cells are usually unable to produce autoantibodies due to lack of appropriate T cell help. Microbial antigens which share similar structures to self-antigens can prime T cells to provide help for autoreactive B cells. These cells are induced to secrete antibodies which can cross react with self and microbial antigens.

with Group A streptococci. Patients with leprosy or tuberculosis often have rheumatoid factors circulating in the blood.

Drugs and chemicals

Administration of L-dopa has been implicated in some cases of SLE and penicillamine can cause a variety of autoimmune diseases such as scleroderma and pemphigus vulgaris. Toxins such as silicon and vinyl chloride have also been associated with scleroderma and cigarette smoking and exposure to hydrocarbon solvents has been linked to the development of Goodpasture's syndrome (see Case Study 15.1). Possible mechanisms whereby environmental agents may trigger autoimmunity are considered in the following section.

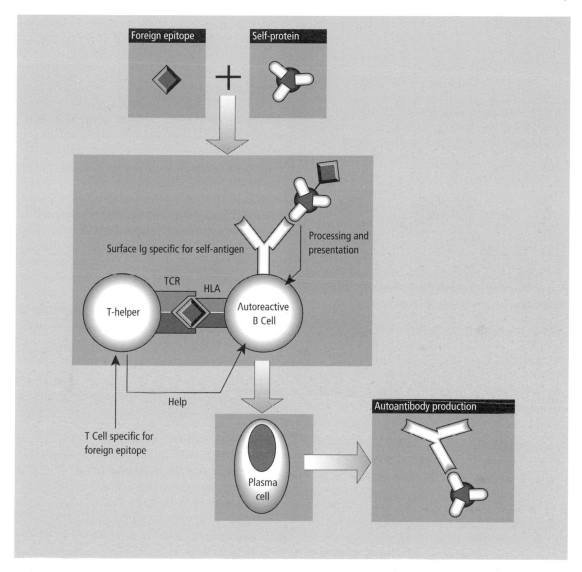

Fig. 13.2(b) Foreign antigens which link to self-antigens may be recognized by T cells which can therefore help the B cells to produce autoantibodies.

Mechanisms of autoimmunity

The stimulation of self-reactive lymphocytes is under tight control of the individual. Precisely how autoimmune disease develops is still uncertain in most instances, but a number of mechanisms have been proposed to explain how these controls might be bypassed either at the level of the T cells (see Fig. 13.1) or B cells.

Molecular mimicry

Some viral and bacterial proteins share antigenic epitopes with proteins of the host. In this way they may 'fool' the immune system into granting them free access because of the maintenance of self-tolerance. On the other hand, an immune response mounted by the host against the epitope of the infectious agent may cross-react with the

113

mimicked host protein sequence leading to auto-immunity (Fig. 13.2a). An example is provided by the association of Group A streptococci with rheumatic heart disease, in which cross-reactivity of anti-streptococcal antibodies with cardiac muscle has been demonstrated.

Provision of foreign T cell epitopes

Another mechanism whereby T cell help may be given to autoreactive B cells is by the linking of foreign antigens containing T cell epitopes to host proteins (Fig. 13.2b). Some drugs and chemicals mentioned in the previous section may exert their effects in this way.

Release of sequestered antigens and exposure of cryptic epitopes

Some self-antigens are not normally exposed to the cells of the immune system and if released during adult life will be seen as 'foreign'. For example autoimmune responses to proteins released from a damaged eye can give rise to sympathetic ophthalmia.

APCs are constantly degrading antigens into peptide fragments for presentation. However, some self-epitopes are never normally exposed to thymic T cells to induce tolerance. These are referred to as *cryptic epitopes* and are essentially recognized as 'foreign', but are usually present at low densities and are therefore unable to activate autoreactive T cells. Responses to cellular stress, infection of APCs and activation of APCs by cytokines might alter the pattern of peptides presented so that cryptic epitopes become dominant and induce autoreactivity.

Failure of suppressive mechanisms

Failure to control autoreactive Th cells may be of major importance in the development of some autoimmune diseases. Controlling factors include T suppressor cells and the suppressive action of hormones and cytokines. Breakdown in one or more of these factors may lead to an autoimmune response. For example, removal of the thymus at birth from OS chickens exacerbates the development of thyroiditis, presumably due to the removal of suppressor T cell control.

Anti-idiotype reactivity

During an immune response, antibodies produced against foreign antigens may stimulate the production of a second wave of antibodies directed against their antigen-binding sites (*idiotypes*). The *anti-idiotypes* may have binding sites which resemble the original epitope. In the case of viral infection, if an antibody is directed at a cell-binding virus component then an anti-idiotype antibody could itself combine with the host cell surface receptor for the virus. Such as anti-idiotype would then be classed as an autoantibody (Fig. 13.3). For example, it has been shown experimentally that anti-idiotypes to antibodies directed against a neuron-binding component of reovirus Type 3 can themselves bind to neurons.

Immunotherapy of autoimmune diseases

The metabolic defects resulting from some organ-specific autoimmune diseases can be corrected by replacing the missing products of the defective organ. For example IDDM can be controlled by administration of insulin, and pernicious anaemia (see Chapter 20) by administration of vitamin B_{12}. Immunosuppressive and cytotoxic drugs are used to dampen down the autoimmune response but, because of the side effects, tend only to be used in progressive or life-threatening disorders.

Newly emerging forms of therapy involve methods for re-establishing tolerance and manipulating T cell recognition of autoantigens. Orally induced tolerance has proved effective in reducing the symptoms of autoimmune disease in animal models. Feeding myelin basic protein to animals with experimental allergic encephalomyelitis can prevent or reverse paralysis, and Type II collagen is effective in delaying the onset of experimental RA. Small scale clinical

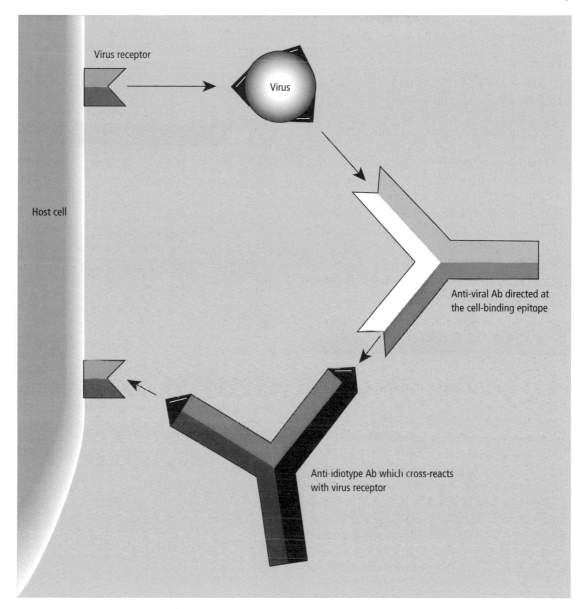

Fig. 13.3 An anti-idiotype antibody, to an antiviral antibody, acting as an autoantibody. In this instance there is 'molecular mimicry' between the idiotype and the autoantigen.

trials on humans have already shown promising results. Peptide epitopes of autoantigens administered experimentally can induce peptide-specific tolerance in neonates and can modify autoimmune responses in adults.

More direct approaches aim to remove the subsets of T cells or cytokines involved in the pathogenesis of autoimmune disease. Monoclonal antibodies against the CD4 molecule of T cells have been used in clinical trials of patients with RA and multiple sclerosis (MS). Unfortunately anti-CD4 therapy is non-specific and might produce general immune suppression if administered over prolonged periods of time. Monoclonal

115

antibodies against cytokines are showing promising results as immunotherapeutic agents. Anti-IFN-γ can prevent experimental autoimmune thyroiditis and diabetes in NOD mice. Collagen-induced arthritis in mice may be prevented by the administration of anti-TNF-α monoclonal antibodies.

Anti-TNF antibodies have proven effective in early clinical trials of patients with RA by helping to block the inflammatory cytokine network. Patients showed a reduction in joint-swelling, stiffness and other clinical symptoms, and a decline in serum levels of rheumatoid factors and markers of inflammation. The antibody was well tolerated by the patients, and repeated therapy following relapse was successful. Based on this data it has been suggested that other diseases may be treated with anti-TNF antibodies.

Summary

Autoimmune disease is the end result of a number of highly complex interconnecting immune reactions. However, considerable advances have been made in recent years in understanding how these autoimmune reactions may arise.

Family studies and HLA gene associations have been useful in identifying those individuals who are at risk of developing disease. The innovation of molecular biology techniques should enable further characterization of these disease susceptibility genes as well as looking for associations elsewhere in the genome. Much emphasis is being placed on the role of the environment in disease induction, particularly with viral infection and by using highly specific molecular analysis it is possible to identify traces of viral DNA that may provide important clues.

The ultimate goal in immunotherapy is to arrest disease and return the individual to a state of tolerance. Considerable research efforts are being focused on the mechanisms of tolerance and how these mechanisms are bypassed or deficient for certain autoantigens. Manipulation of the cyto-kine network using monoclonal antibodies should be useful in increasing our understanding of autoimmune diseases and for the therapy of those diseases where the target autoantigen is not yet known.

Key points

1 A critical feature of the immune system is its ability to discriminate between self and foreign antigens (i.e. exercise self-tolerance). Autoimmunity occurs when mechanisms of tolerance break down.

2 Autoimmune diseases are classified as organ-specific (autoantigen located in one tissue) or systemic (autoantigen is widespread). Animal models have been useful in understanding autoimmune diseases.

3 Autoimmunity develops at the cellular and humoral levels. Autoreactive T cells and the cytokines they secrete are important in the induction of autoimmunity. Autoreactive B cells produce autoantibodies to self-components. These autoantibodies may or may not be directly pathogenic.

4 A number of factors influence the susceptibility of an individual to autoimmune disease. These include genetic, hormonal and environmental (infectious agents and drugs) factors.

5 Mechanisms which lead to autoimmunity include mimicry between foreign and self-antigens, failure of suppressive mechanisms and release of self-antigens not normally exposed to the immune system.

6 Improvements in our understanding of autoimmune pathogenesis are leading to the application of new forms of therapy (e.g. re-establishment of tolerance, or inhibition of the activity of T cells or cytokines).

Further reading

Roitt I., Brostoff J. & Male D. (1993) *Immunology*. Mosby. London

Sercarz, E. & Datta S. K. (1994) Autoimmunity, *Curr. Opin. Immunol*. **6**, 875–958.

Steinman L. (1993) Autoimmune disease. *Sci. Am.* **269**, 74–83.

Immunodeficiency

The immune system is composed of cells (B and T lymphocytes, monocytes and neutrophils) and their secretory products (antibodies, cytokines and serum complement). These function in an integrated manner for host defence against foreign micro-organisms and the generation of inflammatory responses. Although no single component functions without the participation of others, four conceptually different systems for host defence can be identified: *humoral immunity; cell-mediated immunity; phagocytosis* and *complement*. Deficiencies of each of the functional systems occur, some on the basis of genetically determined traits, others due to the effects of the environment such as exposure to drugs (e.g. corticosteroids or cyclosporin A) or viral infections (e.g. the human immunodeficiency virus, measles virus or Epstein–Barr virus).

Understanding the physiological basis of immune deficiency has contributed to an understanding of how the immune system serves to protect the normal host from infection. In fact, the biological significance of many host defence functions has been defined by recognition of the specific problems that occur in patients with inborn errors of individual components of host defence.

This chapter will briefly illustrate how abnormalities of individual components lead to increased susceptibility to infection and other illnesses. Specific examples of immunodeficiency states are selected to illustrate principles. The following sections should therefore be regarded as illustrative rather than comprehensive.

Drug or virus-induced immunodeficiency is not discussed as these topics are considered elsewhere (see Chapter 8 and Case Study 11.2). It is worth noting that some immunodeficiency states are also associated with an increased incidence of certain forms of cancer. This subject is dealt with more fully in Chapter 28.

Deficiency of humoral (antibody-mediated) immunity

X-linked agammaglobulinaemia

X-linked agammaglobulinaemia (XLA) is the prototypic disorder of humoral immunity. XLA results from a deficiency of the enzyme Bruton's tyrosine kinase (Btk) and B lymphocyte development is arrested at the stage of pre-B-cells. Males with this disease do not have mature immunoglobulin-bearing B lymphocytes in peripheral blood, do not have plasma cells or secondary lymphoid follicle formation in lymphoid tissues, and have severe hypogammaglobulinaemia (reduced levels of immunoglobulin in blood). No other compartment of immune function is affected by lack of Btk. In particular, T cell function and cell-mediated immunity is completely intact. Therefore, individuals with XLA serve as a model for discerning the role of antibody in host defence.

The Btk gene has been mapped to the X chromosome, and XLA is therefore not the result of abnormal structural genes on the somatic chromosomes that encode the immunoglobulins themselves. An interesting demonstration of the X chromosome effect on B lymphocyte differentiation is observed in the female carriers of XLA, all of whom are immunologically normal. In normal females, one of the two X chromosomes in each cell is randomly inactivated. This is also observed in all of the cells of XLA carrier women,

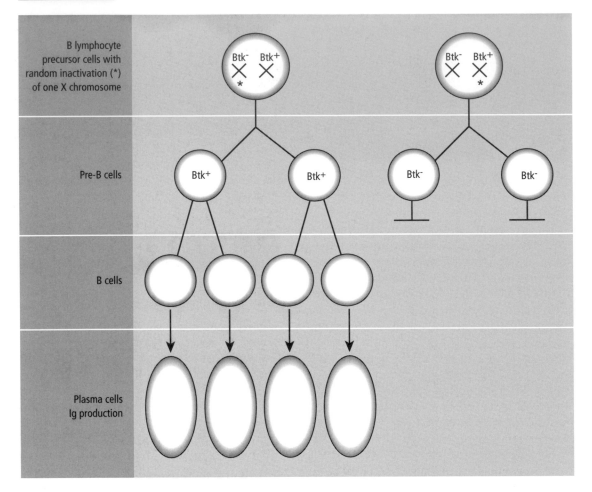

Fig. 14.1 B Lymphocyte growth and differentiation in a female carrier of X-linked agammaglobulinaemia. Early in embryological development, inactivation of one of the X chromosomes occurs in each cell. If the chromosome carrying the abnormal Btk gene (Btk⁻) is inactivated (*), Btk function is normal and subsequent B cell growth and differentiation of the daughter cells occur normally. If the chromosome carrying the normal gene (Btk⁺) is inactivated, Btk function is abnormal and B cell differentiation is blocked. Carrier females are immunologically normal because the surviving B cells can diversify and grow sufficiently for those cells that never develop.

except among their B lymphocytes. The latter cells all inactivate a single X chromosome, the one with the defective Btk gene. Lack of expression of the normal gene blocks B cell differentiation, and therefore only the B cells with the normal X chromosome active are able to fully differentiate (Fig. 14.1). Analysis of X chromosome activation patterns of peripheral blood was used to determine carrier status, even before abnormalities in the Btk gene were identified as the cause of XLA.

The differential diagnosis of hypogamma-globulinaemia in infancy includes transient hypogammaglobulinaemia of infancy, immunoglobulin deficiency with increased IgM, severe combined immunodeficiency disease, and rare cases of HIV infection. Quantitation of B and T lymphocytes in peripheral blood is helpful in distinguishing among these possibilities. Boys with XLA have no detectable B lymphocytes but have normal numbers of T lymphocytes. In contrast, infants with transient hypogammaglobulinaemia

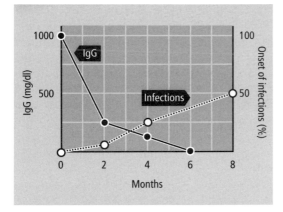

Fig. 14.2 Boys with X-linked agammaglobulinaemia are protected from infection during the first few months of life by transplacentally acquired maternal IgG. As the maternal IgG levels fall (half-life of IgG is approximately 23 days), there is an increasing incidence of infections.

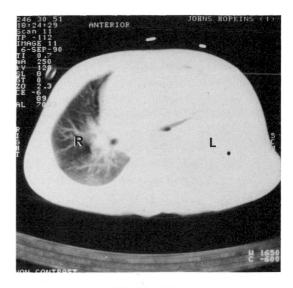

Fig. 14.3 CT scan of a child with X-linked agammaglobulinaemia who presented with pneumococcal pneumonia with empyema predominantly affecting the left lung. The pneumonia in the left lung (L) is represented as a pale area on the CT scan and may be compared with the relatively normal appearance of the right lung (R).

generally have normal numbers of B and T lymphocytes; children with severe combined immunodeficiency have decreased numbers of T lymphocytes with normal, decreased or increased numbers of B cells; and children with HIV infection have decreased numbers of CD4 +ve T lymphocytes.

Boys with XLA are usually protected from infection by transplacentally acquired maternal IgG for their first 3–4 months of life (Fig. 14.2). Thereafter, chronic or recurrent bacterial and viral infections are the predominant clinical manifestation of XLA. Otitis media, pneumonia (Fig. 14.3), diarrhoea and sinusitis occur most often, usually in combination with each other. Infections with heavily encapsulated bacteria such as *Streptococcus pneumoniae* and *Haemophilus influenzae* are common because the host defence against these organisms relies upon the ability of antibody to bind to the polysaccharide capsule with subsequent complement activation and phagocytosis (opsonization). Infections may begin on mucosal surfaces, but are not limited to them because there is absence of serum immunoglobulin. As a result, localized bacterial infections may be spread through the bloodstream to other tissues such as the meninges, joints and bones.

Patients with XLA generally recover uneventfully from viral infections, but not without exception. Enteroviruses (such as coxsackie virus, ECHO virus and poliovirus), which usually cause a self-limiting mild gastro-enteritis in normal children, are prone to cause chronic disseminated infections in XLA patients. Chronic hepatitis, meningo-encephalitis (inflammation of the meninges and brain) and dermatomyositis (co-existent inflammation of skin and muscle) can result from enterovirus infections. These are often fatal, although therapy with gammaglobulin containing virus-specific antibodies may be helpful.

Selective IgA deficiency

This provides an important contrast to XLA. In this disorder, individuals have a complete or almost complete lack of serum and mucosal IgA, but have normal levels of all other immunoglobulin classes and have normal cell-mediated immune function. Many of the clinical features of this disease can be explained by the unique biological properties of IgA. It is the predominant immunoglobulin class on mucosal surfaces, although IgA comprises only 15 percent of immunoglobulin in the serum. IgA is secreted onto mucosal surfaces as a macromolecular complex consisting of two IgA molecules joined to a J chain and a secretory component. The majority of patients with IgA deficiency lack both serum and secretory IgA, but there are rare cases in which there is a deficiency of secretory but not serum IgA.

Unlike the major serum immunoglobulin classes, IgG and IgM, IgA is largely silent as a mediator of inflammatory responses. It does not activate complement or promote opsonization, but functions in antimicrobial defence by inhibiting microbial adherence and by neutralizing viruses and toxins. IgA also has an important role in antigen clearance, preventing soluble antigens from penetrating the mucosa and entering the systemic circulation.

Some patients with selective IgA deficiency have an increased susceptibility to infection, although there is disagreement about the relative risk of infection that IgA deficiency imposes upon the host. Because IgA is the predominant immunoglobulin on mucosal surfaces and only a minor component of serum immunoglobulin, most infections in IgA deficient patients are confined to the mucosal surfaces of the respiratory tract (e.g. otitis media, sinusitis, bronchitis and pneumonia) and gastrointestinal tract (e.g. viral gastroenteritis), and systemic infections such as meningitis and bacterial sepsis are no more common than among the general population.

It is interesting that IgA deficient patients also appear to have an increased susceptibility to atopic and autoimmune diseases (see Chapters 12 and 13). Atopic disorders such as allergic rhinitis, asthma, urticaria, eczema and food allergy, occur in as many as 50 percent of individuals with IgA deficiency. It has been postulated that lack of secretory IgA allows inhaled and ingested antigens to penetrate the mucosal epithelium and to elicit allergic antibody (IgE) responses in the bronchial and gastrointestinal lymphoid tissues. A particu-larly hazardous allergic reaction in IgA deficient patients is the development of anaphylactic reactions following the infusion of plasma or gamma-globulin. The IgA in these products is recognized as a foreign protein in individuals who have no detectable IgA.

A variety of autoimmune diseases have also been associated with selective IgA deficiency. These include juvenile rheumatoid arthritis, systemic lupus erythematosus, autoimmune thyroiditis and pernicious anaemia. The precise mechanisms leading to these clinical manifestations of IgA deficiency cannot be fully explained by the absence of IgA antibodies. It has been hypothesized that disordered immune regulation underlies both IgA deficiency and susceptibility to autoimmune disease. The structural genes for IgA are intact in virtually all IgA-deficient patients, while abnormalities of helper T lymphocytes and cytokine production have been demonstrated. These observations suggest that factors other than the serum IgA level are important in determining the clinical expression of this disease.

Deficiency of cell-mediated (T cell) immunity

DiGeorge's syndrome

This is a genetically determined abnormality (see also Case Study 27.2) that results in a number of defects including abnormal development of the thymus gland. Patients may have thymic hypoplasia (underdevelopment) or aplasia (thymus gland fails to develop). Since the thymus is the gland within which T lymphocytes develop, thymic hypoplasia leads to T lymphocyte deficiency. All T cell sub-populations are affected equally, so that there is deficiency of both CD4 +ve helper cells and CD8 +ve cytotoxic cells. Affected infants have low levels of lymphocytes in the blood circulation (the majority of peripheral blood lymphocytes are T cells) and are depleted of lymphocytes in the paracortical areas of lymph nodes and spleen. The deficiency of cell-mediated immunity results in increased susceptibility to infections with fungi, the protozoan *Pneumocystis carinii*, and *Mycobacterium* spp. because these organisms are intracellular pathogens. That is, they are ingested by monocytes and other phagocytic cells, but are not easily killed without the participation of T lymphocytes. DiGeorge's syndrome patients are also highly susceptible to viral infection because they lack cytotoxic T cells which kill virus-infected host cells (Chapter 8). As a result, relatively common viruses such as varicella zoster (chicken pox) and rotavirus (gastro-enteritis) may cause fatal infections in affected children. Most patients with DiGeorge's syndrome have sufficient residual T cells to allow normal or near normal growth and differentiation of B lymphocytes.

Severe combined immunodeficiency (SCID)

SCID describes a group of disorders, which are characterized by severe functional abnormalities of both B and T lymphocytes. Individuals with this disorder lack virtually all humoral and cell-mediated immune function. They are susceptible to the widest possible array of bacterial, viral, fungal and protozoan pathogens. If untreated, most die of infections within the first year of life.

A number of underlying defects have been identified, each of which is able to produce the SCID phenotype. A congenital absence of lymphoid stem cells leads to complete deficiency of lymphocytes and thus to severe combined immunodeficiency. However, it is interesting that most of the known causes of SCID are the result of defects in T lymphocytes with secondary abnormalities of the B lymphocytes. For example, genetic defects in the production of interleukin-2 (the major T lymphocyte growth factor) or its receptor lead to SCID. In these cases, the near total arrest of T lymphocyte development prevents production of the helper T lymphocyte cytokines that are essential for B lymphocyte growth and differentiation. Such patients can be treated by transplanting T lymphocytes from a normal individual. As the donor T lymphocytes mature, they secrete cytokines and allow the recipient's own B cells to develop. The relationship between T and B lymphocyte deficiences is outlined in Fig. 14.4.

Deficiency of phagocytic cell function

Neutrophils together with monocytes and macrophages are the most important of the body's cells that possess the ability to phagocytose foreign antigens and micro-organisms. Many phagocytic cells are mobile and can move from the bloodstream through tissues to the site of microbial invasion or inflammation, while other phagocytic cells are fixed in the spleen and lymph nodes where they clear micro-organisms and other particulate matter from the blood and lymphatic circulation, respectively.

Monocytes also have the ability to serve as antigen-presenting cells and to secrete a variety of pro-inflammatory substances including cytokines and complement components. In order to function properly, phagocytic cells must attach to a substrate (*adherence*), move through tissues toward the site of microbial invasion (*chemotaxis*), attach to opsonized microbes and ingest them (*phagocytosis*), and kill the microbes (*intracellular killing*). Abnormalities of any of these steps will lead to deficiency in host defence.

Leucocyte adherence deficiency

This is an autosomal recessive trait that results from the lack of expression of the CD11/CD18 family of leucocyte-associated *integrin* molecules [CD11a/CD18(LFA-1), CD11b/CD18 (Mac-1 or complement receptor 3) and CD11c/CD18 (p150,95)] necessary for phagocyte adherence (Table 14.1). The disease results from a defect in the gene encoding the beta chain common to each of these glycoproteins. The inability to adhere to tissue substrate impairs leucocyte mobility. Affected individuals have an increase in the number of circulating blood leucocytes because the cells cannot adhere to vascular endothelium (see Chapter 4). They also have difficulty mobilizing

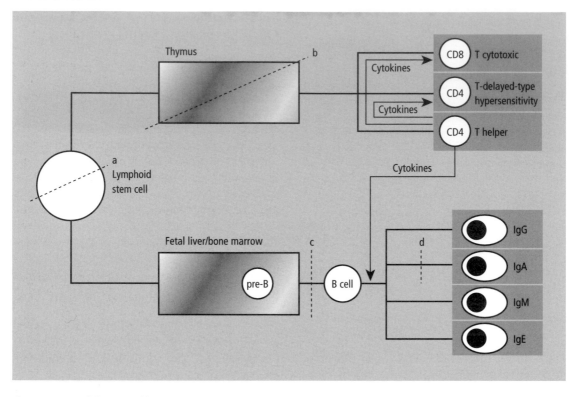

Fig. 14.4 Primary deficiencies of lymphocytes. (a) severe combined immunodeficiency (absence of cell-mediated and humoral immunity) caused by genetically determined absence of lymphoid stem cells; (b) DiGeorge's syndrome (decreased numbers or absence of T lymphocytes) caused by thymic aplasia or hypoplasia. Because T helper lymphocytes produce cytokines that are necessary for B cell development, there may be associated defects in humoral immunity; (c) X-linked agammaglobulinaemia (absence of humoral immunity) caused by deficiency of Btk with block in B lymphocyte differentiation; (d) Selective IgA deficiency, aetiology unknown in most cases.

Table 14.1 Leucocyte adhesion deficiency

Alpha chain	Beta chain	Function
CD11a	CD18	LFA-1 mediates cellular adhesion for interactions of immune cells
CD11b	CD18	CR3 mediates phagocytosis of C3bi-coated targets
CD11c	CD18	p150, 95 mediates adhesion of phagocytes to substrate and to C3bi

Leucocyte adhesion deficiency results from a defect in a gene on chromosome 21 encoding the beta chain (CD18). The gene cluster for alpha chains is on chromosome 16.

those leucocytes to the sites of infection and are unusually susceptible to bacterial infections, especially those that begin along body surfaces such as the skin, gingivae, perirectal area and the lungs.

Chronic granulomatous disease

Chronic granulomatous disease results from a different abnormality of phagocyte function, the inability to kill ingested micro-organisms. In the normal individual, ingestion of a micro-organism by the phagocytic cell results in activation of the myeloperoxidase–H_2O_2–halide system by which molecular oxygen is reduced to superoxide through a series of reactions involving NADPH oxidase. The superoxide in turn undergoes further

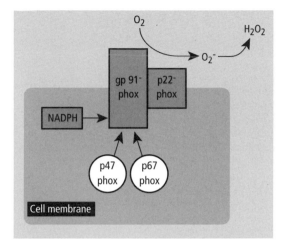

Fig. 14.5 NADPH oxidase system. Chronic granulomatous disease results from mutation in either the gp91-phox (encoded by the X chromosome), p22-phox (chromosome 16), p47-phox (chromosome 7) or p67-phox (chromosome 1) sub-units of the NADPH oxidase assembly. Cytochrome b_{558} is the membrane bound heterodimeric complex of gp91-phox and p22-phox; p47-phox and p67-phox are cytosolic components. When the NADPH oxidase system functions normally, molecular oxygen is reduced to superoxide anion (O_2^-) which leads to the formation of H_2O_2.

reactions leading to the generation of reduced oxygen derivatives such as hydrogen peroxide and hydroxyl radicals. Myeloperoxidase catalyses the reaction of hydrogen peroxide with chloride to create hypochlorite ions. The net effect of these toxic derivatives of reduced molecular oxygen is to kill micro-organisms within the phagocytic vacuole. Individuals with chronic granulomatous disease lack one of the components of the NADPH oxidase system (Fig. 14.5), and are therefore unable to kill most ingested micro-organisms. Their phagocytic cells have normal mobility and normal phagocytosis, and micro-organisms are effectively trapped within phagocytic cells. However, because the micro-organisms cannot be killed, granulomas (see Chapters 4 and 12) and abscesses form within various tissues including the skin, lymph nodes, spleen and liver (Figs. 14.6 and 14.7).

The complement system

The complement system is composed of a large number of serum proteins that act in a cascade to mediate defensive and inflammatory reactions (see Chapter 4). The majority of the biologically significant effects of the complement system are mediated by the third component (C3) and the terminal components (C5–C9). However, in order to perform their biological functions, C3 and C5–C9 must first be activated by other complement components via either the classical or alternate pathway. The classical pathway is

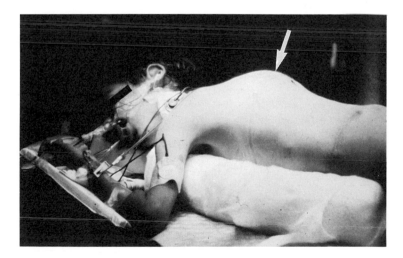

Fig. 14.6 Paravertebral abscess represented by an area of swelling (arrowed) in a boy with chronic granulomatous disease. The abscess in this case was the result of infection with the fungal organism *Aspergillus fumigatus*.

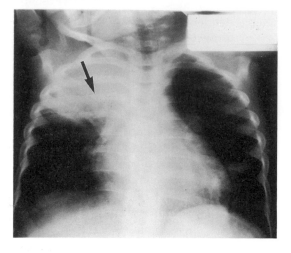

Fig. 14.7 Chest radiograph from a child with chronic granulomatous disease. The patient had previously been immunized with Bacillus Calmette-Guerin (BCG). This is a live attenuated strain of the organism *Mycobacterium bovis* which has been used for the vaccination of children against tuberculosis. The patient developed pneumonia, shown on the radiograph as an area of opacity in the right upper lobe (arrowed). Later, the pneumonia was shown to be the result of infection with the BCG organism. In the normal host BCG is non-pathogenic, however in patients with chronic granulomatous disease it may produce severe, potentially life-threatening, infections.

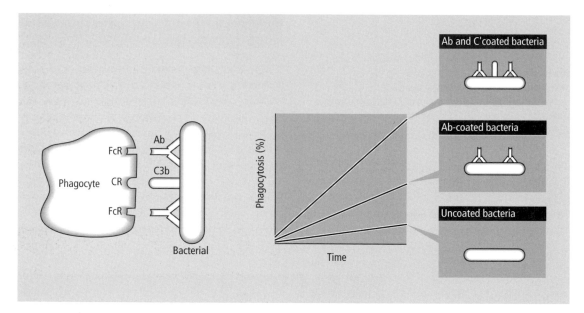

Fig. 14.8 Host defence against encapsulated bacteria involves the co-ordinated interaction of antibody (Ab), complement (C′) and phagocytes. Ab binds to the extracellular capsule, causing a conformational change in the Fc portion of the Ab molecule that allows it to bind to Fc receptors (FcR) on phagocytes (opson-ization). C′ is activated most efficiently via the classical pathway (by bound Ab), but also via the alternate pathway (by bacterial cell wall). In either case, C3b is covalently bound to the bacterial surface. Ingestion of bacteria by phagocytes is enhanced by binding to FcR and complement receptors (CR).

activated by antigen–antibody complexes; the alternate pathway can be activated by molecules with repeating chemical structures such as bacterial polysaccharides or lipopolysaccharides and does not require specific antibody. Once activated, C3 can be covalently bound to the surface of an invading micro-organism, thereby making it more susceptible to phagocytosis (opsonization). C5 can initiate formation of a membrane attack complex, a multimolecular assembly of C5b, C6, C7, C8 and C9, that inserts into cell membranes and thereby lyses the target cell.

Patients with a genetically determined deficiency of a complement component generally have an increased susceptibility to bacterial infection. The kind of bacteria that most often cause these infections depends upon the role of the specific complement component that is missing. For example, deficiencies of the early components (C1, C4, C2 and C3) interfere with the opsonic action of complement, and affected individuals have increased susceptibility to infection from heavily encapsulated bacteria (e.g. *S. pneumoniae, H. influenzae*) for which opsonization is the primary host defence (Fig. 14.8). Individuals with deficiencies of the terminal components (C5–9) have an increased susceptibility to microorganisms against which the bacteriolytic actions of complement are most important. These include Gram-negative bateria, particularly *Neisseria* species. Some individuals with complement deficiency also have a propensity to develop autoimmune disease, including systemic lupus erythematosus (see Chapter 13), and immune complex-mediated disease (see Chapter 12) such as immune complex glomerulonephritis.

Summary

This chapter has described deficiencies of individual components of the immune system. More than 50 genetically determined defects have been identified, affecting virtually all individual components of the immune system. However, it is important to recognize that each of these discrete deficiencies of cells or their products will have multiple effects on immune function because of the interactive nature of the components. For example, deficiency of antibody interferes with activation of the complement cascade via the classical pathway. The secondary deficiency of complement activation, as well as the primary deficiency of antibody, impair opsonization and thereby interfere with the function of phagocytic cells. Study of the primary immunodeficiency diseases has helped our understanding of the complex nature of host immune defence, and its role in the pathophysiology of disease.

Key points

1 Immunodeficiency can be genetically determined or acquired by drug treatment or viral infection (e.g. HIV).

2 Genetically determined deficiencies of each of the four main components of the immune system (T lymphocytes, B lymphocytes, phagocytes and complement) can be identified.

3 Immunodeficiency results in varying degrees of susceptibility to infection and other illnesses. The precise nature of this susceptibility depends upon the nature of the immune defect.

4 Because of the integrated nature of the immune system, a deficiency in one component can affect the function of another.

Further reading

Buckley R.H. (1992) Immunodeficiency diseases. *JAMA*, **268**: 2797–2806.

Primary immunodeficiency diseases: report of a WHO scientific review group. (1992) *Immunodef. Rev.* **3**: 195–236.

Sci. Am. Special Issue, September, 1993.

Case Studies

15.1 Persistent coughing up of blood and ankle-swelling

Clinical features

A 24-year-old man with a 3-week history of persistent haemoptysis (the coughing up of blood) was admitted via casualty after coughing up obvious blood. He had passed only a small volume of blood-stained urine over the last 48 hours.

On examination the patient was hypertensive (blood pressure: 160/90 mmHg). There was some swelling of the ankles which he had only noted over the previous 2 days.

Investigations

Laboratory investigations included those shown in Table 15.1.1.

Table 15.1.1 Investigations performed

Analyte	Value	Reference range
Blood		
Urea	8.2 mmol/l	2.5–6.7
Creatinine	181 µmol/l	70–150
Creatinine clearance	29 mls/min	75–140
Sodium	148 mmol/l	136–145
Potassium	6.5 mmol/l	3.4–5.2
Haemoglobin	10.2 g/dl	13.5–17.5
Albumin	30 g/l	34–48
Urine		
Protein (dipstick)	2+*	0–trace

*2+ reading corresponds to an approximate protein excretion of between 1.5 and 7.5 g per 24 hours.

The clinical features and laboratory results established two immediate clinical problems.
1 Haemoptysis.
2 Significant impairment of renal function. This is indicated by the reduced urine output, raised blood urea and creatinine, and reduced creatinine clearance.

A renal biopsy was performed. Histological analysis of this biopsy revealed that the patient had glomerulonephritis (inflammation of the renal glomeruli) of rapidly progressive type. This form of glomerulonephritis is characterized by infiltration of neutrophils and macrophages within the glomerulus which form 'crescent' shapes leading to the alternative designation of 'crescentic' glomerulonephritis. Immunofluorescent analysis of the tissue showed the presence of IgG distributed in a uniform linear pattern along the glomerular basement membrane. A chest radiograph revealed diffuse interstitial and alveolar infiltrates.

Diagnosis

The presence of haemoptysis and glomerulonephritis suggests either Goodpasture's syndrome or a systemic vasculitis such as Wegener's granulomatosis, polyarteritis nodosa or systemic lupus erythematosus (SLE). Anti-nuclear antibodies could not be detected in this patient and SLE is therefore an unlikely diagnosis. The detection of uniform and linear deposits of IgG within the glomerular basement membrane is a specific feature of Goodpasture's syndrome and is not seen in other forms of glomerulonephritis.

Diagnosis: Goodpasture's syndrome.

Discussion

Goodpasture's syndrome is an autoimmune disease in which autoantibodies are directed towards an antigen found within both glomerular and alveolar basement membranes. The autoantibodies, which are predominantly IgG, may be visualized within these basement membranes by immunofluorescence on tissue sections. They may also be detected in the serum of affected individuals and induce a condition similar to Goodpasture's syndrome when injected into monkeys.

It is now clear that the autoantibodies evoke a Type II hypersensitivity reaction (see Chapter 12), and that this is responsible for the characteristic inflammation and tissue damage. The precise stimulus for the formation of these antibodies is unclear, although it may involve modification of a self-antigen found within basement membranes by either viruses or hydrocarbon solvents, since exposure to these agents has been documented prior to the development of Goodpasture's syndrome. In keeping with the genetic predisposition to autoimmunity (see Chapter 13), there is a high prevalence of the DR2 haplotype in patients with Goodpasture's syndrome.

The clinical course of Goodpasture's syndrome is dominated by recurrent or even life-threatening haemoptysis which is the result of pulmonary haemorrhage secondary to alveolar damage. Renal involvement often appears several weeks after respiratory symptoms and is characterized by the deterioration of renal function over a period of hours or days (acute renal failure) leading to *uraemia* (the retention of waste products, including urea). Although *oliguria* (reduced urine output) or *anuria* (absence of urine production) are frequently seen in acute renal failure this is not always so. *Haematuria* (blood in the urine) may be seen in many other urinary tract diseases and is therefore not specific. *Hyperkalaemia* (raised blood potassium), due to inadequate renal excretion of potassium, may produce life-threatening cardiac dysrhythmias early in the course of acute renal failure.

Oedema, often seen in acute renal failure, is the accumulation of excess fluid in the interstitial space, presenting in this case as swollen ankles. In acute renal failure, oedema is usually the result of inappropriate sodium and water retention which increases extracellular fluid volume. Rarely, if urinary protein losses are great, there may be a significant decrease in plasma protein concentration. This may contribute to the oedema via the resultant passage of water out of capillaries and into the interstitial space.

Treatment and prognosis

Treatment is usually by a combination of plasmapheresis (plasma exchange), which eliminates both circulating autoantibodies and secondary inflammatory mediators, and drug therapy with glucocorticosteroids and cyclophosphamide. Dialysis support may be required for patients in renal failure.

The prognosis for patients with Goodpasture's syndrome is favourable if an early diagnosis is made. Extensive crescent formation within glomeruli is a poor prognostic sign.

Questions

1 What do you think are the likely causes of anaemia in this patient?

Answer: anaemia is not a consistent feature of Goodpasture's syndrome but if blood losses are great an iron deficiency anaemia may result. In chronic renal failure, anaemia may be the result of decreased erythropoietin production by the damaged kidney and the retention of waste products which tend to shorten red cell life span and inhibit red cell production (see Chapter 20).

2 The patient was hypertensive. How do you account for this?

Answer: two mechanisms are operative: (a) renal damage activates the renin–angiotensin–aldosterone system, (b) impaired renal excretion of sodium leading to sodium and water retention, an increase in blood volume and hence an increase in blood pressure (see Chapter 23).

15.2 Breathlessness in a young man

Clinical features

A 23-year-old schoolteacher presented at his family doctor's surgery in early summer complaining of a 3-week history of 'shortness of breath', which was particularly evident after exercise. He was an occasional smoker and had a history of mild eczema and hay fever since childhood but had never suffered any serious illnesses. On examination his doctor noticed mild conjunctivitis and small areas of chronic eczema on the backs of his hands. Examination of his chest was unremarkable except for a few scattered *inspiratory rhonchi* (wheezes) heard throughout his lung fields. His peak flow was reduced at 180 litres per minute.

Given these findings, his family doctor diagnosed asthma, prescribed a salbutamol inhaler and advised the teacher to take two puffs whenever he felt short of breath.

Two weeks later, after a playing in a school cricket match, the teacher became breathless despite taking puffs of his inhaler. He became increasingly wheezy and his chest 'felt tight'. A concerned colleague drove him to hospital.

On admission to the Accident and Emergency Department he was barely able to speak because of his breathlessness. His pulse rate was 120 beats per minute and on examination of his chest the doctor commented that it sounded almost 'silent'. He was given nebulized salbutamol and ipratropium bromide and an intravenous dose of corticosteroids. He was admitted for observation and prescribed a 5-day course of oral steroids.

Table 15.2.1 Investigations performed

Analyte	Value	Reference range
Blood		
Haemoglobin	15 g/dl	13.5–17.5
White blood cell count	8×10^9/l	4–11
Urea	6 mmol/l	2.5–6.7
Sodium	144 mmol/l	136–145
Potassium	3.2 mmol/l	3.4–5.2

Investigations

Laboratory investigations included those shown in Table 15.2.1. These were all normal and did not contribute to the diagnosis. The normal white cell count excluded a chest infection, and a chest radiograph revealed hyperinflated lung fields but no areas of consolidation.

Diagnosis

The patient had presented with acute severe asthma, which is a life-threatening condition. He required emergency treatment and admission to hospital where he remained for several days. The important questions are: why did this happen to a previously healthy individual and could it have been prevented?

Diagnosis: acute severe asthma.

Discussion

Although this patient suggested to his doctor that his breathlessness was a new symptom, it should have been tied in with the background history and clinical features of conjunctivitis which clearly define an atopic tendency. The association with exercise was noted but a more detailed history would have elicited that exercise in winter months was not associated with symptoms and therefore this was more likely to be associated with the patient's recognized pollen allergy (hay fever). Had the seasonal nature of the symptoms been recognized, a more appropriate therapeutic strategy might have been instituted which would have prevented the need for hospital admission.

Adequate history-taking is the key to identifying likely allergens in the atopic individual. In addition, the appropriate use of laboratory investigations can be informative. In this case the patient was followed up as an outpatient and had some further investigations. Total serum IgE was raised at 544 U/l (reference range: 1.5–120 U/l) and pulmonary function testing showed a moderate obstructive pattern which reversed with beta-2 agonists. The consultant immunologist who saw him performed skin-testing which demonstrated strong reactions to grass and tree pollens.

Testing for allergen-specific IgE was not performed as it was not felt that this would add any useful information. Tests for allergen-specific IgE are only indicated where skin-testing is not possible due to: the risk of an anaphylactic response; the presence of severe eczema; the need for anti-histamine therapy, which cannot be withdrawn; or occasionally in young children.

Treatment and prognosis

Preventative therapy was instituted in this case. Inhaled disodium cromoglycate was prescribed as a mast cell stabilizer. This must be taken regularly on a daily basis and acts by preventing the immediate release of mast cell mediators in response to allergen. In addition, the patient continued to carry his salbutamol inhaler and take it prior to participating in any outdoor activities.

The simple approach was adequate in this case; in more refractory cases regular beta-2 agonists would be required with the possible addition of inhaled corticosteroids.

Questions

1 Why were the investigations listed in Table 15.2.1 performed?

Answer: The results of the emergency investigations were consistent with acute severe asthma. They were also important in excluding other possible predisposing causes of his condition, including infection or *spontaneous pneumothorax* (air in the pleural cavity due to leakage of air from the lungs).

2 Why were corticosteroids administered and what is the mechanism of their action?

Answer: corticosteroids were used to prevent a 'late phase' response which could have developed 4–6 hours after his initial treatment. They are thought to act by blocking the synthesis of arachidonic acid metabolites and hence preventing the formation of the late phase or newly formed mediators (see Chapter 12).

Part 5
Nutritional and Gastrointestinal Disorders

Nutritional Disorders

Introduction

In order to grow, to develop mentally and physically, and to maintain all aspects of health, the body requires a regular supply of nutrients (proteins, minerals and vitamins) and energy (carbohydrates and fats). We have to bear in mind that we eat food, not nutrients, which means that the supply of nutrients must come from sources that not only fit the traditional, cultural and social background, but also suit the taste and preferences of the individual.

This chapter considers the contribution of nutrition to the maintenance of health and the potential ill effects of selected nutritional deficiency states.

Good and bad foods?

There is a popular desire for extreme simplification of dietary information, as exemplified by attempts to list foods as 'good' and 'bad', or 'junk' and 'healthy'. There is no such distinction since it is the quantity consumed which matters. There are certainly good and bad diets but even a food rich in a whole range of nutrients will make an insignificant contribution if the amount eaten is small. Equally a food poor in nutrients, or even a toxin, may have no harmful effect if only a little is consumed.

A good or adequate diet is one that supplies all the required nutrients. Since no single food supplies the whole range, this calls for a variety of foods—the greater the variety, the greater the chance of obtaining the 50 or so nutrients needed. At the same time, an excess of one nutrient can lead to problems. It does not seem likely that such high levels of any nutrient could arise from the consumption of everyday foods. However, the use of concentrated supplements containing an excess of one nutrient can interfere with the absorption and utilization of other nutrients. It is also believed that 'too high' an intake of saturated fats is an adverse factor in so-called 'diseases of affluence' (e.g. atherosclerosis, see Chapter 22).

How much do we need?

We know with certainty *what* we need—proteins (or their 20 constituent amino acids), certain types of fats (essential fatty acids), 13 vitamins and about 20 minerals. What we do not know is *how much* of each is required by the individual. In addition, individuals differ in their needs.

Estimates of average needs are derived from the three sources listed below.

1 Observation of the incidence of nutrient deficiency diseases in population groups and comparison of the amount of the nutrient being ingested with that in population groups free from such diseases.

2 Animal experimentation. This yields relatively precise information of the amounts needed to prevent or cure the disease, but leaves the problem of how to scale up for human beings.

3 In the earlier days of investigation, direct experiments were carried out on human subjects by feeding them a range of dose levels to ascertain the amount needed to prevent or cure the disease.

More recently, the administration of labelled isotopes has permitted a measure of the turnover of a given nutrient in the body. The amounts needed to maintain the body pool of the nutrient may also be estimated, but the optimum size of such pools may not be known.

The objective is to prepare tables of 'estimated daily requirements' allowing for differences in, for example, age, work output, etc. in order to be able to plan food supplies and to monitor the nutrient intake of population groups. These are variously called *recommended daily allowances* or *intakes* (RDA or RDI) or, in the UK, *dietary reference values* (DRV). Because of inadequate data, some of these figures are provisional and conclusions are often a matter of opinion. There are differences in figures reached in different countries and even then they are frequently revised.

RDAs are average daily requirement figures for each nutrient with a statistical margin of safety of two standard deviations (2sD). They apply to population groups and not to individuals, as individuals differ considerably in their requirements. However, if the average intake of a population group reaches RDA then it is likely that all in the group will reach their individual requirements. The UK tables provide three levels. The middle figure is the *estimated average requirement* (EAR) derived from measurements outlined above.

With the addition of 2sD the value is termed *reference nutrient intake* (RNI) and is equivalent to RDA. A lower value, 2sD below EAR, is the *lower reference nutrient intake* (LRNI) and may be used to assess the adequacy of the diet of the individual. If the intake of a nutrient falls below this level there is a possible risk to health, and although there may be adaptive mechanisms which reduce the risk of disease, these may not be fully effective for some time.

Deficiency diseases

Severe and prolonged shortages of any vitamin or mineral give rise to a specific disease, and eventually to death (Table 16.1). Although the cause and cure are well known, nutrient deficiency diseases are still common in 'developing' countries. They are due to chronic shortage of food (*undernutrition*—which would result in multiple deficiencies) and/or dependence on a limited variety of poor quality foods (*malnutrition*).

Table 16.1 Some vitamin and mineral deficiency disorders

Vitamin/mineral	Deficiency disorders
Vitamin A	Xerophthalmia, night blindness
Thiamin (B_1)	Beri beri
Riboflavin (B_2)	Fissured mouth (cheilosis) and eye lesions
Niacin	Pellagra, skin, gut and CNS lesions
Vitamin B_{12}	Megaloblastic anaemia
Folic acid	Megaloblastic anaemia, neural-tube defects
Vitamin C	Scurvy
Vitamin D	Rickets, osteomalacia
Vitamin K	Coagulation factor deficiencies
Iron	Microcytic anaemia
Iodine	Hypothyroidism
Zinc	Growth defects and poor wound-healing

While there are virtually no signs of malnutrition in the Western world we do not know the long-term effect of marginal shortages. There is evidence of biochemical deficiencies of several vitamins (shown by biochemical measurements of tissues) in 5–10 percent of groups of people examined in several European countries, but it is not known whether this gives rise to functional defects.

Protein-energy malnutrition

The two types of protein-energy malnutrition (sometimes called protein-calorie malnutrition or PCM), *marasmus* and *kwashiorkor*, are major causes of delayed development and ultimately death in many regions of the 'developing' world. The simplest form of this and perhaps the easiest to correct when food aid is available, is marasmus. Marasmus is due to a severe shortage of all nutrients especially food energy (calories) and young children are most susceptible because of their relatively high requirements for energy to support growth and development (around 100 calories per kilogram of body weight in infants compared to 30 in adults).

The situation is more complex when energy intake is adequate but other nutrients (especially protein) are lacking, resulting in the condition known as kwashiorkor. In kwashiorkor, the diet is low either in total protein or in high quality protein (or both), producing the familiar pattern of children with stunted growth and pot bellies.

Of the 20 amino acids, eight cannot be synthesized from other sources and have to be obtained from the diet. The biological value of a protein depends on how much of these *essential* amino acids it contains. Protein foods containing all eight essential amino acids in the amounts required (e.g. egg and human milk) have a biological value close to 100 percent, but many sources of cereal protein have biological values of 60 percent or less. Quantity of protein can compensate for relatively poor quality. Reliance on a single staple cereal food in times of shortage can therefore lead to deficiency states, whereas combining a variety of foods provides high quality protein overall.

Kwashiorkor is often accompanied by other deficiency states, particularly of the B group vitamins, thiamin and niacin, and of vitamin A producing beri beri, pellagra and xerophthalmia respectively. Furthermore, severe malnutrition leads to increased susceptibility to infection, and infection exacerbates the problem of malnutrition by increasing demands for nutrients.

Malnutrition in 'developing' countries is often due to weaning infants onto unsuitable foods. The obvious solution is to make available nutritionally adequate baby foods. However, when they are made available, those who need them frequently cannot afford them, and those who can afford them may not need them.

Xerophthalmia

It is ironic that a shortage of vitamin A, the first of the vitamins to be named and one of the earliest ones to be made available on a factory scale, is a major public health problem in many parts of the world. About a quarter of a million children worldwide go blind each year due to *xerophthalmia* resulting from vitamin A deficiency. Eight to nine million develop other deficiency signs in the eye and many, in some areas 50 percent, die. Xeroph-

thalmia is most often seen in conjunction with other deficiency states, notably severe protein-energy malnutrition.

Vitamin A is present in the diet in two forms, as ready-made vitamin A (*retinol*) from animal sources, and as *carotene* in plant foods. Carotene is a deep orange-red in colour, as is obvious in carrots, and to a lesser extent, in orange-yellow fruits, but it is also present in all green parts of plants where the colour is masked by the green of the chlorophyll.

Scurvy

Deficiency of Vitamin C has not been a major public health problem in most 'developed' countries for many centuries. *Scurvy* is characterized by easy bruising, bleeding gums and poor wound healing, and in children may cause skeletal malformation. The disorder was first recognized in the middle of the 17th and 18th centuries when scurvy was a principal cause of death among sailors who did not have access to fruits and vegetables for long periods. On land, scurvy occurred towards the end of the winter during which there had been few fruits and vegetables available.

Vitamin B$_{12}$ and folate deficiencies

There are several complicating factors that help to bring about deficiency diseases. For example, *pernicious anaemia* is not due to a dietary deficiency of vitamin B$_{12}$ but to an inability to absorb it through lack of 'intrinsic factor' in the stomach (see Chapter 20).

A shortage of folic acid also gives rise to megaloblastic anaemia but a more common problem arises from the increased requirements for folic acid also in the early stages of pregnancy. Folic acid deficiency in early pregnancy is thought to contribute to neural-tube defects in the newborn, including spina bifida.

Vitamin D deficiency

Rickets is a childhood disorder characterized by disturbance of normal ossification marked by bending and distortion of the long bones. The condition is due to a shortage of vitamin D, is associated more with lack of exposure of the skin to sunlight which effects vitamin D synthesis rather than to a simple dietary deficiency. It was once very common in the slum areas of industrial cities in the UK, and reappeared among Asian immigrants in the 1960s and 1970s. The adult equivalent, *osteomalacia*, is characterized by the loss of calcium from bones, which is not uncommon among housebound, elderly people.

Iron deficiency

Iron-deficiency anaemia is the most common nutrient deficiency disease in Western countries. It is often due to poor absorption; the iron may be present in a chemical form that is poorly absorbed or there may be inhibitory substances present in foods eaten at the same time as the iron-containing food.

In 'developing' countries the problem is aggravated by chronic blood loss due to intestinal parasites and by a poor supply of meat products from which iron is relatively well absorbed (see also Chapter 20).

Iodine deficiency

Goitre (enlargement of the thyroid gland) caused by deficiency of iodine affects some 200 million people worldwide and, until recent years, was found in limited localities in many Western countries. For example, in Derbyshire, UK, enlargement of the thyroid gland due to iodine deficiency is often referred to as 'Derbyshire neck'. The cause is a low iodine content of the soil water which is reflected in the food grown there. In children, the resulting severe hypothyroidism gives rise to *cretinism*.

Although goitre has disappeared in some countries through the practice of enriching foods with iodine, its disappearance from the UK appears to have been due to the availability of a wider variety of imported foods grown in suitable soils.

Enrichment of food

There are three solutions to the problem of simple dietary deficiency diseases: (i) popularization of the 'better' foods, (ii) provision of dietary supplements or medical administration and (iii) enrichment of specified foods with the missing nutrients. The first two present considerable difficulties and have not been very successful; enrichment has achieved limited success.

In many Western countries, margarine is enriched by law with vitamins A and D because it replaces butter which is a source of these vitamins. This was not effected in response to an outbreak of any deficiency disease (apart from a problem in Denmark in 1916) but as a precaution. Similarly, white bread is enriched with vitamin B_1, thiamin and iron, again, not as a result of any public health problem but as a precaution to replace milling losses (*restoration*).

In some countries, vitamin B_2 and calcium are also added; since these are present in whole grain only in small amounts, this is an example of *fortification* as a public health precaution.

Enrichment of foods in the 'developing' countries, where there are obvious deficiency diseases, is not often practicable because of lack of technical expertise, the difficulty in finding a suitable food that would convey the nutrient to the target group and lack of means of enforcement. In a few areas, vitamin A, some of the B vitamins and iodine have been added to some foods, but it is generally considered that the best means of preventing deficiency diseases is to promote the consumption of those foods that are particularly rich in the missing nutrients.

Historically, where deficiency diseases have disappeared, this has largely been due to an overall improvement in standards of living which result in a more varied diet, rather than to enrichment or clinical treatment.

Not too much of anything

As deficiency diseases have disappeared from the well fed countries of the world they have been replaced by the so-called 'diseases of affluence' – coronary heart disease, stroke and certain forms of cancer.

An important dietary factor appears to be 'too high' an intake of saturated fatty acids. In countries where the incidence of these diseases is high there is a relatively high intake of saturated fats. Where the incidence is low, while the total fat intake might be the same (40 percent of energy intake) the fatty acids are largely mono-unsaturated (mostly oleic acid from olive oil) and often include long chain fatty acids from fish oils (eicosapentaenoic acid and docosohexaenoic acid) which appear to exercise a beneficial effect.

Sugar, which contributes only energy and no nutrients to the diet, often accounts for 15–30 percent of the total energy intake. Apart from its effect on dental decay and perhaps on encouraging obesity through an excessive intake of food, sugar 'dilutes' the nutrients in the diet. Furthermore, there has been a general reduction in energy expenditure concomitant with modern life styles and therefore of average food intake, which has the effect of reducing the intake of nutrients.

There is evidence that too high an intake of salt can be a cause of hypertension (high blood pressure) in some people (see Chapter 23). About 500 mg of sodium per day is essential in the diet but the average intake is about 10 times as much.

Anti-oxidant nutrients

An adequate diet is one that supplies enough of all the nutrients, 'enough' being based on the prevention of deficiency diseases. However, there is evidence that greater intakes of some nutrients may help to prevent certain forms of cancer and even delay ageing.

During the course of normal metabolic reactions, a number of highly reactive molecules, known as *free radicals*, are formed. They can react with and damage the membranes of cells but are rapidly destroyed or blocked ('*quenched*') in the body by a series of protective mechanisms including action by anti-oxidants.

Several nutrients function as anti-oxidants, including vitamins A, C and E, carotene and selenium. For example, the incidence of cancer of the lung (and some other forms) is lower when the diet is rich in fruits and vegetables, and higher when their intake is low. This is supported by measurements of blood levels of these nutrients. The greater part of dietary carotene is converted into retinol (vitamin A) in the walls of the intestine but a small amount appears to escape this process and reaches the bloodstream. A larger intake of carotene results in a higher level in the blood and appears to offer protection. While intervention trials have been undertaken in which supplements of beta-carotene have been administered it is not clear whether other, non-nutritional substances in fruits and vegetables (such as lycopene in tomatoes) are also effective or whether there is a need for the whole battery of substances that are present in these foods.

Summary

Although the Western world appears to be adequately fed, nutritional advice generally includes reduced consumption of saturated fatty acids, salt and sugar, and increased consumption of fruits, vegetables and whole grain cereal products. This would tend to ensure a greater variety of foods than is present in many diets and avoid the excesses that are risk factors in a range of diseases. In 'developing' countries severe problems of undernutrition (inadequate supplies of food) and malnutrition (deficiencies of certain nutrients) are relatively common for reasons of poverty, reliance on a limited range of locally grown foods and climatic disasters.

Key points

1 Varied diets are necessary to provide the full range of nutrients to maintain health.

2 Estimated daily requirements of individual nutrients are calculated for population groups. Individual requirements are likely to differ from these estimates to some extent.

3 Deficiency disorders are not always due to dietary lack. Malabsorption, increased losses, higher demand and chronic infection can all contribute to specific deficiency states.

4 In 'developed' countries, certain 'diseases of affluence' appear to be linked to dietary imbalance.

5 Anti-oxidant nutrients may give some protection against certain forms of cancer and diseases of ageing.

Further reading

Bender A.E. & Bender D.A. (1982) *Nutrition for Medical Students*. Wiley, Chichester.

Bender D.A. (1993) *Introduction to Nutrition and Metabolism*. UCL Press, London.

Passmore R. & Eastwood M.A. (1986) *Human Nutrition*. Churchill Livingstone, London.

Report on Health and Social Subjects 41. (1991) *Dietary Reference Values for Food, Energy and Nutrients for the United Kingdom*. Report of the Panel on Dietary Reference Values of the Committee on Medical Aspects of Food Policy. HMSO, London.

Jaundice and Liver Disease

Introduction

Jaundice is a clinical sign and should be regarded as an indication of disease, rather than as a distinct disease. This chapter considers the ways in which haematological, liver and biliary tract disorders can each cause jaundice.

Jaundice is the result of an increase in the concentration of *bilirubin* in the blood and is characterized by a distinctive yellow colouration of the skin and the sclerae. The reference range for total bilirubin concentration in the blood is wide, typically 2–16 µmol/l, although minor increases above 16 µmol/l are often not clinically evident. Jaundice is usually clinically apparent only when the plasma concentration of bilirubin exceeds 30 µmol/l.

Bilirubin metabolism

Bilirubin production

Bilirubin is constantly produced as a natural breakdown product of haemoglobin. Erythrocytes have a limited life span in the circulation and when they are no longer viable, red cells are destroyed and the haemoglobin they contain is degraded. The haemoglobin molecule contains four *haems* (each consisting of a porphyrin ring structure and iron) and four *globin chains* (see Chapter 20). During haem breakdown (*catabolism*) which occurs in the spleen, iron is removed from the molecule and the porphyrin ring opens out to form the yellow-green pigment bilirubin. Bilirubin enters the blood circulatory system and is transported to the liver, where it is metabolized.

Haemoglobin catabolism

Haemoglobin is broken down in the following stages.

1 The globin chains are hydrolysed to individual amino acids which enter the general amino acid pool to be used in further protein synthesis.

2 Iron is released from haem and re-utilized, initially becoming bound to transferrin for transport either to iron stores or back to the bone marrow for further incorporation into developing red blood cells.

3 The remaining porphyrin component of haem is degraded to protoporphyrin, which is then converted to a linear tetrapyrrole, bilirubin (Fig. 17.1).

An overview of bilirubin metabolism

Each day approximately 400–500 µmol of bilirubin are formed; around 80 percent of which is derived from red blood cells which have reached the end of their life span. The remaining 20 percent comes from other sources, including ineffective erythropoiesis (see Chapter 20) and the breakdown of myoglobin, cytochrome enzymes and peroxidase.

When it is first formed, bilirubin is lipid soluble, and is transported in a complex with plasma albumin. During hepatic uptake, bilirubin is released from albumin, enters hepatocytes and is bound to intracellular-binding proteins. Bilirubin then undergoes further chemical change, becoming conjugated with glucuronic acid to form a water soluble substance, *bilirubin glucuronide*. Most of the conjugated bilirubin then passes from the liver into the biliary system and enters the small intestine in the bile.

Hepatic uptake, conjugation and secretion of

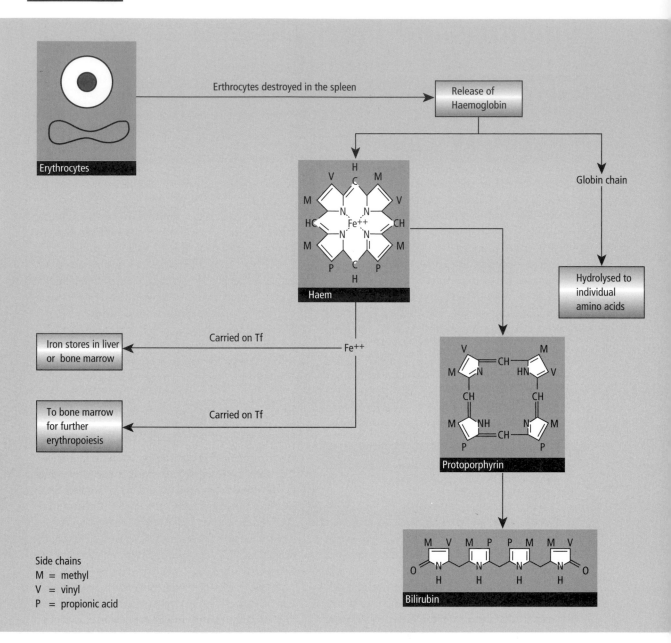

Fig. 17.1 Formation of bilirubin. Erythrocytes are destroyed in the spleen at the end of their life span. Haemoglobin is released from the cells and is catabolized into haem and globin. The amino acids from the globin chains enter the amino acid pool to take part in further protein synthesis. Iron is released from haem, is carried in the plasma attached to transferrin (Tf), and is incorporated into newly synthesized haem or is deposited in iron stores as ferritin or haemosiderin. The protoporphyrin ring from haem opens to form a linear tetrapyrrole, bilirubin.

bilirubin is normally very rapid—studies with radioisotope-labelled bilirubin indicate that the whole process can take less than 3 minutes.

Conjugation of bilirubin

Dissociation of the albumin–bilirubin complex takes place when it arrives at hepatocyte membrane receptors, facilitating transport of bilirubin across the cell membrane in a process involving intracellular-binding proteins.

Conjugation with glucuronic acid occurs at the propionic acid side chains on the bilirubin molecule and is catalysed by bilirubin–UDP–glucuronyl transferase located in the endoplasmic reticulum of hepatocytes. Three types of bilirubin glucuronide are formed—two are monoglucuronides, together comprising approximately 25 percent of conjugated bilirubin and the other is a diglucuronide forming the remaining 75 percent of the bilirubin found in bile.

The movement of conjugated bilirubin from hepatocytes into the biliary system occurs against a concentration gradient and is thought to be due to active carrier-mediated transport. A proportion is concentrated in the gall bladder and is released into the duodenum shortly after a meal.

Bilirubin in the intestinal tract

After entering the small intestine, reabsorption of bilirubin glucuronides is minimal. Subsequently, some is converted to stercobilinogen by normal flora in the large bowel. Most stercobilinogen is oxidized and excreted in the faeces as stercobilin, which is largely responsible for the dark brown colour of faeces. A small proportion of stercobilinogen is absorbed to enter the enterohepatic circulation and is then re-excreted by the liver. Some also appears in the urine as colourless urobilinogen which oxidizes spontaneously to brown urobilin.

Causes of jaundice

The characteristic yellow colouration of the skin and sclerae in jaundice becomes clinically evident only when the concentration of bilirubin in the blood is substantially increased above the reference range. There are three major types of jaundice, each of which has a different underlying cause. These can be differentiated to a limited extent by observation of the colour and appearance of the urine and faeces and by consideration of basic laboratory data. The three principal types of jaundice are outlined below.

1 *Pre-hepatic (haemolytic) jaundice* is due to an increase in the rate of production of bilirubin caused by an increase in the rate of red blood cell destruction. The hyperbilirubinaemia (increased blood bilirubin) of haemolytic anaemia (see Chapter 20) typifies pre-hepatic jaundice.

2 *Post-hepatic (obstructive) jaundice* is due to a decrease in the rate of excretion of bilirubin, usually caused by biliary obstruction. Gall stones are a common cause of post-hepatic jaundice.

3 *Hepatocellular jaundice* is due to disease of, or damage to, hepatocytes which limits bilirubin conjugation, and may also affect bilirubin uptake and secretion.

Pre-hepatic jaundice

Pre-hepatic jaundice is the result of increased bilirubin presented to the liver for conjugation, and occurs when large numbers of red blood cells are destroyed before they reach the end of their normal life span (approximately 120 days), a condition known as haemolytic disorder. In addition, haematological disorders (e.g. megaloblastic anaemia; see Chapter 20) associated with an increase in ineffective erythropoiesis can also produce pre-hepatic jaundice. Very occasionally, mild jaundice due to haem breakdown follows substantial bleeding into tissues such as muscle.

The liver is usually able to metabolize moderate increases in production of bilirubin from red cell breakdown, so a relatively mild reduction in erythrocyte life span generally does not cause jaundice. However, if large numbers of red blood cells are destroyed *extravascularly* (i.e. outside the circulatory system, usually in the spleen) over short periods of time, the amount of bilirubin produced may exceed the capacity of the liver to conjugate bilirubin.

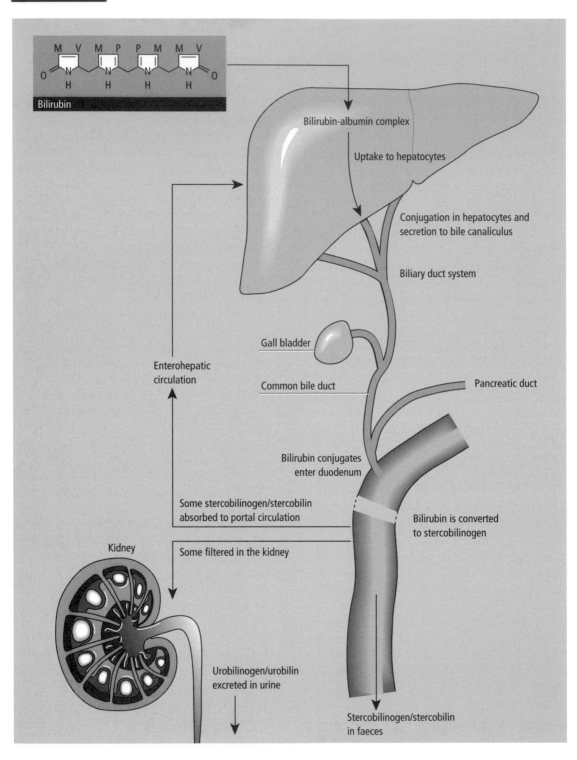

Bilirubin

Bilirubin-albumin complex

Uptake to hepatocytes

Conjugation in hepatocytes and secretion to bile canaliculus

Biliary duct system

Gall bladder

Enterohepatic circulation

Common bile duct

Pancreatic duct

Bilirubin conjugates enter duodenum

Some stercobilinogen/stercobilin absorbed to portal circulation

Bilirubin is converted to stercobilinogen

Kidney

Some filtered in the kidney

Urobilinogen/urobilin excreted in urine

Stercobilinogen/stercobilin in faeces

In pre-hepatic jaundice the excess bilirubin in the blood is of the *unconjugated type*. Since this is not water soluble, and is complexed with albumin in blood plasma, unconjugated bilirubin cannot be filtered by glomeruli and does not appear in the urine. This is the origin of the term 'acholuric jaundice' which used to describe these disorders ('acholuric' means the absence of bilirubin in urine). The liver functions at high capacity to conjugate increased amounts of bilirubin for excretion into the alimentary canal and the stools remain dark, due to the relatively high concentrations of stercobilinogen and stercobilin in the gut. More stercobilinogen and stercobilin are absorbed, and eventually appear in the urine as an increased concentration of urobilinogen and urobilin.

People with inherited haemolytic disorders, such as hereditary spherocytosis (see Chapter 20), produce large amounts of bilirubin throughout their lives and have a tendency to develop both anaemia and mild jaundice. Bilirubin conjugation and excretion occur at a high rate, and bile pigments can become highly concentrated. This predisposes some patients to the formation of gall stones composed of bile pigments which occasionally cause biliary obstruction. Thus some patients with congenital haemolytic anaemia causing a mild pre-hepatic jaundice may also develop post-hepatic (obstructive) jaundice.

Post-hepatic (cholestatic) jaundice

Conjugated bilirubin normally leaves the liver and passes to the intestine via the bile ducts. An obstruction preventing bilirubin from entering the duodenum causes post-hepatic (*cholestatic*) jaundice. In the case of complete biliary obstruc-

Fig. 17.2 Schematic diagram of bilirubin metabolism. Bilirubin is carried in the blood plasma complexed with albumin. The bilirubin is then taken up by hepatocytes, becomes conjugated to glucuronic acid and is secreted into the biliary system. The molecule is converted to stercobilinogen in the gut and most of this passes out with the faeces, although some is reabsorbed into the portal circulation and a small proportion is excreted in the urine.

tion, bilirubin cannot enter the intestine and the stools are very pale, often having a light clay colour. Because bilirubin cannot be excreted it accumulates in the blood. Some of the bilirubin will become conjugated and is detected in the blood as the water soluble bilirubin glucuronide.

Post-hepatic jaundice is usually characterized by the passing of a deep yellow urine which froths when shaken. This is due to the presence of bilirubin which, in its water-soluble form, readily undergoes glomerular filtration. In contrast, the concentration of urobilinogen/urobilin in the urine is reduced because less is available for absorption from the intestinal tract. An increase in conjugated bilirubin in the blood is often accompanied by severe itching, and there may be fat malabsorption due to the absence of bile salts in the proximal small intestine.

There are several causes of obstructive jaundice including tumours of the head of pancreas which can press on the bile ducts preventing bile flow. More commonly, gall stones cause obstructive jaundice if the stones block the common bile duct. In some cases, obstructive jaundice results from intra-hepatic cholestasis due to dysfunction of bile secretion at the bile canaliculi. This form of jaundice may be a feature of certain types of hepatocellular damage, that due to primary biliary cirrhosis for example, and can be difficult to classify as either hepatocellular or post-hepatic solely on the basis of routine biochemical tests.

Hepatocellular jaundice

Hepatocellular jaundice occurs when the hepatocytes, which are normally responsible for uptake, conjugation and secretion of bilirubin are damaged by toxins or disease. Causes of hepatocellular damage include various forms of infective hepatitis, abuse of alcohol or other drugs, cirrhosis and certain autoimmune disorders.

Hepatocellular jaundice may be broadly subdivided on the basis of whether the defect is due to abnormal uptake, conjugation or secretion of bilirubin, as outlined below.

Impaired uptake

Impaired uptake of bilirubin results in an increase in the concentration of plasma unconjugated bilirubin. This form of hepatocellular jaundice is seen in some patients with hepatitis (inflammation of the liver) or cirrhosis and may also be a feature of Gilbert's syndrome (see below).

Conjugation defects

Failure to conjugate bilirubin occurs in Gilbert's syndrome, and is due to a congenital deficiency of the glucuronyl transferase enzyme. Inability to conjugate bilirubin efficiently is also a feature of other types of hepatotocellular damage associated with cirrhosis, hepatitis and some drugs.

Secretion defects

A third type of hepatocellular jaundice is due to failure to secrete conjugated bilirubin into the bile. This occurs in the rare congenital *Rotor* and *Dubin–Johnson* syndromes, but can also be a feature of acquired hepatocellular damage.

In practice, these abnormalities are often not clearly differentiated and may merge into one another: viral hepatitis, alcohol abuse or cirrhosis can each be associated with defects in hepatic uptake, conjugation or secretion of bilirubin. In addition, post-hepatic jaundice due to physical obstruction may cause hepatocellular damage, due, in part, to increased back-pressure from biliary accumulation of bile pigments.

Hepatocellular jaundice does not always result in a distinctive pattern of routine laboratory test results, and can show features of other types of jaundice. If there is accompanying biliary obstruction, or a secretion defect, levels of conjugated bilirubin in the blood are high and bilirubin appears in the urine as a consequence, whereas conjugation defects result in an increase in unconjugated bilirubin in the blood.

Jaundice in the newborn

Jaundice may develop in the first few days of life.

The erythrocyte count is normally very high at birth due to the presence of fetal haemoglobin (HbF) which has high oxygen affinity. As production switches predominantly to the lower oxygen affinity adult haemoglobin (HbA), large numbers of red blood cells are destroyed. This results in the production of substantial amounts of unconjugated bilirubin. In some neonates, the liver (which may have not yet fully matured) lacks sufficient glucuronyl transferase to conjugate this relatively high concentration of bilirubin, and the plasma concentration of unconjugated bilirubin increases. It is essential to monitor jaundice carefully in newborn babies because if the levels of lipid soluble unconjugated bilirubin become too high, a form of brain damage known as *kernicterus* may ensue.

A more severe form of jaundice with a different underlying cause is present at birth in *haemolytic disease of the newborn* (HDNB). This condition is usually the result of the presence of maternal IgG rhesus antibodies with anti-D specificity, which cross the placenta and react with their corresponding antigens on the baby's erythrocytes. This results in erythrocyte destruction and affected babies are born with anaemia and jaundice. In severe cases, exchange blood transfusion is required. HDNB is less commonly seen today than in the past because prophylactic measures are now available to prevent the development of rhesus (anti-D) antibodies in the maternal circulation.

Investigation of jaundice

Clinical investigation

Simple clinical observation often gives valuable clues as to the type of jaundice. For example, splenomegaly (enlarged spleen), anaemia, dark stools and an absence of bilirubin in urine are typical of pre-hepatic jaundice. Deep jaundice with severe itching, bright yellow urine and pale stools is typical of post-hepatic jaundice.

One of the principal functions of bile acid in the gut is to aid fat digestion and absorption, so many patients with biliary obstruction experience intolerance of dietary fat; lipid rich meals cause nausea and some patients become anorexic (see Chapter 18). Fat malabsorption may result in deficiency of the lipid soluble vitamins A,D,E and K. Blood coagulation factors II, VII, IX and X (see Chapter 21) depend on adequate concentrations of vitamin K for their synthesis, so reduction in these is common in many liver diseases. This is rarely severe enough to result in spontaneous bleeding, but it does cause a slight prolongation of the prothrombin time test.

Laboratory investigation

Certain basic biochemical tests have already been mentioned: estimation of plasma bilirubin (unconjugated and conjugated) and detection of urobilinogen/urobilin and bilirubin in urine. In addition to these tests, routine haematological tests (full blood count and reticulocyte count) and investigations for haemolytic disorders may be indicated.

Typical results of basic biochemical tests in jaundice are shown in Table 17.1, though these should be regarded as preliminary investigations only which give no indication of the underlying cause. Furthermore, in practice, the pattern of laboratory results is often equivocal and additional investigations are required to enable a preliminary classification of jaundice. These usually include further biochemical tests in addition to clinical investigations such as liver biopsy, ultrasound scans of the abdomen or endoscopic retrograde cholangiopancreatography (ERCP).

Enzymes in liver disease

The measurement of certain enzymes in the blood plasma assists the differentiation of jaundice. When cells are damaged they release their contents into the surrounding fluids of the body and, in the case of liver disease, raised plasma concentrations of a number of liver enzymes are seen. These enzymes include alkaline phosphatase, gamma-glutamyl transferase (gamma-GT) and the transaminases, aspartate aminotransferase (AST) and alanine aminotransferase (ALT). Increased plasma concentrations of these enzymes indicate, with varying specificity, liver damage.

One of the more specific enzymes is gamma-GT which is sensitive to acute liver cell damage and is particularly useful in the diagnosis of alcoholic liver disease (see Case Study 19.3). Of the transaminases, raised ALT concentrations are rather more specific for liver damage than AST: for example, a rapid rise in serum ALT concentration is typical in viral hepatitis. However, an AST concentration of more than twice the ALT is regarded by some as indicative of chronic hepatocellular disease (for example cirrhosis due to alcohol abuse).

An increase in alkaline phosphatase is much less specific for liver disease, but a disproportionate rise in this enzyme is typical in post-hepatic jaundice. However, results of these tests are indicative, not diagnostic, and must be considered in the light of other clinical and laboratory data.

Other laboratory tests

Other tests of value in the investigation of hepatocellular jaundice include detection of viral antigens or antibodies (particularly in hepatitis B viral infection) and the demonstration of circulating autoantibodies to various tissue components. Antimitochondrial antibodies are present in the serum of most patients with primary biliary

Table 17.1 Typical laboratory findings in the principal types of jaundice

Type of Jaundice	Serum bilirubin		Urine	
	Conjugated	Unconjugated	Bilirubin	Urobilin/ urobili- nogen
Pre-hepatic	Normal	Raised	Absent	Increased
Hepatocellular	Variable	Normal/raised	Variable	Variable
Post-hepatic	Raised	Normal/raised	Present	Low

Key points

1 Lipid soluble unconjugated bilirubin is derived from the breakdown of haem. This is transported to the liver bound to plasma albumin and forms the majority of plasma bilirubin under normal conditions.

2 Conjugated bilirubin (formed from water soluble bilirubin glucuronides) is excreted into the duodenum, via the biliary system, and is later converted to stercobilinogen and stercobilin in the lower gut where it passes out in the faeces. Some stercobilinogen is reabsorbed from the small intestine and circulates in the blood plasma to be re-excreted in the bile. A small amount is filtered in the kidney and appears in the urine as urobilinogen and urobilin.

3 The major features of pre-hepatic jaundice are: increased plasma concentration of unconjugated bilirubin; increased urinary urobilinogen and urobilin;

no urinary bilirubin; and dark stools. Clinical features include possible anaemia and a relatively mild jaundice.

4 The major features of post-hepatic jaundice are: increased plasma concentration of conjugated bilirubin; reduced urinary urobilinogen and urobilin with the presence of bilirubin in the urine; and pale stools. Clinical features commonly include severe jaundice with itching, fat intolerance and fat malabsorption.

5 Hepatocellular jaundice: hepatocellular damage may induce a defect in uptake, conjugation or secretion of bilirubin. Intra-hepatic cholestasis may also result from acute hepatocellular damage and is similar to post-hepatic jaundice. Thus, the results of basic laboratory investigations in hepatocellular hyperbilirubinaemia may resemble those of pre-hepatic or post-hepatic jaundice, or both.

cirrhosis, whereas anti-smooth muscle cell antibodies are present in the sera of approximately half of patients with chronic active hepatitis.

Summary

This chapter has described the origin and classification of jaundice and has considered some clinical and laboratory investigations in liver disease. Jaundice indicates a variety of possible clinical and metabolic defects, and its cause requires thorough investigation. This usually includes examination of the chemical constituents of the urine, the estimation of bilirubin, of certain enzymes in the blood plasma, and a variety of clinical investigations, often including liver biopsy.

Further reading

Bateson M. & Bouchier I. (1988) *Clinical Investigations in Gastroenterology.* Kluwer Academic, London.

Whitby C.G., Smith A.F. & Beckett G.J. (1988) *Lecture Notes on Clinical Chemistry.* (4th edn.). Blackwell Scientific Publications, Oxford.

Gastrointestinal Disorders

Introduction

The primary function of the gut is the absorption of fluid and nutrients from the diet, separating useful nutritional factors from potential toxins, and the final excretion of waste products. Food taken by mouth passes down the oesophagus to the stomach, where the acid environment kills many contaminating bacteria. Most digestion takes place after food has entered the duodenum. The addition of bile and pancreatic secretions in the duodenum facilitate nutrient absorption in the jejunum and ileum. Intestinal contents pass from the terminal ileum into the large intestine (colon), which continues to reabsorb fluid until solid faecal waste is excreted.

Many different disease processes act upon the gut but the symptoms and clinical effects are often similar and not specific to any disorder. In this chapter the major influences on disease in each area of the gastrointestinal tract will be discussed, although in many situations the causes are not known. In the stomach and duodenum, for instance, control of stomach acid relieves many symptoms, although rarely cures the underlying condition. Malabsorption is frequently the result of small intestinal disease but does not signify a particular aetiology. Colonic diseases are characterized by bowel disturbance, particularly diarrhoea, but the complaint has many causes. This chapter reviews some clinically important disease processes in the gastrointestinal tract.

Acid-related disorders

Physiology of gastric secretion

Eating food, or even just the thought, sight or smell of it, stimulates the stomach to produce hydrochloric acid and pepsin to begin the process of digestion. Acid is secreted by the parietal cells in the body of the stomach while the chief cells produce *pepsinogen* which is converted to the active enzyme, *pepsin*, by acid.

Cephalic stimulation of acid secretion results from anticipation of food and is mediated by the activation of fibres within the vagus nerve which innervates the stomach. Acetylcholine released from these neurones directly stimulates the parietal cells to produce acid via cholinergic receptors. However, the same neurones also induce acid secretion by releasing the neurotransmitter histamine from small endocrine cells in the gastric mucosa, the *enterochromaffin-like* or ECL cells. Histamine also activates receptors in the parietal cells. These receptors are structurally different from histamine receptors elsewhere in the body and are designated H2 receptors.

Once food enters the stomach, acid secretion is primarily controlled by the hormone *gastrin* which is secreted from the G cells of the stomach antrum, near the outlet to the duodenum. Gastrin is released in response to food in the stomach, but its release is inhibited by a pH below 3 (negative feedback). Gastrin also stimulates acid secretion by initiating release of histamine from the ECL cells which then act upon the H2 receptors of the parietal cell. Histamine therefore has a central role in the control of acid secretion.

Acid pump of parietal cells

After a histamine or acetylcholine molecule has bound to a parietal cell receptor, a complex series of intracellular mechanisms activates the final common pathway of acid secretion, the $H^+K^+ATPase$ enzyme or proton pump. The

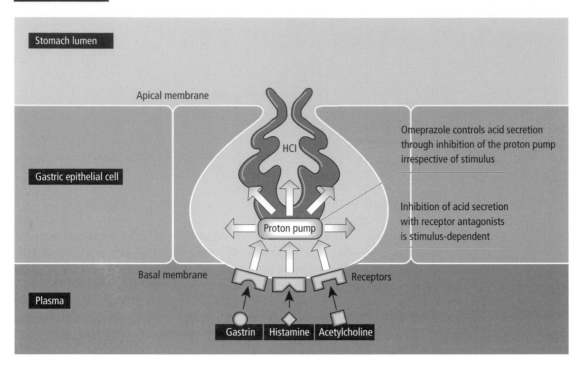

Stomach lumen

Apical membrane

HCl

Gastric epithelial cell

Omeprazole controls acid secretion through inhibition of the proton pump irrespective of stimulus

Proton pump

Inhibition of acid secretion with receptor antagonists is stimulus-dependent

Basal membrane   Receptors

Plasma

Gastrin | Histamine | Acetylcholine

proton pump exchanges H^+ ions (protons) from the cell cytoplasm for K^+, ions which re-enter the cell, so producing acid and lowering pH in the stomach lumen (Fig. 18.1).

Pharmacological intervention

An understanding of the physiology of acid secretion allows effective pharmacological intervention. Specific reversible blocking of histamine H2 receptors reduces acid secretion and drugs such as cimetidine and ranitidine act in this manner. Profound anacidity can be achieved by blocking the final common pathway of acid secretion with proton pump inhibitors. Drugs such as omeprazole and lansoprazole act in this way. Acid suppression relieves many symptoms of upper gastrointestinal disease and these drug groups are now among the most widely prescribed in the world.

Mucosal defence mechanisms

To counteract the corrosive forces of acid and pepsin in the lumen, the stomach is protected from

Fig. 18.1 Various stimuli act via the proton pump to regulate acid secretion. Omeprazole regulates the proton pump.

self-digestion by a mucosal defensive barrier. A thick mucus layer traps bicarbonate ions secreted from epithelial cells, so neutralizing luminal acid. If superficial mucosal injury does occur, a rapid repair and healing mechanism acts to reconstitute surface cell continuity. Important mediators of this response are local prostaglandins, particularly prostaglandin E_2 and prostacyclin, which may act by increasing mucosal blood flow. Increased cell proliferation to make good the cell deficit may be stimulated by hormonal factors such as epidermal growth factor and local peptides. In the duodenum, alkaline secretions, including those from the pancreas, neutralize stomach acid and raise pH.

Peptic ulceration

Failure of the defensive barrier in the stomach or duodenum leads to mucosal injury. This may be precipitated by excess acid secretion, poor stomach emptying or bile reflux. Infections and drugs, particularly non-steroidal anti-inflammatory drugs (NSAIDs) may also lead to local inflammation. At the most extreme, mucosal injury penetrates the underlying layers to produce a benign peptic ulcer. Ulcers may occur in the stomach (gastric ulcer) or duodenum (duodenal ulcer), but both together are termed *peptic ulcer*. Hereditary factors producing a familial tendency may combine with environmental influences, such as smoking, diet, NSAID ingestion or *Helicobacter pylori* infection, to influence an individual's risk of developing peptic ulcer. No consistent pathophysiological defect explains the development of all peptic ulcer cases. Duodenal ulcer patients as a group have higher peak acid secretion and serum pepsinogen than controls, while in gastric ulcer patients these levels are normal or reduced. These observations suggest that duodenal ulcer is due to excess 'aggressive' factors (pepsin, HCl) while gastric ulcers are due primarily to impaired mucosal defence.

While the underlying disease mechanisms are complex, acid suppression in many upper gastrointestinal diseases is effective in healing inflammation and particularly ulcers. For example, effective anacidity produced by a proton pump inhibitor will heal 90 percent of peptic ulcers in 4 weeks. However, when pharmacological treatment ceases, recurrence is very common, reaching 80–90 percent within 1 year.

Helicobacter pylori

In 1983 a Gram-negative organism, subsequently named *Helicobacter pylori*, was isolated from gastric biopsies of patients with peptic ulcer. The organism is now known to be present in over 90 percent of duodenal and 80 percent of gastric ulcer cases. Eradication of the organism by antibiotics reduces the ulcer relapse rate. The mechanism of the association remains unclear. *H. pylori* secretes a urease enzyme which tends to raise the local pH of the gastric mucosa and this may lead to excess gastrin production and hyperacidity.

H. pylori infection is also associated with gastric malignancy. Inflammation in the stomach associated with *H. pylori*, together with mutagens produced by bacterial action on dietary products, may induce a change in the gastric mucosa towards a cell type more commonly found in the small intestine. This is called *intestinal metaplasia* and is the major predisposing factor for development of gastric malignancy.

Physiology of digestion

Protein absorption

Between 70 and 180 grams of protein enter the small intestine daily in an adult, and only 1–2 grams of nitrogen, representing 6–12 grams of protein, is excreted in the faeces. Dietary protein is first hydrolysed in the stomach by pepsin which breaks down peptide bonds within proteins. However, most protein hydrolysis occurs in the small intestine and is catalysed by pancreatic proteolytic enzymes. These enzymes – trypsin, chymotrypsin, elastase and the carboxypeptidases – are secreted by the pancreas as inactive precursors. Each functions differently, hydrolysing peptide bonds between particular amino acids or at a specific site on the amino acid chain. Free amino acids are then absorbed by group-specific transport systems, while an independent mechanism transports the remaining small peptide chains.

Carbohydrate absorption

Around 50 percent of energy intake in the Western world consists of carbohydrates, predominantly in the form of starch, sucrose and lactose. Starch is a glucose polymer, digestion of which begins in the mouth by the action of salivary amylase. Most starch degradation, however, occurs in the alkaline pH of the duodenum and jejunum and is catalysed by pancreatic amylase. The final products of luminal digestion of starch are maltose (2 glucose molecules), maltotriose (3 glucose molecules) and short chain dextrins (4–8 glucose molecules).

Hydrolysis by specific enzyme complexes on the intestinal mucosal cells breaks down these products and the dietary disaccharides, sucrose and lactose, into their constituent monosaccharides, glucose, galactose and fructose. Active absorptive mechanisms then transfer the monosaccharides into the mucosal cell.

Fat absorption

Most of the average daily 70 gram fat intake is triglyceride; usually long-chain fatty acids combined with glycerol. Lipolysis, the breakdown of triglyceride to free fatty acid (FFA) and monoglyceride, is performed predominantly by pancreatic lipase in the small intestine. An essential step in fat absorption is an increase in the water solubility of fats, which facilitates mucosal diffusion. This is achieved by combining FFA and monoglyceride with bile acids secreted by the liver into water soluble 'micelles'. The process of micelle formation increases fat diffusibility over 100-fold allowing absorption into the mucosal cell where the triglycerides are reconstituted. The triglycerides are then transported from the gut to the circulation via the lymphatics.

Bile acid synthesis

Bile acids, derived from cholesterol in the liver, are conjugated with glycine or taurine and excreted via the bile duct into the duodenum. The main bile acids synthesized are cholic acid and chenodeoxycholic acid. The gall bladder acts as a reservoir for bile acids, and empties in response to the hormone cholecystokinin. After assisting fat absorption, 95 percent of bile acids are actively reabsorbed by the distal ileum into the portal circulation and re-excreted by the liver back into the bile. This cycle is referred to as the 'entero-hepatic' circulation and acts to conserve bile acids. The remaining five percent of bile acids are dehydroxylated by bacteria and lost in the stools.

Malabsorption

Malabsorption is a disturbance of transfer of nutrients from the gut into the circulation. Malab-

sorption may affect only a single nutrient, as in iron deficiency, or may be a more general process interfering with the absorption of a range of substances to a greater or lesser degree. Nevertheless, the clinical features of malabsorption disease may be limited to a few poorly absorbed nutrients or to a particular dietary component (for example, a presenting feature in coeliac disease is often iron deficiency anaemia).

Causes of malabsorption

Effective absorption depends upon an adequate supply of nutrients which are effectively digested. This in turn depends upon sufficient time in contact with an intact and functional gut mucosa for absorption to occur. A defect in any of these stages may lead to malabsorption. Nutrients which are poorly absorbed, rapidly metabolized or which depend upon complex digestive steps are amongst those most likely to be affected by malabsorption. The main causes of malabsorption are given in Table 18.1.

Impaired digestion

Pancreatic deficiency

Chronic damage to the pancreas, often due to alcohol abuse or cystic fibrosis (see Chapter 25), results in reduced levels of pancreatic enzymes. Without pancreatic enzymes, absorption, particularly of fat, is impaired, leading to malabsorption.

Luminal bile acid deficiency

The presence of adequate bile acids in the gut is essential for fat absorption. Liver damage may result in inadequate production and secretion of bile acids, while obstruction of the bile ducts will prevent bile entering the gut (see Chapter 17). Bile acid reabsorption into the enterohepatic circulation may be reduced if the terminal ileum has been surgically removed or is diseased, as seen in Crohn's disease (see later). Drugs may also interfere with bile acid reabsorption. The resin, cholestyramine, binds bile acids, resulting in their

Table 18.1 Causes of malabsorption

IMPAIRED DIGESTION	
Pancreatic deficiency	Chronic pancreatitis
	Cystic fibrosis
Luminal bile acid deficiency	
Decreased excretion	Severe liver disease
	Bile duct obstruction
Decreased ileal	Ileal resection
reabsorption	Crohn's disease
	Drugs (cholestyramine)
Excess deconjugation	Bacterial intestinal overgrowth
RAPID INTESTINAL TRANSIT TIME	Post-surgery
	Hypolactasia (lactase deficiency)
DEFICIENT MUCOSAL ABSORPTION	Surgical resection/short bowel
	Coeliac disease
	Infection: Giardiasis
	Tropical sprue
	Crohn's disease
	Irradiation damage

faecal loss. If sufficient bacteria colonize the small intestine, bile acids are deconjugated to a greater extent, also reducing reabsorption and increasing faecal loss. All these processes deplete the bile acid pool and can produce malabsorption.

Rapid intestinal transit time

The intact small intestine has an excess of absorptive capacity such that all but the most poorly absorbed nutrients can be adequately absorbed unless transit time is extremely rapid. Nevertheless, after surgery or when the gut cannot hydrolyse certain sugars, commonly lactose (the disaccharide in milk), there may not be sufficient contact time for absorption to take place.

Deficient mucosal absorption

The length of the small bowel is approximately 6 metres, but most nutrients can be absorbed if only 1 metre remains. Nevertheless, if surgery or disease produces a small bowel of substantially

shorter length, malabsorption may occur (short gut syndrome).

Small intestinal mucosal disease may reduce absorptive capacity. A common cause worldwide is infection with the protozoan *Giardia lamblia*, the cause of giardiasis. In the UK, coeliac disease is the most frequent mucosal cause of malabsorption. (See Case Study 19.1). Coeliac disease is a result of hypersensitivity to gluten in wheat and is characterized by loss of intestinal villi, so reducing the surface area available for absorption (Figs. 18.2 and 18.3). Small intestinal damage from other causes, including Crohn's disease and irradiation, can also result in loss of absorptive function.

Symptoms and signs of malabsorption

Weight loss and diarrhoea are frequent in malabsorption. *Steatorrhoea* describes the characteristic diarrhoea of fat malabsorption with pale, bulky, offensive, fat-laden stools. Fat soluble vitamins, particularly vitamin D, may also be deficient resulting in osteomalacia. Deficiency of other vitamins, minerals and trace elements may also occur. Iron and folic acid deficiency are characterized by tiredness and anaemia (see Chapter 20). Serum albumin is reduced, partly through protein malabsorption and partly because albumin may be lost into the gut, resulting in oedema of the legs and abdomen. In children, malabsorption may be difficult to diagnose, the only clues being 'failure to thrive' (that is, inadequate weight or growth gain).

Intestinal adaptation

The functional reserve of the small intestine is such that up to 75 percent can be lost with little consequence. If part of the intestine is lost, the remainder quickly responds by increasing mucosal mass and absorption. Whilst specialist absorptive mechanisms, such as vitamin B_{12} transport (see Chapter 20) cannot be replaced, much of the general absorptive capacity is recovered. This process is referred to as 'intestinal adaptation' and is mediated partly by the presence of food in

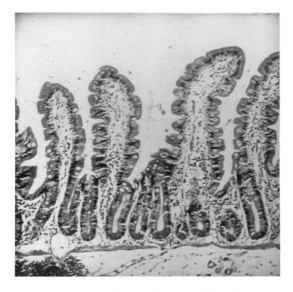

Fig. 18.2 Normal jejunal mucosa showing well-formed finger-like villi projecting above shorter crypts.

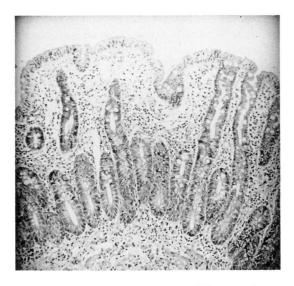

Fig. 18.3 In coeliac disease, the projecting villi have been lost and the mucosa appears flat.

the gut which stimulates intestinal cell proliferation and partly by the secretion of trophic (growth-accelerating) hormones, particularly enteroglucagon, and pancreato-biliary secretions.

Inflammatory bowel disease

Inflammation in the gut may occur in response to a wide variety of stimuli. The term 'inflammatory bowel disease' (IBD) usually refers to two specific chronic inflammatory diseases whose main pathological site is the intestine. These diseases are *Crohn's disease* and *ulcerative colitis*. Despite intensive research, no cause has been found for either condition.

Ulcerative colitis

Ulcerative colitis (UC) is a chronic disease characterized by inflammation of part or all of the large intestine. The diffuse inflammatory process always affects the most distal part of the bowel, the rectum, and can remain localized to this site. However, the disease often spreads proximally to a variable extent and in severe cases affects the entire colon. In contrast to Crohn's disease, inflammation does not occur elsewhere in the gut. Ulcerative colitis is essentially a mucosal disease characterized by an acute inflammatory infiltrate (see Chapter 4). Only rarely does the inflammatory process involve the deeper layers below the muscularis mucosae.

Clinically, patients complain of diarrhoea mixed with blood and associated abdominal pain. In severe cases the colon may dilate in a potentially life-threatening complication known as 'toxic dilatation'. Diseases associated with UC can occur in organs remote from the gut. Skin disorders, acute arthritis, spinal and eye inflammation and liver disease are all recognized extra-intestinal manifestations of UC. These features suggest that UC is a general or systemic condition not confined to the large bowel.

Crohn's disease

The inflammatory process in Crohn's disease may occur not just in the colon but in any part of the gastrointestinal tract. The most frequently affected site is the terminal ileum. Unlike UC, the disease is not continuous but patchy with 'skip

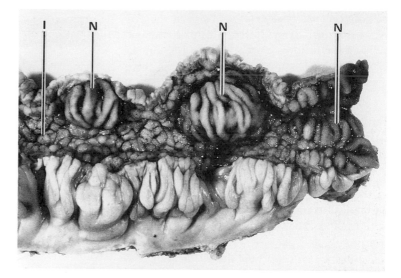

Fig. 18.4 Crohn's disease in large bowel. Large bowel opened longitudinally to show areas of normal (N) and inflamed (I) mucosa. The appearance of patchy areas of inflamed mucosa within normal bowel (skip lesions) is characteristic of Crohn's disease.

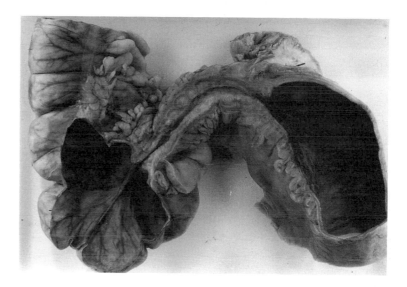

Fig. 18.5 Tight intestinal stricture caused by Crohn's disease.

lesions' of disease separated by normal mucosa (Fig. 18.4). The inflammation in Crohn's disease penetrates through all layers of the bowel wall, resulting in deep fissuring ulcers and a fibrotic reaction (resulting in the deposition of collagen fibres) leading to stricture formation and ultimately obstruction (Fig. 18.5). The inflammatory process differs from UC in that it is transmural (is present throughout all layers of the bowel wall) and is composed of lymphocytes, plasma cells and macrophages which often congregate to form granulomas (see Chapter 4).

Symptoms in Crohn's disease depend upon disease location. Weight loss, abdominal pain and diarrhoea are most common, but the transmural ulceration in Crohn's disease produces a tendency for involvement of adjacent tissues in the inflammatory process. The result is sometimes abnormal communications or *fistulae* between the diseased bowel and other organs, particularly the skin, bladder, genital tract or other parts of the gut. Abscess formation and infection are also frequent. While these features are not seen in UC, similar extra-intestinal complications occur in both diseases.

Pathogenesis of inflammatory bowel disease

The precise causes of both Crohn's disease and ulcerative colitis remain unknown. Molecular biological techniques for detecting specific DNA have failed to identify an infective agent. No dietary factor has been reliably implicated in either disease.

The most favoured hypothesis for both conditions is that disordered immunoregulation leads to inappropriate immune responses, which initiates the inflammation. Support for this theory has come from the detection of anti-neutrophil cytoplasmic antibodies in the serum of 50 percent of UC patients. Abnormal immunity and in particular a pathogenic role for neutrophils in the gut wall has also been postulated for Crohn's disease.

While underlying mechanisms remain uncertain, it is clear that inflammatory mediators are abnormal in IBD tissue. Pro-inflammatory cytokines, such as interleukin-1 (IL-1), IL-8 and tumour necrosis factor are released by mucosal macrophages while activated lymphocytes release immunoregulatory cytokines such as IL-2 and IFN-gamma. The tissue injury and inflammation is also associated with increased levels of oxygen free radicals and leukotrienes (see Chapter 4). It is difficult in this complex situation to separate fundamental disease causes from the local effects of active inflammation.

Two major groups of drugs are used in the treatment of IBD. The 5-aminosalicylic acid (5-ASA) derivatives probably act by reducing the production of inflammatory mediators. Corticosteroids are also effective in the treatment of both Crohn's disease and ulcerative colitis.

Gastrointestinal malignancy

Malignancy occurs throughout the gastrointestinal tract but is particularly frequent in the oesophagus, stomach and colon. Small intestinal cancer is rare. The incidence of gut malignancies varies widely throughout the world and even in different regions of the same country. This suggests that major environmental factors are important in their cause. However, various influences may determine each individual's risk within these populations. A recurrent finding is that long-term inflammation of the gut predisposes to malignant change.

Colorectal cancer

Colorectal cancer is now second only to lung cancer as a cause of death from malignant disease in the UK. Furthermore, the incidence is increasing in Western societies but remains rare in rural Africa. This again suggests a causal environmental factor and the high-fat, low-fibre diets consumed in Europe and North America have been suggested to predispose individuals to the disease, although this has not been proven. Chronic inflammation in the colon predisposes individuals to malignant change, particularly in chronic UC. The risk of malignancy increases with increasing disease duration and extent of inflammation.

Malignant colonic disease is believed to begin in an area of *dysplastic* or abnormal epithelium. In the colon this may produce an *adenoma* (a benign tumour of glandular epithelial cells) which is often also referred to as a 'polyp'. As the adenoma grows, the dysplasia may progress in severity and eventually invasion of the muscularis mucosae of the polyp stalk occurs, producing an overt malignancy. This 'adenoma-carcinoma' sequence is believed to underlie all colonic cancers (see Chapter 29).

Genetic influences are important in colonic carcinoma and contribute to at least 6 percent of cases. *Familial adenomatous polyposis* (FAP) is an example (see Case Study 27.1). In this syndrome, hundreds and sometimes thousands of colonic

Key points

1 Mucosal injury and ulceration in the upper gastro-intestinal tract is the result of excessive aggressive factors, such as acid and pepsin, that overwhelm the mucosal defences. Suppression of acid secretion allows the mucosa to heal. Chronic infection with the bacterium, *Helicobacter pylori*, is associated with both peptic ulceration and gastric malignancy.

2 Malabsorption is a clinical syndrome not a specific diagnosis. A wide variety of diseases may interfere with the complex mechanism of nutrient absorption. The most common in the UK is coeliac disease, a hypersensitivity to gluten found in wheat.

3 There are two types of specific chronic inflamma-tory bowel disease – Crohn's disease and ulcerative colitis. Ulcerative colitis is limited to the colon while Crohn's disease may effect the entire gut but commonly occurs in the terminal ileum. Both diseases may cause abdominal pain, weight loss and diarrhoea and have similar extra-intestinal complications.

4 Colorectal cancer is the second most frequent cause of death from cancer in most 'developed' countries. Several factors appear to predispose individuals to colorectal cancer including chronic inflammation, genetic factors and environmental influences, including diet.

polyps are formed, beginning in the teenage years. Progression to malignancy is inevitable in untreated cases, with death before the age of 40. Inheritance is autosomal dominant and the defective gene has now been identified, allowing genetic diagnosis with DNA markers in almost all cases.

Colonic cancer at a young age also occurs in *hereditary non-polyposis colon cancer*. In this autosomal dominant condition, fewer adenomas occur than in FAP but malignancy may also occur elsewhere, particularly in the endometrium. Other than in these well described genetic syndromes, the increased frequency of colonic cancer in close relatives of index cases suggests that genetic as well as environmental influences are important in the aetiology of the disease.

The clinical effects of peptic ulceration, malabsorption, gut inflammation and malignancy are described. The underlying biological mechanisms leading to each disease have not yet been fully clarified.

Summary

In this chapter, the most important disorders of the gastrointestinal system have been presented.

Further reading

Bouchier I.A.D., Allan R.W., Hodgson H.J.F & Keighley M.R.B. (1993) *Gastroenterology: Clinical Science and Practice*. Saunders, London.

Bray J.J., Cragg P.A., MacKnight A.D.C, Mills R.G.& Taylor D.W. (1984) *Lecture Notes on Human Physiology*, 3rd edn. Blackwell Scientific Publications, Oxford.

Ganong W.F. (1983) *Review of Medical Physiology*, 16th edn. Lange Medical, Connecticut.

Pounder R.E. (Ed.) (1992) *Recent Advances in Gastroenterology* No. 9. Churchill Livingstone, London.

Case Studies

19.1 Diarrhoea and abdominal distension

Clinical features

A 50-year-old woman presented with diarrhoea. She gave a 10-year history of intermittent diarrhoea and tiredness but symptoms had worsened considerably in the last 2 weeks. The diarrhoea was up to five times daily, described as creamy-white and associated with wind and abdominal distension. She was not on any medication.

On examination the patient was pale and her abdomen was distended. There was marked ankle swelling.

Investigations

Laboratory investigations included those shown in Table 19.1.1.

Colonoscopy, gastroscopy and small bowel barium meal x-ray were all normal. A jejunal biopsy was performed. This showed a flat mucosal surface with a total loss of villi (subtotal villous atrophy). A chronic inflammatory infiltrate was present within the lamina propria.

Diagnosis

The histological appearance of the jejunal biopsy showed subtotal villous atrophy consistent with coeliac disease. The laboratory findings are also consistent with a malabsorption syndrome. Low serum albumin, anaemia with low folate and ferritin levels but a normal vitamin B_{12} concentration all suggest malabsorption.

Diagnosis: coeliac disease.

Discussion

Adult coeliac disease can be defined as a condition in which there is an abnormal jejunal mucosa which improves when treated with a gluten-free diet and relapses when gluten is reintroduced. The highest incidence of coeliac disease in the world is found in the west of Ireland where 1 in 300 of the population are affected. In the UK, the incidence is around 1 in 2000. There is a familial tendency which may be explained in part by the association of coeliac disease with HLA DQw2.

Coeliac disease is the result of a sensitivity to gluten which is a constituent of wheat, rye and barley. More specifically, the responsible protein is contained in the alcohol-soluble fraction of gluten; known as gliadin. The precise mechanisms of the damage to the small intestine are unknown but are thought to be due to a local immunological reaction to gliadin.

Table 19.1.1 Investigations performed

Analyte	Value	Reference range
Blood		
Haemoglobin	10.1 g/dl	11.5–15.5
Serum folate	0.6 µg/l	1.9–14
Red cell folate	84 µg/l	100–640
Vitamin B_{12}	255 ng/l	200–900
Ferritin	6 µg/l	10–300
Albumin	18 g/l	34–48
Thyroid-stimulating hormone	40.8 mU/l	0.3–4.0
Free thyroxine	9.8 pmol/l	9–24

Recently, it has been proposed that there are two stages in the development of the disease. Firstly, a genetically determined state of inappropriate immunity (hypersensitivity) to gliadin is induced in local intra-epithelial T lymphocytes. This does not produce overt disease until exposure to a second factor occurs. The nature of the second factor is unknown but may be sudden exposure to gliadin or to an infectious agent. Exposure to the second factor activates the damaging immunological mechanisms and disease results.

Coeliac disease primarily affects the proximal small bowel. Loss of normal villi results in a mucosae which appears flat with elongated intestinal crypts. There is often an infiltrate of inflammatory cells present within adjacent connective tissue (the *lamina propria*) and numbers of intra-epithelial lymphocytes are increased.

The clinical features of coeliac disease are common to all types of malabsorption and include weight loss, weakness and diarrhoea due to fat malabsorption. The stools are pale, bulky and offensive. In addition to deficiencies of iron and folate, there may also be *hypocalcaemia* (low serum calcium concentration), due to vitamin D malabsorption which, if long standing, may result in *osteomalacia* (a decrease in calcified bone due to poor mineralization).

A number of other diseases are associated with coeliac disease including chronic liver diseases and certain endocrine abnormalities. The high thyroid-stimulating hormone (TSH) concentration in this patient is indicative of *hypothyroidism*. The thyroid deficiency was rapidly corrected by replacement therapy with thyroxine.

Treatment and prognosis

A gluten-free diet combined with oral folic acid and iron supplementation produced a remarkable clinical response in this patient. Within 4 months all the laboratory indices, including the serum albumin had returned to normal. Life-long dietary gluten exclusion is recommended for adult pa-

tients. Rarely, coeliac disease can be complicated by the development of intestinal lymphoma.

Questions

1 Explain the typical finding of folate and iron deficiency in coeliac disease.

Answer: malabsorption of a wide range of nutrients occurs in coeliac disease and deficiencies of nutrients with relatively low body stores become apparent at an early stage. Iron and folate are absorbed mostly in the proximal small intestine, the area of the gut mainly affected by coeliac disease. Haemopoietic tissues have high demands for folate and iron, so anaemia soon follows the development of deficiency states. Anaemia may be predominantly due to iron deficiency (microcytic and hypochromic), to folate deficiency (macrocytic, normochromic) or may show features of both types of anaemia (see also Chapter 20).

2 Explain the significance of the increased concentration of thyroid-stimulating hormone in hypothyroidism.

Answer: thyroid-stimulating hormone is secreted by the anterior pituitary gland in response to the action of thyrotropin-releasing hormone (TRH) from the hypothalamus. TSH stimulates the production of thyroid hormones and their release from the thyroid gland. Hypothyroidism (reduced activity of the thyroid gland) is characterized by reduced synthesis of the thyroid hormones, thyroxine (T_4) and tri-iodothyronine (T_3). The secretion of TSH is normally controlled by a negative feedback loop involving thyroxine, in which high levels of thyroxine depress TSH secretion. TSH levels increase in hypothyroidism in an attempt to stimulate the thyroid gland to secrete sufficient thyroxine for the maintenance of normal metabolic rate.

19.2 Abdominal pain and diarrhoea

Clinical features

A 46-year-old woman complained of right-sided colicky abdominal pain and diarrhoea for 6 weeks. She had lost 2 stones in weight but passed no blood in the stools. On examination, she was pale and had mouth ulceration. A tender mobile mass was felt in the lower abdomen.

Investigations

Laboratory investigations included those shown in Table 19.2.1.

Table 19.2.1 Blood investigations

Analyte	Value	Reference range
Total white cell count	11.9×10^9/l	4.0–11.0
Red cell count	4.14×10^{12}/l	3.8–5.8
Haemoglobin	9.3 g/dl	11.5–15.5
Haematocrit	0.302	0.37–0.47
Mean cell volume	73.0 fl	82–92
Mean cell haemoglobin	22.46 pg	27.0–32.0
Platelet count	400×10^9/l	150–400
Erythrocyte sedimentation rate	103 mm/hour	0–20

Blood film
White blood cell differential
Neutrophils	76%
Lymphocytes	17%
Monocytes	5%
Eosinophils	2%
Basophils	0%

The total leucocyte (white cell) count is slightly high, with a mild neutrophilia.
Erythrocyte morphology: microcytic (cells reduced in size) and hypochromic (staining intensity reduced). Normal erythrocytes would appear normocytic and normochromic–see Chapter 20. The erythrocyte sedimentation rate (ESR) is very high, reflecting active inflammatory disease.

Examination of the colon by sigmoidoscopy and abdominal ultrasound tests were normal. A small bowel barium meal x-ray showed narrowing and thickening of the distal ileum consistent with Crohn's disease.

Diagnosis

The combination of weight loss and diarrhoea over a short period of time suggests significant bowel pathology. This is supported by the iron deficiency anaemia (indicated by the low mean cell volume or MCV) and raised ESR (erythrocyte sedimentation rate). Active inflammation or malignant disease are most likely to produce these results while the normal sigmoidoscopy makes colitis unlikely. Typical Crohn's disease was shown by the small bowel barium meal x-ray. The distal ileum is the most common site of presentation.

Diagnosis: Crohn's disease.

Discussion

Each year, in most 'developed' countries, Crohn's disease is diagnosed in approximately five people in every 100 000. The disease affects more women than men, often presents before the age of 30, and tends to occur more frequently in certain families, suggesting genetic susceptibility in some people. Typical symptoms of Crohn's disease and other inflammatory bowel disorders (notably ulcerative colitis), include colicky abdominal pain, diarrhoea, fever, weight loss and anorexia. Fistula formation is relatively common in Crohn's disease and may require surgical intervention. Changes associated with Crohn's disease may extend beyond the affected area indicated by radiography or laparotomy (exploratory abdominal surgery). Abnormalities in proximal small intestinal permeability to folic acid and sugars have been demonstrated in patients in whom disease was apparently confined to the distal ileum and colon.

It can be difficult to make a precise diagnosis in inflammatory bowel disease because the clinical features of Crohn's disease and ulcerative colitis are similar. In both conditions, there may also be systemic complications, including iritis (inflammation of the iris), arthritis and in some long standing cases, sclerosing cholangitis (inflammation and fibrosis of the bile ducts).

The causes of Crohn's disease (and ulcerative colitis) are as yet unknown. Recently, it has been suggested that patients born during measles epidemics are more likely to develop Crohn's disease than those who were not. There was no such association with ulcerative colitis. The significance of this finding remains to be established.

Treatment and prognosis

The patient was commenced on high dose corticosteroids. Initially there was a good response to treatment. However, 3 months later the patient returned with fever and right-sided pain. An abscess obstructing the right kidney was diagnosed and surgical resection was performed.

As with many other chronic inflammatory diseases, Crohn's disease is characterized by periods of remission and relapse. Remission is induced by high dose steroids which are then gradually reduced. Aminosalicylates are beneficial in ulcerative colitis and may be combined with corticosteroids in Crohn's disease with colonic involvement.

Inflammatory bowel disease affecting the colon is associated with an increased risk of colorectal cancer.

Questions

1 Can you explain the haematological findings?

Answer: the microcytic hypochromic anaemia could indicate iron deficiency due either to chronic blood loss or malabsorption of iron. Alternatively, chronic inflammatory disorders can produce a similar haematological picture, with hypochromic and microcytic red blood cells. Iron deficiency is characterized by low serum iron, low serum ferritin and a raised serum transferrin concentration. The causes of anaemia due to chronic inflammation are complex, but the anaemia is probably due, at least in part, to a defect in the utilization of iron (see Chapter 20). In anaemia associated with chronic inflammation serum iron is also low, but serum ferritin is normal or high and serum transferrin is usually low. This patient's anaemia was probably due to a combination of chronic blood loss and inflammatory disease.

The ESR is a non-specific test which is raised in a wide variety of conditions, notably inflammatory and malignant disorders. Occasionally, especially in elderly patients, the ESR is raised and despite extensive investigations no cause is found. The measurement of plasma viscosity gives much the same information, and is subject to fewer variables, so is offered by some laboratories as an alternative to the ESR.

The raised leucocyte count, the majority of cells being neutrophils (neutrophilia), is consistent with an inflammatory disorder.

2 How does Crohn's disease differ from ulcerative colitis?

Answer: clinically, Crohn's disease can be difficult to distinguish from ulcerative colitis since both diseases cause chronic inflammation and ulceration in the gut. However, whereas Crohn's disease can affect any area of the gut from the mouth to the anus, ulcerative colitis is confined to the colon. In addition, in Crohn's disease the inflammatory process typically extends through the gut wall, whereas, usually, in ulcerative colitis the mucosa and sub-mucosa only are affected. Non-caseating granulomas (see Chapter 4) are a characteristic histological finding in Crohn's disease.

19.3 Recurrent epigastric pain with abnormal liver function tests

Clinical features

A 52-year-old publican was admitted to hospital with severe epigastric pain (pain in the upper central region of the abdomen radiating to the back). The pain had developed with increasing intensity over 6–8 hours and the patient had also experienced retching and vomiting.

This patient had been seen in the Outpatients Department three months previously for investigation of recurrent epigastric pain and steatorrhoea (the passage of bulky greasy stools due to fat malabsorption). Typically the abdominal pain lasted for 3–4 days, was accompanied by nausea, and could be eased slightly by sitting forward. An abdominal radiograph had revealed pancreatic calcification and after further investigations a diagnosis of chronic pancreatitis had been made.

Investigations

On admission to hospital the patient's blood pressure was moderately raised at 175 mm systolic, 95 mm diastolic. A full blood count, ESR and blood biochemistry were requested. The results are shown in Table 19.3.1.

Diagnosis

The most likely cause of the acute onset of epigastric pain in this case is acute exacerbation (sudden increased severity) of chronic relapsing pancreatitis. However, it is important to exclude other, unrelated, conditions for which surgery might be indicated. Damage to the exocrine pancreas results in the release of pancreatic enzymes into body fluids, so the very high serum amylase

Table 19.3.1 Blood investigations performed on first admission

Analyte	Value	Reference range
Total white cell count	12.6×10^9/l	4.0–11.0
Haemoglobin	14.2 g/dl	13.5–17.5
Haematocrit	0.42	0.40–0.50
Mean cell volume	100 fl	82–92
Platelet count	180×10^9/l	150–400
Erythrocyte sedimentation rate	20 mm	0–10

Blood film
White blood cell differential

Neutrophils	79%
Lymphocytes	16%
Monocytes	4%
Eosinophils	1%
Basophils	0%

Biochemistry

Random blood glucose	3.6 mmol/l	3.5–8.9
Total bilirubin	30 µmol/l	2–16
Aspartate aminotransferase	68 U/l	5–40
Alanine aminotransferase	115 U/l	0–40
Gamma glutamyltransferase	190 U/l	2–50
Serum amylase	1600 U/dl	0–200

is indicative of acute pancreatitis. However, serum amylase levels also rise in perforated peptic ulcer, acute intestinal obstruction and acute biliary obstruction, but peak levels are usually less than five times the upper range of normal. In acute pancreatitis serum amylase usually increases to at least five times the upper reference range within 24 hours. Other pancreatic enzymes such as trypsin and lipase also increase in acute pancreatitis. In this case the serum amylase was approximately eight times the upper reference range.

The most common cause of pancreatitis is chronic alcohol abuse but other possible causes include hyperparathyroidism, protein-energy malnutrition and trauma. High levels of bilirubin and transaminase enzymes together with red cell macrocytosis (see Chapter 20) indicate liver damage, again possibly due to alcohol abuse. In some cases of pancreatitis there is cholestatic jaundice, due to pressure from the swollen head of pancreas on the common bile duct (see Chapter 17), but jaundice may also be due to hepatocellular damage.

Pancreatitis can also affect the endocrine pancreas, causing diabetes mellitus. In this case blood glucose was normal, indicating that diabetes mellitus had not developed.

Diagnosis: chronic relapsing pancreatitis, with liver damage due to alcohol abuse.

Treatment and prognosis

The patient was treated conservatively with bed rest and a low fat diet and the acute condition resolved. On further direct questioning, the patient admitted to excess alcohol intake, and he was counselled to abstain. He was discharged from hospital and was eventually referred to a psychiatric clinic and to self-help groups when it became apparent that he was continuing to drink heavily.

Discussion

The patient continued to drink heavily, began to neglect himself and eventually lost his job. He attended his family doctor's surgery every 3 months to collect a prescription for vitamins and on each occasion he would claim to be in control of his drinking. One day, the patient collapsed at home, vomited material resembling coffee grounds and an emergency admission to hospital was arranged. On admission to hospital

Table 19.3.2 Blood investigations

Analyte	Value	Reference range (female)
Total white cell count	11.5×10^9/l	4.0–11.0
Red cell count	3.90×10^{12}/l	4.5–6.5
Haemoglobin	9.6 g/dl	13.5–17.5
Mean cell volume	108 fl	82–92
Platelet count	120×10^9/l	150–400

haematemesis (vomiting of blood) due to upper gastrointestinal bleeding was confirmed, and gross abdominal *ascites* (accumulation of fluid in the abdominal cavity) was noted. An endoscopic examination revealed *oesophageal varices* (see later). Laboratory results on this occasion are shown in Table 19.3.2.

The white cell differential count on this occasion revealed an absolute neutrophilia. The haemoglobin concentration and red cell count were low due to acute blood loss.

Bleeding persisted and the patient was transfused. Despite this, the haemoglobin remained low, indicating continued bleeding. Blood coagulation tests were requested.

The prothrombin time was prolonged (17 seconds, normal control 13 seconds). The activated partial thromboplastin time was also prolonged (60 seconds, normal control 41 seconds). Because most coagulation factors are synthesized in the liver, these abnormalities reflect hepatocellular damage. Vitamin K and fresh frozen plasma were administered in an attempt to correct the coagulation defect and the bleeding was eventually controlled.

The patient was discharged from hospital, but he died at home 6 weeks later. At post mortem examination, the liver was found to be enlarged to a weight of 2165 grams. On slicing, the liver was rather yellow-coloured and greasy in texture. Histological examination showed that many of the hepatocytes were swollen and that large vacuoles were present in their cytoplasm. A frozen section was taken, and when stained appropriately showed that the vacuoles were full of lipid.

The liver in this patient showed the appearances of so-called 'fatty change' or *steatosis*. This is not a feature specifically related to alcohol abuse and can occur under the influence of numerous other agents.

Alcohol abuse accounts for substantial worldwide morbidity, causing a range of medical, psychological and sociological problems. In addition the consequences of alcohol abuse include substantial mortality from disease or trauma. Although most attention focuses on the effects of alcohol on the liver and gastrointestinal tract, there are also wide-ranging adverse effects on the central nervous and cardiovascular systems and on mental health (see Chapter 32).

Questions

1 What is the cause of red cell macrocytosis in liver disease?

Answer: erythrocyte mean cell volume (MCV) is often high in alcoholic liver disease. This is sometimes due to folate deficiency resulting from poor diet, but may also be due to liver damage. The precise mechanisms causing macrocytosis in alcoholic liver disease are not yet established. It has been suggested that acetaldehyde generated by oxidation of ethanol by bone marrow macrophages damages erythrocyte precursors causing enlargement of mature erythrocytes (see Chapter 20).

2 Why was the prothrombin time prolonged in this patient?

Answer: the liver synthesizes most coagulation factors, so when there is hepatocellular damage,

synthesis of blood coagulation factors is often reduced. In addition, if there is cholestasis there is also malabsorption of fat, thus reducing absorption of fat soluble vitamins including vitamin K. Vitamin K is necessary for the synthesis of coagulation factors II, VII, IX and X, so in vitamin K deficiency their concentrations fall, thereby prolonging the prothrombin time and other coagulation tests (see Chapters 17 and 21).

3 What are the likely causes of gastrointestinal bleeding in alcoholic liver disease?

Answer: inflammation of the gastric mucosa and peptic ulceration are associated with alcohol abuse, and bleeding may occur in either condition. Furthermore, in cirrhosis, pressure in the hepatic portal vein rises and a collateral circulation becomes established in other vessels to bypass the liver. One effect of this is that the veins of the lower oesophagus become dilated and distended (a condition known as oesophageal varices) and may bleed. Bleeding is often exacerbated by reduced levels of blood coagulation factors, so the administration of vitamin K or the replacement of missing coagulation factors by transfusion of fresh frozen plasma may be indicated.

Part 6
Blood and Circulatory Disorders

Anaemia

Introduction

Anaemia is not a single disease entity. It is a consequence of one of a number of disorders underlying defective erythrocyte (red blood cell) production or excessive loss of erythrocytes from the circulation. Therefore, whenever a patient is found to be anaemic it is essential to investigate the underlying cause. This chapter considers the fundamental causes of different types of anaemia and concludes with an overview of the basic laboratory investigations used to classify anaemia.

Blood formation

Red cell formation

Haemopoiesis (blood cell production) takes place in the bone marrow. All blood cells (erythrocytes, leucocytes and platelets) are derived from a single clone of primitive cells—the *pluripotent stem cell*. Stem cells have the ability to divide and differentiate under the influence of specific cytokines. Initially they form *myeloid* and *lymphoid* stem cells (Fig. 20.1). Myeloid stem cells give rise to the progenitors of the three principal cell lines outlined below.

1 The myeloid–monocyte series (producing granulocytes and monocytes).
2 The megakaryocyte series (producing platelets).
3 Erythroid progenitor cells (producing red blood cells).

Erythropoiesis is the component of haemopoiesis which produces mature red blood cells. Erythropoiesis takes place in several stages as the erythroid precursor cells develop from relatively undifferentiated early pronormoblasts to late normoblasts, which then lose their nucleus before being released into the circulation as *reticulocytes* (young red blood cells).

Haemoglobin synthesis

Haemoglobin (Hb, molecular weight 68 000) is the oxygen-carrying component of erythrocytes. Each red cell contains over 600 million Hb molecules. The Hb molecule is a tetramer of four haem groups (Fig. 20.2) and four globin chains. Normal adult haemoglobin contains two types of globin chain—two *alpha chains* (each 141 amino acids) and two *beta chains* (each 146 amino acids).

The assembly of haem takes place in mitochondria in the cytoplasm of erythrocyte precursor cells in bone marrow. Four haem molecules each combine with alpha or beta globin chains synthesized in ribosomes in the cell cytoplasm to form haemoglobin (Fig. 20.3). Several factors can interfere with the synthesis of haemoglobin including lack of essential nutrients (as in iron deficiency), certain inherited structural abnormalities or defects in the efficient assembly of haemoglobin molecules.

Causes of anaemia

Anaemia is defined as a reduction either in the concentration of haemoglobin in the blood or in numbers of circulating erythrocytes. Usually if one of these is reduced then the other is reduced also, because haemoglobin is contained within erythrocytes. However, there are circumstances in which haemoglobin concentration may be mildly reduced with a normal red cell count. This occurs particularly in the early stages of iron deficiency anaemia and some *thalassaemia syndromes* (see later). In such cases, despite a normal red cell

166

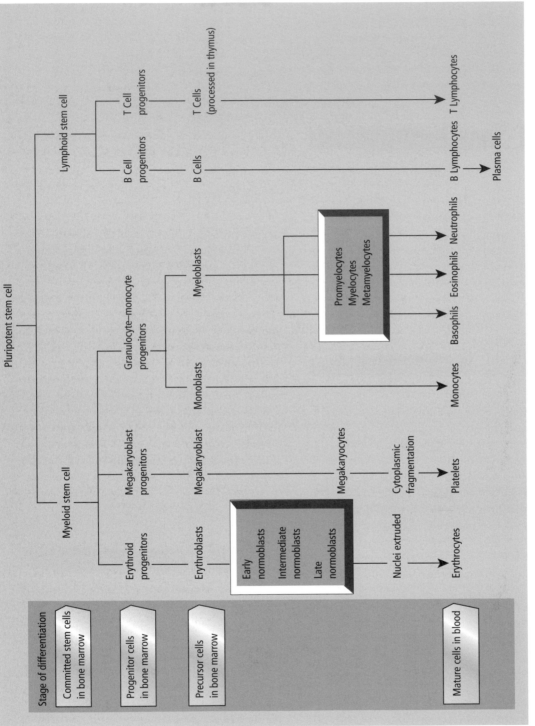

Fig. 20.1 Haemopoiesis. All mature blood cells are derived from pluripotent stem cells. Haemopoietic stem cells have the ability to divide and differentiate under the influence of specific growth factors. Lymphoid stem cells give rise to B and T cell lines. B lymphocytes undergo further differentiation into plasma cells for antibody production. T lymphocyte precursors are processed in the thymus to produce T cells—T helper, T suppressor and cytotoxic T cells. Myeloid stem cells give rise to three types of progenitor cell which produce erythrocytes, platelets or cells of the monocyte and granulocyte series.

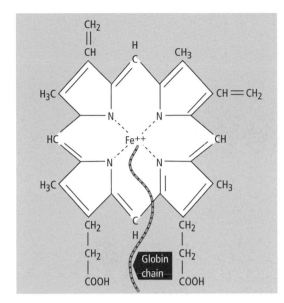

Fig. 20.2 The structure of haem. Each haem is formed from a porphyrin ring into which is inserted ferrous iron. An alpha- or beta-globin chain attaches to each haem, four of which combine to form each haemoglobin molecule.

Table 20.1 Principal causes of anaemia

- defective haemoglobin synthesis
- diminished erythrocyte production
- excessive erythrocyte destruction
- blood loss

Defective haemoglobin synthesis

Defective haemoglobin synthesis falls into two groups—defects of haem synthesis and defects of globin synthesis. Defects in haem synthesis can be due to failure of enzyme-mediated assembly of porphyrin rings, or due to lack of available iron at the site of synthesis. Defective globin chain synthesis may be *qualitative* (resulting in structurally abnormal haemoglobins) or *quantitative* (resulting in delayed synthesis of one or other globin chain). Defects in haemoglobin synthesis often result in red blood cells which are smaller than normal and contain reduced amounts of haemoglobin.

Porphyrias

Defects in assembly of porphyrin rings are known as *porphyrias*. Porphyrias are a rare group of inherited disorders characterized by deficiencies of enzymes controlling haem synthesis. The rate-limiting step in haem synthesis, the condensation of glycine and succinate to form 5-aminolaevulinic acid (ALA), is catalysed by ALA synthase (see Fig. 20.3). Product inhibition normally controls ALA synthase activity, so faulty haem synthesis results in overproduction of porphyrins or their precursors. Clinical effects of the porphyrias include photosensitivity, dermatitis and neurological disorders resulting from accumulation of porphyrins in the tissues. A type of anaemia characterized by abnormal accumulation of iron in erythrocyte precursors (*sideroblastic anaemia*), which can be congenital or acquired, is usually due to a similar defect in haem synthesis. Exposure to high concentrations of lead, which inhibits several stages of porphyrin synthesis, may be accompanied by a similar form of mild anaemia.

count, individual cells are reduced in size and contain a decreased amount of haemoglobin. Most other types of anaemia are characterized by reduction in both total haemoglobin concentration and red cell count with erythrocytes of normal or increased cell size.

The preliminary diagnosis of anaemia is based on establishing a reduction in total blood haemoglobin concentration, though this gives no indication of the cause. The reference range for haemoglobin concentration differs for males and females—it is usual for adult females to have rather lower haemoglobin levels than their male counterparts. Furthermore, a low haemoglobin concentration does not always signify anaemia: an increase in plasma volume can cause an apparent anaemia (*pseudo-anaemia*), although the total haemoglobin circulating content is normal. This is seen, for example, in pregnancy (in which a mild reduction in haemoglobin concentration is normal) and can be difficult to differentiate from genuine anaemia in pregnancy. The causes of anaemia are summarized in Table 20.1.

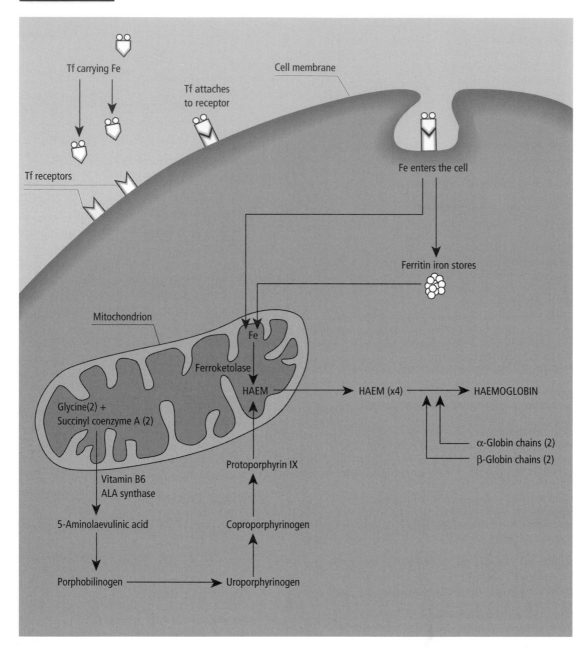

Fig. 20.3 Haemoglobin synthesis in developing erythroblasts. The essential components for the synthesis of haem are pyrrole rings and iron, together with the enzymes which assemble these into iron-containing porphyrin rings. Iron is transported to developing red blood cells in the bone marrow by the carrier protein transferrin (Tf). Tf attaches to specific receptors on the cell membrane and the whole complex (iron, Tf and receptor) is taken into the cell. The iron then either enters cellular iron stores (as ferritin) or passes to mitochondria where it combines with protoporphyrin IX to form haem. Four haems then combine with globin chains to form haemoglobin. After Hoffbrand and Pettit (1993).

Iron deficiency

Iron deficiency, the cause of the commonest nutritional anaemia, results in diminished haem synthesis, and hence reduced haemoglobin within erythrocytes. Iron deficiency anaemia also occurs when the rate of erythropoiesis increases to compensate for blood loss or the demands of pregnancy. Dietary sources of iron may be adequate to support a normal rate of erythropoiesis but are often insufficient to maintain a higher rate.

An important cause of iron deficiency anaemia is chronic blood loss. During haemorrhage, iron is irretrievably lost from the body and dietary sources of iron are insufficient to compensate for the loss. Malabsorption of iron (as in coeliac disease, see Case Study 19.1) is another potential cause of deficiency. Iron deficiency is characterized by low serum iron, low serum ferritin (reflecting depleted iron stores) and a raised concentration of serum transferrin.

Causes of *apparent* iron deficiency (blood count results which mimic those of iron deficiency with low serum iron) include defects in plasma iron transport in chronic inflammatory diseases such as rheumatoid arthritis. Serum ferritin concentrations are often normal or high and serum transferrin is usually low. This type of anaemia is normally unresponsive to iron therapy.

Inherited defects in globin chain synthesis

Qualitative globin chain defects (*haemoglobinopathies*) are usually due to base substitutions (*point mutations*) in the DNA which codes for the polypeptide globin chains, resulting in single amino acid substitutions. Such changes have variable outcomes, depending on the nature and site of the amino acid substitution, ranging from no clinical effect to severe consequences such as altered oxygen affinity, or destabilization of the haemoglobin molecule resulting in reduced erythrocyte life span.

Sickle cell disease

One of the most important of the single amino acid substitution defects is the replacement of glutamic acid by valine at position 6 in the beta chain of HbA to produce sickle haemoglobin (HbS). When inherited as a homozygous condition, under conditions of low oxygen tension, HbS precipitates as long filaments, distorting the shape of the erythrocytes. The resulting sickle-shaped cells lodge in small blood vessels causing painful *infarctions* (death of surrounding areas of tissue following sudden deprivation of blood supply) and reduction in red cell life span (see also Chapter 25 for more details of the molecular biology of sickle cell disease). Sickle cell disease is relatively common in West African populations.

Thalassaemia syndromes

Quantitative globin chain defects (*thalassaemias*) are associated with an imbalance in the rate of synthesis of alpha and beta globin chains, usually due to depression of synthesis of one or other chain. The effects are variable, depending on the degree to which globin chain synthesis is suppressed, but can be life-threatening.

Two closely linked genes on the short arm of chromosome 16 code for alpha globins, so synthesis of alpha chains is controlled by four genes in each cell. *Alpha thalassaemia* is characterized by deletion or alteration of one or more of these genes, the severity of the clinical outcome varying with the number of genes affected. Severe forms of alpha thalassaemia, with deletion of all four genes, are invariably fatal, and pregnancy with an affected fetus frequently fails to reach full term. Less severe forms of alpha thalassaemia (deletion of three of the four genes) are associated with variable survival and quality of life. Typically there is moderate anaemia and the formation of unstable beta chain tetramers (HbH) may be a feature. Alpha thalassaemia traits (deletion of one or two genes) are of little clinical significance to affected individuals, but genetic counselling is essential for affected partners in a child-bearing relationship.

Beta globin chains are coded for on the short arm of chromosome 11. Severe *beta thalassaemia* is associated with profound anaemia from the first year of life and dependence on regular transfusions. Iron overload due to these transfusions becomes a problem, though the risk of this can be reduced by the use of iron-chelating agents. Beta thalassaemia minor is much less severe, with a blood picture superficially similar to that of iron deficiency.

The precise cause of anaemia in the different haemoglobinopathies and thalassaemia syndromes is complex and varies, but increased haemolysis leading to reduction in erythrocyte life span and ineffective erythropoiesis (see later) both contribute.

Diminished erythrocyte production

In this group of anaemias, haemoglobin synthesis is normal, but erythropoiesis is reduced. Defects in erythropoiesis may be due to nutrient lack, bone marrow *hypoplasia* (underactivity), infiltration of bone marrow with malignant cells or to various chronic disease states.

Nutrient lack

Certain vitamins and other nutrients are essential for normal blood formation. Of particular importance in erythropoiesis are the B group vitamins, vitamin B_{12} and folate, which are essential for DNA synthesis. A deficiency of either of these vitamins is associated with disordered maturation of erythrocyte precursors (normoblasts) in the bone marrow. In prolonged vitamin B_{12} or folate deficiency, erythrocyte precursor cells display a characteristic morphological alteration in which nuclear maturation lags behind that of the cytoplasm (*megaloblastic change*). These abnormal cells are known as *megaloblasts*. The mature erythrocytes resulting from megaloblastic erythropoiesis are much larger than their normal counterparts and are known as *macrocytes*, although they are reduced in number. Deficiencies of vitamin

B_{12} and folate have three major causes—dietary insufficiency, malabsorption and metabolic interference.

Dietary deficiency of vitamin B_{12} is rare, but since the vitamin is present only in foods of animal origin, strict vegetarians are susceptible. Absorption of vitamin B_{12} from the intestinal tract requires the presence of a glycoprotein, *intrinsic factor* (IF), secreted by parietal cells in the fundus and body of the stomach. IF binds to vitamin B_{12} and the complex is absorbed in the distal ileum, so lack of IF results in vitamin B_{12} malabsorption. The most common disorder associated with vitamin B_{12} malabsorption is *pernicious anaemia*, an autoimmune condition characterized by the presence of autoantibodies to parietal cells and/or intrinsic factor. Disturbance of vitamin B_{12} metabolism is rare but prolonged exposure to nitrous oxide anaesthesia has been shown to cause megaloblastic change.

Folate deficiency may arise due to dietary lack, particularly in times of increased requirements, such as in pregnancy, or in disorders associated with rapid cell turnover (psoriasis, neoplastic and haemolytic disorders). Malabsorption of folate is a feature of some digestive tract disorders, for example coeliac disease (see Case Study 19.1), and serum or red cell folate assays may be used to monitor progress and response to treatment in coeliac disease patients. Finally, the drug methotrexate, which is mainly used in the treatment of leukaemia, competes with folate for the enzyme *folic acid reductase*, reducing purine synthesis and causing megaloblastic change in the bone marrow.

Bone marrow hypoplasia

Reduced erythropoiesis can also be due to bone marrow damage, leading to *hypoplastic* or *aplastic anaemia* (anaemia due to reduced haemopoietic activity) with a resulting pancytopenia (reduction in all blood cell types). There are several known potential causes of aplastic anaemia, although many cases are of unknown aetiology. Some are *iatrogenic* (physician-induced), caused by exposure to cytotoxic drugs or radiotherapy. Thyroid, liver or renal disease, or viral infection may also result in bone marrow hypoplasia.

Ineffective erythropoiesis

Ineffective erythropoiesis (IE) is a failure of erythrocyte precursor cells to reach maturity, resulting in their destruction in the bone marrow. Some degree of IE occurs in normal haemopoiesis, affecting up to 1 in 8 erythrocyte precursor cells. An increase in IE contributes to many forms of anaemia, including those seen in the thalassaemia syndromes, megaloblastosis and some leukaemias.

Malignant blood disorders

Leukaemias and other malignant blood diseases are an important cause of anaemia due to reduced erythropoiesis. Leukaemias are categorized as *acute* or *chronic* and are further subdivided according to the particular haemopoietic cell line involved (see Case Study 31.1). Characteristically, the bone marrow contains large numbers of leukaemic cells which replace normal haemopoietic cells, and there may also be some megaloblastic change. Most leukaemias, particularly the acute forms, are characterized by anaemia, which is often severe, *thrombocytopenia* (reduction in blood platelet count) and *neutropenia* (reduction in circulating neutrophils), the latter causing the patient to be highly susceptible to bacterial infection.

Chronic disease states

Inflammatory or neoplastic disease may cause diminished red cell production, though in certain chronic inflammatory disorders (e.g. rheumatoid arthritis), anaemia may also be due to a defect in iron utilization. Chronic renal failure is associated with impaired erythropoiesis because the kidney is a major source of the hormone *erythropoietin*, necessary for optimal red cell production.

Excessive erythrocyte destruction (haemolytic disorders)

The normal red cell has a mean life span in the circulation of 110–120 days. Reduced erythrocyte life span may result in anaemia, though this is not always the case because the bone marrow is usually able to increase production of erythrocytes to compensate for the premature loss. Despite this, if red cell life span is very short or the defect is permanent, premature cell death may not always be fully compensated by an increase in the rate of erythropoiesis and anaemia results. There are two major groups of haemolytic disorder—those due to *intrinsic* or *extrinsic* erythrocyte defects.

Intrinsic erythrocyte defects

Intrinsic erythrocyte defects leading to haemolytic disorders are often congenital and can be subdivided into three categories. These are defects of: (1) *haemoglobin*; (2) *intracellular enzymes* and (3) *the erythrocyte membrane*.

1. Alterations in haemoglobin structure can cause reduction in erythrocyte life span due to instability of the haemoglobin molecule itself or its defective interaction with other cell structures.

2. Deficiencies or structural defects of intracellular enzymes, such as *pyruvate kinase* (PK) or *glucose-6-phosphate dehydrogenase* (G_6PD), affect the ability of erythrocytes to metabolize nutrients and provide for their energy needs. The cells do not survive for their normal duration in the circulation, particularly, in the case of G_6PD deficiency, if exposed to oxidative stress.

3. Erythrocyte membrane defects, usually associated with abnormalities of the cytoskeleton, become clinically significant if they alter the biconcave disc shape and reduce erythrocyte deformability. This reduces the ability of the cells to enter and pass through small blood vessels. The affected cells become trapped in the splenic sinusoids and are removed from the circulation prematurely.

One example of this group of disorders is *hereditary spherocytosis*. In this condition, an inherited defect in the *spectrin* group of cytoskeletal proteins results in spherical erythrocytes which have a reduced life span. The rate of erythropoiesis increases to compensate for this, but if the rate of production fails to keep pace with the rate of destruction then anaemia results. There is normally a substantial reserve capacity in the bone marrow which can compensate for reduced red blood cell life span, although periodically the bone marrow may fail to compensate fully, particularly if the patient has an infection or health is compromised in some other way.

Extrinsic erythrocyte defects

Extrinsic defects are usually acquired and affect erythrocytes which are not intrinsically abnormal in any way. Examples include infection with malarial parasites (see Chapter 10), other systemic infections, severe trauma or burns, or heart valve defects. The development of autoantibodies to antigens on the red cell surface (such as those of the rhesus system) is a cause of *autoimmune haemolytic anaemia*, which can be triggered by exposure to certain drugs. Immune-mediated haemolytic transfusion reactions, though rare, also cause significant reduction in erythrocyte life span.

Nutritional aspects of haemolytic disorders

In most haemolytic disorders, haemoglobin is broken down extravascularly and the iron and globin chains are recycled within the body. For this reason, there is not usually any iron deficiency in uncomplicated haemolytic disorders. However, folic acid is often administered in chronic haemolytic disorders to avoid megaloblastic changes which can arise due to folate depletion resulting from high rates of erythropoiesis.

Blood loss

Blood loss causes erythrocytes to leave the circulation prematurely, though the effects of *acute* and *chronic* blood loss differ. Acute blood loss leads to a fall in total blood haemoglobin over the first 24 hours. Normally, the bone marrow makes up the deficit in red cell numbers within a few weeks, as long as bleeding does not continue.

In prolonged (chronic) blood loss there is often insufficient iron available from dietary sources to compensate for that which has been lost from the body. Thus, in chronic blood loss of a degree sufficient to cause anaemia, the eventual outcome is invariably iron deficiency. Lack of iron leads to impaired haemoglobin synthesis and this, added to the requirement for increased erythropoiesis to replace lost red blood cells, results in anaemia.

Chronic blood loss, including that due to menstruation, is an important cause of iron deficiency anaemia. However, (as mentioned earlier) iron deficiency may also be due to malabsorption or to poor diet (see also Chapter 16).

Classification of anaemia

When a patient is first recognized to be anaemic the underlying cause is not always immediately apparent, so laboratory data are used as a basis for further investigations. Anaemia is initially classified on the basis of erythrocyte size and morphology. The average size of the erythrocytes, measured as *mean cell volume* (MCV) is most useful in defining the type of anaemia, which is provisionally classified as *normocytic* (normal MCV), *microcytic* (reduced MCV) or *macrocytic* (high MCV).

Mean cell haemoglobin (MCH) (the amount of haemoglobin in the average erythrocyte) and erythrocyte morphology on stained blood films are also important. If staining intensity is reduced

Table 20.2 Laboratory classification of anaemia

	Hb	RBC	MCV	MCH
Microcytic hypochromic	Low	Variable	Low	Low
Normocytic normochromic	Low	Low	Normal	Normal
Macrocytic normochromic	Low	Low	High	Normal/high

the red cells are described as *hypochromic*, which usually correlates with a low mean cell haemoglobin. Measurement of total haemoglobin concentration, *erythrocyte count* (RBC), MCV and MCH enable different types of anaemia to be described as microcytic hypochromic, macrocytic normochromic, and normocytic normochromic (Table 20.2, p. 172).

Classification of anaemia on the basis of cell size gives little information on the specific underlying cause(s) in individual cases. However, it does indicate some possible groups of causes and helps to exclude others, so that further investigations to identify the precise aetiology of the anaemia may be initiated. As with other disorders, the aetiology of anaemia can be multifactoral, and the precise cause is not always obvious. Table 20.3 shows some possible causes of microcytic, normocytic and macrocytic anaemias.

Table 20.3 Classification of anaemia

MICROCYTIC ANAEMIA
Reduced mean cell volume (MCV <80 fl approx)

May be
Hypochromic or sometimes normochromic

Examples
Iron deficiency anaemia
Anaemia of chronic inflammatory disease (e.g. rheumatoid arthritis)
Thalassaemia

MACROCYTIC ANAEMIA
Increased mean cell volume (MCV >95 fl approx)

Two types – megaloblastic or non-megaloblastic:
Megaloblastic (macrocytosis due to megaloblastic erythropoiesis)
Examples
Vitamin B_{12} or folate deficiency
Acute leukaemia with megaloblastic changes in the bone marrow

Non-megaloblastic (macrocytosis without megaloblastic change)
Examples
Some cases of liver disease
Alcoholism (but note that folate deficiency may have a role)
Some haemolytic anaemias

NORMOCYTIC ANAEMIA
Normal mean cell volume (usually normochromic, and normocytic anaemia)

Examples
Acute blood loss
Some haemolytic anaemias
Some anaemias of chronic duration (e.g. chronic renal failure),
Hypoplastic or aplastic anaemias, malignancy, pregnancy

Summary

The aim of this chapter has been to review the major causes of anaemia. In this volume, it is only possible to give an overview, and readers wishing to consider the subject in greater depth are advised to refer to the texts listed for further reading.

Key points

1 The four basic causes of anaemia are defective haemoglobin synthesis, diminished erythrocyte production, excessive erythrocyte destruction and blood loss.
2 Iron deficiency anaemia can arise from poor diet, malabsorption or from chronic blood loss.
3 The haemoglobinopathies and thalassaemia syndromes are inherited conditions affecting haemoglobin synthesis and structure.
4 Erythropoiesis is reduced in aplastic anaemia and in leukaemic infiltration of bone marrow.
5 Vitamin B_{12} and folate deficiencies cause megaloblastic changes to erythropoiesis.
6 Haemolytic disorders may be inherited or acquired. Some inherited haemolytic disorders have a high incidence in certain population groups.
7 Anaemia may be provisionally classified on the basis of cell size and morphology.

Further reading

Hoffbrand A.V. & Pettit J.E. (1993) *Essential Haematology*, 3rd edn. Blackwell Scientific Publications, Oxford.
Hughes-Jones N.C. & Wickramasinghe S.N. (1991) *Lecture Notes on Haematology*, 5th edn. Blackwell Scientific Publications, Oxford.

Disorders of Haemostasis

Introduction

The haemostatic system helps to ensure that blood is confined to, and flows freely within, the circulatory system. The process of normal haemostasis involves: platelets; vascular endothelium; the blood coagulation cascade; and a wide range of substances which promote or inhibit clot formation. Haemostatic mechanisms thus contribute to the maintenance of efficient blood flow, and to the arrest of bleeding from injured blood vessels.

This chapter considers those circulatory disorders that result from defects in haemostatic mechanisms.

An overview of haemostasis

Complex haemostatic processes have evolved to prevent excessive blood loss after injury and to maintain circulatory system integrity. These processes depend upon the interaction of the three factors outlined below.

1 The blood vessel wall, in which endothelial damage initiates clotting processes.
2 Circulating blood platelets, which are activated by vessel wall injury or other tissue damage.
3 The blood coagulation and fibrinolytic mechanisms, and their respective inhibitors.

Disturbance of any aspect of haemostasis can lead to either bleeding or *thrombosis* (formation of a clot within the vascular system). Expressed very simply, most bleeding disorders are due to underactive haemostasis, and many thrombotic disorders are due, at least in part, to overactive haemostatic mechanisms.

The arrest of bleeding

The physiological mechanisms underlying the arrest of bleeding are two-fold, and are explained below.
1 *Vasoconstriction* (narrowing of blood vessels) to help prevent further blood loss.
and
2 Formation at the site of injury of a *haemostatic plug* (a 'clot') derived from platelets and fibrin strands, in which erythrocytes and leucocytes become trapped. The fibrin strands are formed by activation of the blood coagulation cascade, culminating in the conversion of fibrinogen to fibrin (Fig. 21.1).

Because this process is so potent, control mechanisms are required to prevent extension of a clot once it has formed. These control mechanisms include *blood flow* (which washes away activated coagulation factors), *prostacyclin production* by vascular endothelium (which inhibits platelet activity), *fibrinolysis* (which dissolves clots) and inhibitors of plasma coagulation factors.

Platelet structure and physiology

Platelets are cytoplasmic fragments derived from megakaryocytes and are able to survive in the circulation for up to 10 days. Electron microscopy of platelets reveals three zones (Fig. 21.2) as listed below.
1 The *outer zone*, which is membrane-associated. This has a role in platelet adhesion and aggregation and interacts with the blood coagulation cascade. Platelet membrane phospholipid participates in blood coagulation and several plasma coagulation factors, including fibrinogen, are present on the platelet surface.
2 The *sol gel zone* (*cytosol*) which contains contractile proteins, microfilaments and microtubules.

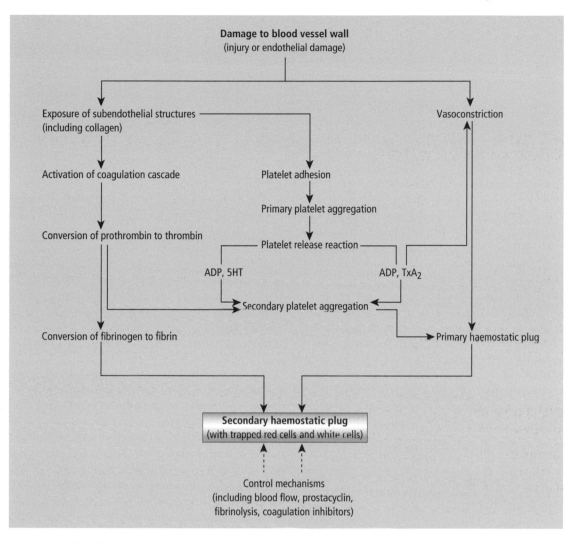

Fig. 21.1 Principles of haemostasis showing involvement of blood vessels, platelets, the blood coagulation cascade, and control mechanisms. Vascular injury and exposure of the subendothelium cause vasoconstriction and activation of platelets and the blood coagulation cascade. Complex interactions between these three mechanisms result in the conversion of fibrinogen to fibrin, and the formation of primary and secondary haemostatic plugs. Control mechanisms limit any unnecessary extension of the clot. (Key ADP, adenosine diphosphate; TxA$_2$, thromboxane A$_2$; 5HT, 5 hydroxytryptamine.)

The cytosol contents contribute to platelet shape change, adhesion, aggregation, and the 'release reaction' (see below).

3 *Platelet organelles* (dense bodies, alpha granules and lysosomes), containing a variety of haemostatically active compounds which are released when platelets are activated.

Once activated, normal platelets adhere to the damaged vessel wall, aggregate to one another and release their granule contents—which include adenosine diphosphate (ADP), 5 hydroxytryptamine (5HT also referred to as serotonin), adrenaline and thromboxane A$_2$ (TxA$_2$). Release of these components further potentiates platelet activity.

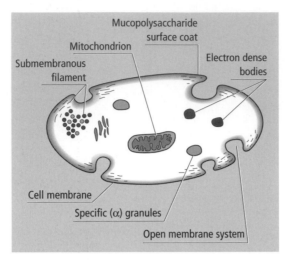

Fig. 21.2 Platelet ultrastructure. A diagrammatic representation of a blood platelet in section. The outer zone consists of a mucopolysaccharide surface coat, submembranous filaments and open and closed membrane systems which provide phospholipid for participation in the coagulation cascade. Within the cytosol are further membrane systems, microfilaments and microtubules. Electron-dense bodies contain adenosine diphosphate (ADP), serotonin and calcium, all of which participate in the platelet release reaction. Specific (alpha) granules contain growth factors, fibrinogen and other pro-coagulant substances. Platelets are rich in mitochondria which satisfy their high demand for energy.

This phase culminates in the formation of a *primary haemostatic plug* at the site of injury. Simultaneous activation of the coagulation cascade, initiated in part by platelet activation, results in the incorporation of fibrin into a *secondary haemostatic plug*.

Prostaglandin metabolism in platelets and blood vessels

Platelet aggregation is stimulated by exposure to a range of substances including *collagen* and *thrombin*, the latter being formed in the coagulation cascade. Thrombin binds to receptors on the vascular endothelium and on platelet membranes. This causes release of arachidonic acid which is metabolized by cyclo-oxygenase to prostaglandin G_2 (PGG_2). PGG_2 is further metabolized to TxA_2 in platelets, and to prostacyclin (PGI_2) in the vascular endothelium.

TxA_2 and PGI_2 have opposing effects on platelet adenylate cyclase: PGI_2 stimulates activity of this enzyme causing an increase in cyclic AMP, thus lowering free calcium ion concentrations and reducing platelet adhesion and aggregation. In addition to its inhibitory effect on platelets, PGI_2 is a vasodilator, whereas TxA_2 has the opposite effect, acting as a vasoconstrictor and a potent inducer of platelet aggregation (Fig. 21.3).

Regular ingestion of low dose aspirin (acetylsalicylic acid) is thought to have some protective effect against arterial thrombosis in susceptible patients. Aspirin inhibits platelet cyclo-oxygenase, thereby reducing TxA_2 production for the life of those platelets in circulation at the time. The inhibition of endothelial cyclo-oxygenase is transient, so the overall effect is an excess of PGI_2 over TxA_2, thus reducing platelet activity.

The blood coagulation cascade and its control

The *blood coagulation cascade* exhibits the typical features of other biological cascades—i.e. amplification, specificity and control. This potent mechanism is balanced by several naturally occurring inhibitors (notably the *serine protease inhibitors* or SERPINS) and the fibrinolytic system which digests clots once they are formed.

The intrinsic and extrinsic coagulation systems

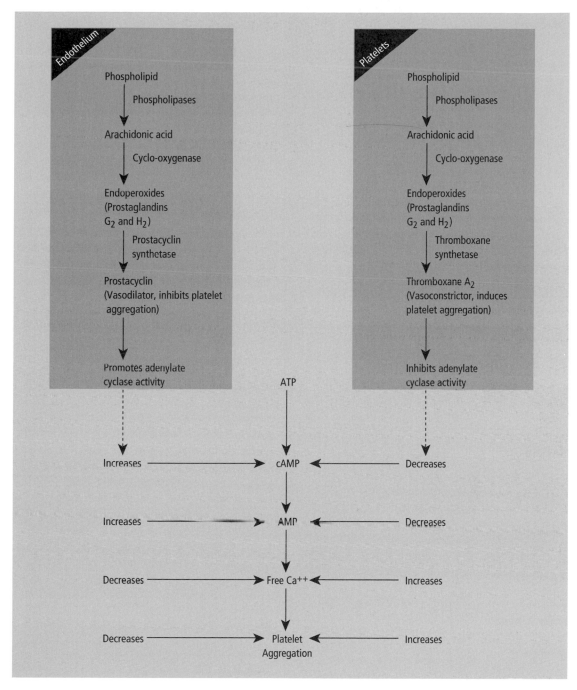

Fig. 21.3 The synthesis of prostaglandins in vascular endothelial cells and in platelets. Arachidonic acid metabolism follows different paths in vascular endothelial cells and platelets. In endothelial cells prostacyclin synthetase catalyses the conversion of endoperoxides to prostacyclin, whereas in platelets the equivalent reaction is catalysed by thromboxane synthetase to form thromboxane A_2. Prostacyclin and thromboxane A_2 have opposing actions on blood platelets.

are often depicted as separate, quite distinct mechanisms and can be demonstrated as such *in vitro*, enabling differentiation of a range of coagulation factor defects. However, there is evidence that, *in vivo*, there is integration of extrinsic and intrinsic coagulation cascades, interaction with platelets (via membrane phospholipid) and also a relationship to inflammatory events (via the complement and kinin systems, see Chapter 4). In addition, there are several examples of feedback within the coagulation cascade, and a simultaneous activation of the fibrinolytic system (Fig. 21.4).

Role of the vascular endothelium in haemostasis

Healthy vascular endothelium opposes coagulation by producing prostacyclin, which inhibits platelet aggregation. Other substances opposing clot formation include tissue plasminogen activator (tPA) which stimulates fibrinolysis, and the coagulation inhibitors anti-thrombin III and thrombomodulin.

Conversely, endothelial cells synthesize *von Willebrand factor*, a procoagulant protein which promotes platelet adhesion and aggregation, and acts as a carrier for the factor VIII coagulation factor. Thus, healthy vascular endothelium contributes to both promotion and inhibition of blood coagulation.

Haemostatic involvement in thrombotic and bleeding disorders

Factors contributing to bleeding and thrombosis

Bleeding

Most bleeding (*haemorrhagic*) disorders arise from deficiencies in platelets or plasma coagulation factors, although increases in fibrinolysis or coagulation inhibitors may also be implicated.

Thrombosis

During the 19th century, Virchow described three factors contributing to the onset of thrombosis, which later became known as *Virchow's triad*. These were: damage to the inner surface of the vessel wall; disturbed blood flow and altered 'blood mechanisms'.

Virchow's 'blood mechanisms' are now known to be haemostatic systems involving complex interaction between the vascular endothelium, platelets and the blood coagulation cascade. One or more of the three factors described by Virchow contribute to most arterial and venous thromboembolic disorders.

Clinical conditions arising from disturbed haemostasis

Activation of haemostasis may result from the following damage.
1 Trauma or other physical damage requiring activation of haemostatic mechanisms to prevent blood loss.
2 Endothelial damage, often associated with atherosclerosis, causing abnormal haemostatic activation which can result in vessel occlusion.
Thus, haemostatic disorders may be divided into two categories.
1 Disorders of underactivity—bleeding disorders such as *haemophilia A, Christmas disease*, or *thrombocytopenic purpura*.
2 Disorders of overactivity—thrombotic disorders such as *thrombotic stroke*; *coronary heart disease*; and *deep venous thrombosis* (Table 21.1). However, it must be emphasized that many additional factors contribute to the pathogenesis of thrombotic disorders, particularly lipid imbalances associated with atherosclerosis (see Chapter 22).

Bleeding disorders

Abnormal bleeding may arise from defects in platelets, blood coagulation factor disorders (either congenital or acquired) or defects in the vascular wall. Of these, platelet defects are the

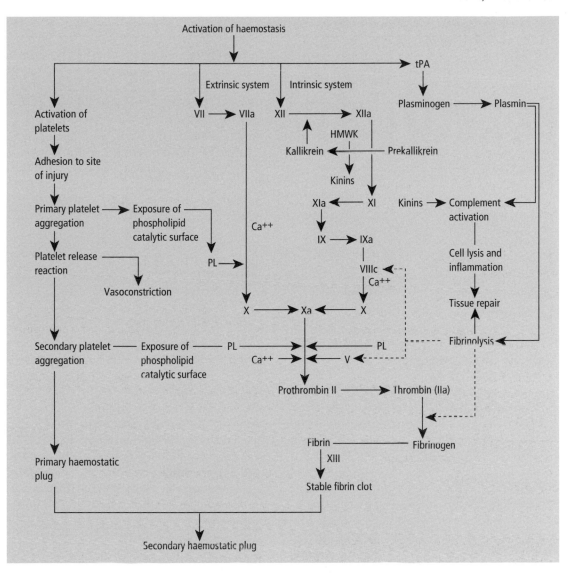

Fig. 21.4 An overview of haemostasis (showing integration of the blood coagulation cascade with other haemostatic mechanisms). Vascular injury activates the coagulation cascade, platelets and fibrinolysis. Activation of coagulation factor XII causes generation of kallikrein and kinins, which initiate complement activation and inflammation. The conversion of plasminogen to plasmin causes both complement activation and fibrinolysis. Platelet activation results in release of a range of procoagulant substances, particularly platelet phospholipid, which provides a catalytic surface for the coagulation cascade. The extrinsic and intrinsic systems of the coagulation cascade are shown as distinct entities, but there is thought to be interaction between the two *in vivo*. Proenzymes are XIII, XII, XI, IX, X, VII, II. Activated serine proteases are XIIa, XIa, IXa, Xa, VIIa, IIa. Cofactors are VIIIc and V.

PL, platelet phospholipid; tPA, tissue plasminogen activator; HMWK, high molecular weight kininogen.

Table 21.1 Haemostatic involvement in bleeding and thrombotic disorders

HAEMOSTATIC ACTIVITY	REDUCED	INCREASED
POSSIBLE CLINICAL CONSEQUENCE	BLEEDING	THROMBOSIS
Contributory haemostatic factors		
Abnormalities of the vessel wall	Cut/rupture	Atheroma Exposure of subendothelium
Platelets	Reduced numbers Reduced function	Increased numbers Increased reactivity?
Coagulation factors	Reduced concentration Abnormal structure	Increased concentration
	Increased inhibitors of coagulation	Reduced inhibitors of coagulation (Anti-thrombin III, protein C or S)
	Increased fibrinolysis	Reduced fibrinolysis
Other causes		Reduced blood flow Increased blood viscosity Hyperlipidaemia

most common, followed by coagulation factor disorders. Bleeding due primarily to disorders of the vascular wall is rare.

Platelet disorders

Platelet disorders are usually acquired. *Thrombocytopenia* (reduction in platelet numbers) usually presents with superficial bleeding (*petechiae* or *bruising*) and may be due to failure of platelet production or shortened platelet survival. Most cases of *idiopathic thrombocytopenic purpura* (ITP) are now recognized to be autoimmune in origin and in such cases circulating IgG autoantibodies to platelets can be identified. Drugs can also induce an autoimmune response to platelets, resulting in thrombocytopenia, although some drugs also depress megakaryocyte production. Other conditions that produce thrombocytopenia include aplastic anaemia (see Chapter 20) and leukaemia.

Defects in platelet function rarely cause major spontaneous bleeding, though they may increase blood loss after dental extraction or surgery. Ingestion of aspirin or other non-steroidal anti-inflammatory agents blocks the activity of platelet cyclo-oxygenase, causing a characteristic transient defect in platelet function. However, this is rarely sufficient to cause bleeding alone, but may exacerbate bleeding from other lesions, for example, tumours.

Congenital coagulation disorders

The best known of the congenital bleeding disorders are *haemophilia A* and *haemophilia* B (*Christmas disease*) which are due to deficiencies of factor VIIIc and factor IX respectively. The inheritance of both conditions is X-linked and both are characterized by painful spontaneous bleeding into joints and muscles. *Von Willebrand's disease* is a rare inherited autosomal bleeding disorder due to deficiency of von Willebrand factor, resulting in reduced factor VIII coagulant activity and abnormal platelet function.

Acquired bleeding disorders

Examples of acquired coagulation factor disorders are seen in liver disease and *disseminated intravascular coagulation* (DIC). In liver disease there is often a reduction in several blood coagulation factors, particularly those that depend on vitamin K for their synthesis (see Chapter 17). DIC is characterized by widespread deposition of *microthrombi* (small blood clots) with consequent depletion in platelets and coagulation factors, and a high risk of spontaneous bleeding. DIC is often associated with leukaemias, other malignant blood disorders, and may occur as a complication in pregnancy or childbirth.

Thrombotic disorders

It appears that different components of the haemostatic system may predominate in venous and arterial thrombosis. In general, venous *thrombo-embolism* (see below) is often triggered by changes in blood coagulation factors or their inhibitors together with reduced or sluggish blood flow, while arterial thrombosis is usually associated with damage to the vascular endothelium and increased platelet activity. However, these are not mutually exclusive—for example, increased blood fibrinogen concentration has been linked to increased risk of coronary artery occlusion, and platelets are undoubtedly involved in the pathogenesis of venous thrombosis.

Venous thrombo-embolism

An *embolus* is defined as a clot (or other form of solid material, such as fat, or an air bubble) that is transported in the circulatory system. *Thrombo-embolism* is the occlusion of a blood vessel by a clot which originated in a larger vessel and which has been carried in the circulatory system from its original site.

Typically, venous thrombi form initially in the deep veins of the leg(s) following surgical operations with prolonged bed rest. This is associated with relative stasis of blood flow and the post-operative *hypercoagulable state*, which is character-

ized by raised concentrations of some blood coagulation factors. The fibrinolytic system is activated and gradually dissolves any clots, but fragments may break off to form emboli. These pass through the vena cava and the right chambers of the heart, but lodge in the pulmonary circulation resulting in *pulmonary embolism* (PE). PE results in reduced perfusion of the lungs, varying in severity depending on the site and size of the occluded vessel. Acute chest pain and *haemoptysis* (coughing up of blood-stained sputum) are among the typical clinical features. Small pulmonary emboli may produce few signs and symptoms whereas large emboli can result in sudden death.

Although the causes of most venous thrombosis, for example that following surgery, can be readily explained, in a small proportion of patients other factors are thought to be responsible. For example, unexplained or recurrent venous thrombosis is sometimes associated with oestrogen therapy or various malignant diseases.

Deficiencies of coagulation inhibitors, particularly protein C, its cofactor protein S, and antithrombin III, although rare are increasingly recognized as potential causes of venous thrombosis.

Arterial thrombosis

Atheroma (see Chapter 22) undoubtedly predisposes to arterial thrombosis. Interaction between blood platelets and atheromatous deposits appears to be fundamental to the development of thrombotic arterial occlusion. These events are briefly summarized as follows.

1 Atheromatous damage to the arterial intima or exposure of subendothelial structures triggers platelet activation.

2 This is followed by adhesion of platelets to the site of injury, platelet shape change and primary aggregation, the platelet release reaction and further aggregation.

3 Platelets secrete *platelet-derived growth factor* (PDGF) during the release reaction. PDGF causes mitotic division of intimal smooth-muscle cells, and migration of medial smooth-muscle cells to

the arterial intima. Thus, localized activation of platelets exacerbates damage to the intima of the blood vessel.

4 Simultaneous activation of the blood coagulation cascade also occurs, enhanced by the platelet release reactions, and fibrin becomes associated with the platelet aggregates, trapping red cells. The resulting thrombus may extend, partially or fully occluding the vessel, though fibrinolytic mechanisms are also activated to limit this spread.

The precise aetiology of arterial atheromatous change has not yet been clearly elucidated. Fatty streaks are common in young people and may be reversible, though they may progress to form *atheromatous plaques*, which are less easy to reverse and are associated with intimal damage. The cause of this initial endothelial damage is unclear, though it has been postulated that atheroma may form as a reaction to free radical damage (see Chapter 22). As aforementioned, complete vascular occlusion is one possible consequence of atheromatous change.

The clinically important result of haemostatic activation in atherosclerosis is vessel occlusion. This denies an area of tissue of its blood supply (causing *ischaemia*). If this occurs in the coronary arteries which supply the heart muscle (*myocardium*), reduced blood flow results in myocardial ischaemia, and this in turn can lead to chest pain on exertion (*angina pectoris*). Complete coronary artery occlusion results in the death of an affected area of heart muscle, a condition known as *myocardial infarction* (MI). Among predisposing factors for MI are: high blood lipids and atherosclerosis (see Chapter 22); increased platelet activity; raised blood coagulation factors; hypertension (see Chapter 23); and vasoconstriction or arterial spasm.

Summary

This chapter has briefly reviewed some haemostatic imbalances which contribute to bleeding and thrombosis. Efficient haemostasis depends on a complex interaction of compounds released from vascular endothelium, blood platelets, and the coagulation cascade and all their integrating, promoting and inhibitory factors.

Our current concepts of the detailed contribution of haemostatic mechanisms to the aetiology and pathogenesis of bleeding and thrombotic disorders are constantly being refined, with important developments in understanding currently taking place.

Key points

1 Activation of haemostatic mechanisms involving blood platelets and the coagulation cascade follows damage to the vascular endothelium.

2 Following physical or traumatic damage, haemostatic mechanisms are triggered to prevent excessive blood loss.

3 Disorders of haemostasis cause a number of bleeding disorders, both congenital and acquired.

4 Haemostatic imbalance is also associated with certain arterial and venous thrombo-embolic disorders.

5 Reduced blood flow and venous stasis, together with raised coagulation factor concentrations (particularly post-operatively), or reduced coagulation inhibitors, predispose to venous thrombo-embolism.

6 In arteries, where endothelial injury is associated with atheromatous deposits, haemostatic activation appears to exacerbate the damage, often resulting in thrombus formation.

Further reading

Ball M. & Mann J. (1988) *Lipids and Heart Disease—A Practical Approach*. Oxford University Press, Oxford.

Hoffbrand A. V. & Pettit J.E. (1993) *Essential Haematology*. Blackwell Scientific Publications, Oxford.

Atherosclerosis

Introduction

Coronary heart disease (CHD) is a major cause of disability and death in the Western world. In the past decade, over 160 000 people in the UK have died each year from CHD and more significantly 30 000 of the men who died each year were aged less than 65. The causes of CHD are multifactorial, but the principal pathological process associated with CHD is *atherosclerosis*, which means hardening of the arteries and is caused by *atheroma*. The term atheroma describes a degenerative accumulation of lipids, collagen and smooth muscle fibres on the inner surface of an artery. This chapter considers the major factors believed to contribute to the pathogenesis of atherosclerosis.

Overview

The pathogenesis of atherosclerosis is complex, probably multifactorial and is not yet completely understood. Atherosclerosis is characterized by a progressive accumulation within the arterial wall of cholesterol-containing particles, cells, cell fragments and support matrix materials such as fibrin. Over a period of years this results in the development, on the inner surface of the artery, of *atheromatous plaques* composed of these elements. In time, this can result in narrowing of the arterial lumen which may become life-threatening. Blood flow may be compromised to such an extent that vital organs are deprived of oxygen, resulting in the development of *ischaemia* (reduced oxygen supply) in the tissues supplied by the affected arteries.

Clinical examples of the effects of ischaemia are *angina pectoris* (chest pain on exertion due to ischaemia affecting heart muscle) or *intermittent claudication* (pains in the calves of the legs when walking). Furthermore, thrombosis (see Chapter 21) may develop at the site of an atheromatous plaque. If this occurs in the coronary arteries that supply the myocardium, the resultant ischaemia may lead to death of myocardial tissue (myocardial infarction) producing the clinical effects of a heart attack.

Although the precise causes of atherosclerosis have not yet been fully elucidated, it is known that certain other diseases or particular lifestyles confer a high risk of development of atherosclerosis. Typical 'risk factors' include hypertension (see Chapter 23), cigarette smoking and diabetes mellitus, each of which is discussed in more detail later in the chapter.

The aetiology and pathogenesis of atherosclerosis

The normal human artery is composed of several layers (Fig. 22.1), as described below.

1 The *tunica intima*, an inner smooth uninterrupted monolayer of endothelial cells overlying a thin layer of connective tissue matrix, scattered within which are small numbers of smooth-muscle cells, together with collagen and *glucosaminoglycans* (GAG). The intima is bounded by elastic tissue (the internal elastic lamina).

2 The *tunica media*, a thick layer of smooth-muscle cells separated by small amounts of elastin, collagen and GAG.

3 The *tunica adventitia*, an external layer of connective tissue, separated from the media by the external elastic lamina. The adventitia consists of collagen, fibroblasts and GAG.

Atheromatous plaques usually arise in the arterial intima, typically causing narrowing of the

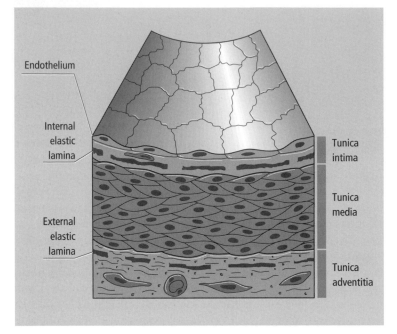

Fig. 22.1 Structure of a normal human artery. The main layers of the arterial wall are the intima, media and adventitia, with the internal elastic lamina and the external elastic lamina separating these layers.

Endothelium

Internal elastic lamina

External elastic lamina

Tunica intima

Tunica media

Tunica adventitia

lumen. This may eventually lead to complete occlusion of the vessel lumen, particularly if there is also secondary activation of haemostasis, resulting in thrombus formation (see Chapter 21). Many factors are thought to contribute to the development of atherosclerosis, and two hypotheses of current interest will be discussed in some detail. These are the *lipid hypothesis* and the *endothelial injury hypothesis*.

The lipid hypothesis

Lipids (fats) are transported in the bloodstream in a variety of particles containing greater or lesser amounts of cholesterol and triglyceride. The major particles which transport lipids are: *chylomicrons* (and chylomicron remnants which are triglyceride rich); *very low density lipoproteins* (VLDL, triglyceride rich); *low density lipoproteins* (LDL, cholesterol rich) and *high density lipoproteins* (HDL, cholesterol rich). A schematic diagram of plasma lipoprotein metabolism is shown in Fig. 22.2.

Despite the popular view that all forms of blood lipid are 'harmful', not all of these lipid transport molecules are implicated in the development of atherosclerosis. For example chylomicron metabolism has not been shown to have any relationship to atherosclerosis. However, LDL is the major carrier particle for cholesterol in plasma, and much of the mechanistic evidence relating it to the development of atherosclerosis is strong. The major precursor particle for LDL, VLDL, which is triglyceride rich may also be linked to the development of atherosclerosis, but the evidence of a causal relationship with this particle is less strong.

HDL is secreted from the liver as a protein-rich particle which contains small amounts of cholesterol. Once in the circulation, the HDL particle has the ability to acquire and exchange cholesterol from other circulating lipoprotein particles (including LDL) and can directly take up cholesterol from arterial intima. The importance of HDL is that its plasma concentration is inversely related to the risk of heart disease. By comparison, the risk of heart disease is directly related to the concentration of cholesterol in LDL. Thus, high plasma concentrations of LDL cholesterol confer a relatively higher risk of CHD, whereas the

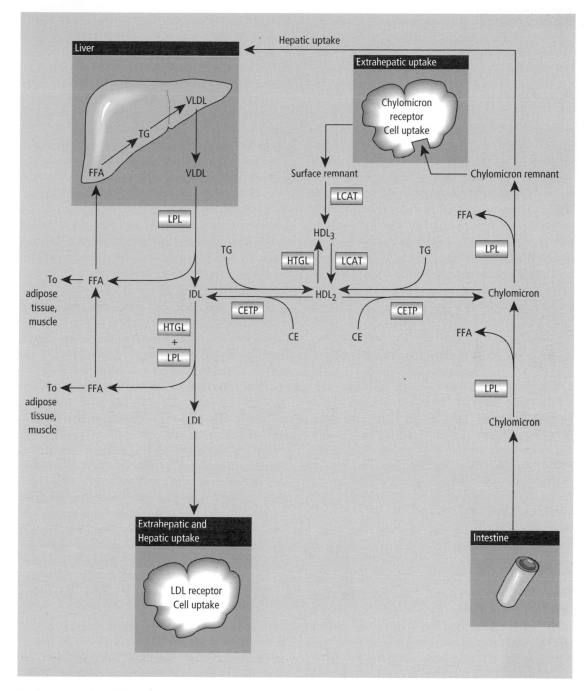

Fig. 22.2 An overview of lipoprotein metabolism. Dietary fats and cholesterol are absorbed from the gut and assembled as triglyceride-rich chylomicrons. Lipoprotein lipase (LPL), in the capillary walls of muscle or adipose tissue, releases free fatty acids (FFA) and monoglycerides. As the fats are removed, the chylomicrons reduce in size, their density increases and the remaining cholesterol is carried as high density lipoprotein (HDL). HDL circulates in the blood and is taken up by liver cells where some is metabolized to VLDL. Circulating VLDL is a substrate for lipoprotein lipase and is converted via intermediate density lipoprotein (IDL) to HDL or LDL. Specific cell receptors allow capture of LDL for cell membrane synthesis and energy requirements. Excess LDL in the blood predisposes to atheroma formation. (Lipid subfraction: CE, cholesterol; FFA, free fatty acids; TG, triglycerides; VLDL, very low density lipoprotein; HDL, high density lipoprotein. Enzymes: LPL, lipoprotein lipase; CETP, cholesterol esterase transfer proteins; HTGL, hepatic triglyceride lipase; LCAT, lecithin cholesterol acyl transferase.)

reverse is true for high concentrations of HDL cholesterol.

Lipoprotein tissue uptake

Uptake of LDL into cells is by one of two mechanisms these being the *classical receptor-mediated pathway* and *non-receptor uptake of LDL*.

The classical receptor-mediated uptake pathway described by J. L. Goldstein and M. S. Brown (1979) involves a receptor (the *apolipoprotein B100 receptor*) present on cell membranes (for example in liver) which recognizes apolipoprotein B100 on LDL particles. The receptor and the bound lipoprotein are taken up by the cell and the lipoprotein particle is broken down by *lysosomal degradation*, resulting in the release of free cholesterol. The release of free cholesterol completes a feedback loop which prevents further biosynthesis of cholesterol within tissues that are capable of *de novo* synthesis.

Non-receptor-mediated uptake occurs by endocytosis in a variety of cells in the presence of high concentrations of LDL. In addition there is uptake of 'modified' LDL by phagocytic cells, particularly monocytes and macrophages. LDL particles undergo modification, including oxidation by free radicals, which allows them to bind to the modified LDL receptor (or 'scavenger' receptor) on macrophages. The susceptibility of LDL particles to free radical damage (including oxidation, acetylation or butylation) may also directly induce endothelial damage.

The interaction of LDL with monocytes which have migrated to the intima, initiates the transformation of these cells into lipid-laden macrophages and ultimately they become 'foam cells' packed with lipid. These foam cells in the intima are typical findings in early atherosclerosis.

The endothelial injury hypothesis

Although it is clear that lipid accumulation is one of the important early events in the development of atherosclerosis, other pathological mechanisms also have a role. The *endothelial injury hypothesis* (advanced as long ago as 1949 by J. B. Duguid,

from a model first proposed in 1856 by R. Virchow), is also likely to be of primary importance in the development of atheromatous lesions. The deposition of lipids within the intima early in atherosclerosis produces fatty streaks within the artery which are visible macroscopically. Fatty streaks result in endothelial disruption and when this occurs a variety of other cellular constituents in blood are activated. The coagulation cascade and other haemostatic mechanisms (see Chapter 21) are stimulated by local cell injury. Tissue factors are released and these further activate blood coagulation, resulting in the generation of thrombin and fibrin, the activation of platelets and the secretion of local growth factors from endothelial cells.

The presence of fibrin promotes the secretion of growth factors that stimulate the proliferation of smooth-muscle cells in the arterial intima. Fibrin may also bind lipoproteins. The migration of smooth-muscle cells to the subendothelial layers and their subsequent mitotic division is partly under the influence of *platelet-derived growth factor* (PDGF) released from platelets activated during haemostasis (see Chapter 21).

Collagen fibres are also laid down within the tunica media and at this stage the fatty streak can be identified as an atheromatous plaque. Other major components of the plaque are soft tissue, cholesterol (from LDL) within foam cells and GAG. The production of tissue growth factors activates more macrophages and activation of the coagulation cascade is further perpetuated.

Progression of atherosclerosis

If the atherosclerotic plaque progresses, it changes from a *simple lesion* to a *complicated lesion*, so called because it becomes unstable as haemorrhage and ulceration of tissue adjacent to the plaque occur. Although the surface of the plaque may be fibrous, the centre of the lesion can become necrotic and liquify as coagulation factors and LDL continue to accumulate (Fig. 22.3). The plaque may develop in one of the following three directions.

1 The necrotic centre can stabilize and produce an ever widening and protruding fibrous plaque.

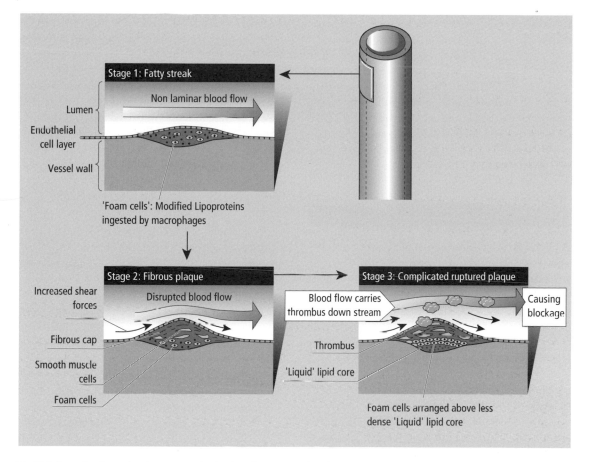

Fig. 22.3 Stages in atherosclerosis. Fatty streaks develop when macrophages containing LDL and triglycerides (foam cells) accumulate in the subendothelium. There is minimal effect on blood flow at this stage. Subsequently, smooth-muscle cells and fibroblasts migrate to the area, and a fibrous cap forms over the lesion (which is now termed a fibrous plaque). Blood flow is disturbed and shear forces increase. Any rupture of the fibrous plaque is associated with activation of platelets and the blood coagulation cascade which causes thrombus formation. This may itself cause local vessel occlusion or the thrombus may dislodge to form an embolus which is carried in the blood, eventually to lodge in a smaller vessel, causing occlusion at this distant site.

With gradual evolution the plaque can slowly occlude the arterial lumen.

2 A more catastrophic end-point is the rupture of the necrotic centre through the middle of the fibrous plaque into the arterial lumen. The release of contents from the necrotic centre can activate coagulation, causing thrombus formation and leading to blockage within that part of the lumen.

3 Alternatively, the arterial flow may take the contents and/or any thrombus to an area distal to the rupture, where occlusion can occur, an event known as *embolism*.

The postulated role of lipoprotein(a)

The lipid hypothesis and the endothelial injury hypothesis are not mutually exclusive and both are likely to contribute to the atherosclerotic process. A further link between the lipid and the endothelial injury hypotheses is the 'rediscovery' of *lipoprotein(a)* (Lp(a)), a particle which contains LDL linked by a disulphide bridge to *apolipoprotein(a)*. Apolipoprotein(a) shows remarkable similarities to *plasminogen* (a fibrinolytic pro-enzyme) and contains the same binding domain. Plasminogen receptors are usually exposed in areas where blood coagulation has been activated, for example at the site of a thrombus.

It is thought that Lp(a), binds to plasminogen receptors, inhibiting the formation of plasmin and thus preventing dissolution of the clot. Furthermore, the binding of Lp(a) to plasminogen receptors in areas where there is thrombus formation, introduces further lipid (especially cholesterol), which can be modified and taken up to perpetuate intimal damage.

Other factors in atherosclerosis

While it is clear that high plasma lipid concentrations contribute to the production of the fatty streak and ultimately to the atheromatous plaque, the high incidence of heart disease in the Western world cannot be explained simply by raised plasma cholesterol concentrations. Other major risk factors for coronary artery disease include smoking, hypertension and diabetes mellitus.

Smoking

Smoking causes a variety of changes within the arterial circulation. These include: *vasoconstriction* (as a direct result of the action of nicotine), *reduced metabolism of VLDL* and an *increase in the production of lipoprotein particles* that are intermediate in density between the VLDL and LDL (and are therefore called intermediate density lipoproteins or IDL). These intermediate particles are potentially important in the development of atherosclerosis since they are not taken up by the classical apolipoprotein B100 receptor-mediated pathway and are susceptible to oxidation because of their high concentrations of cholesterol. Another of the changes associated with smoking is *an increase in plasma fibrinogen concentrations*. This promotes platelet aggregation and initiates activation of the coagulation cascade in areas already affected by vascular damage.

Hypertension

The result of hypertension is to produce smooth muscle hypertrophy (thickening of the medial layers of the arteries). This in turn causes a restriction in the arterial lumen size. Increased pressure of blood acts on the arteries to cause hydrodynamic stress and this produces increased *shear* (i.e. the difference between blood flow in the centre of the lumen of an artery and that at the wall). These high shear forces within arteries cause direct mechanical injury to the arterial endothelium and subsequent activation of coagulation processes.

Diabetes mellitus

Diabetes mellitus causes a variety of tissue changes which are the result of high concentrations of plasma glucose (see Case Study 24.3). Glycation of proteins, both in plasma and in cells, may cause alteration of their properties and activate haemostasis. Furthermore, diabetes potentiates the modification of lipoprotein particles, increasing the amount of intermediate density lipoproteins and altering the structure and composition of LDL particles, making them more susceptible to oxidative damage.

Summary

Atherosclerosis develops over a period of years, and can eventually cause complete arterial occlusion. Endothelial injury, hyperlipidaemia, activation of the blood coagulation cascade and activation of platelets all contribute to its pathogenesis. At present, the most effective strategy to reduce the incidence of coronary heart disease is prevention of atherosclerosis. Risk factors for atherosclerosis should be identified in individual patients. Treatment aims to reduce risk factors, principally by modification of lifestyle, and focuses on: (i) cessation of smoking; (ii) identification and treatment of individuals with hypertension; (iii) reduction of fat content in the diet; (iv) identification and treatment of diabetes mellitus and; (v) modification of haemostatic mechanisms in patients at high risk of thrombosis.

Key points

1 Coronary heart disease (CHD) is a disorder causing substantial morbidity and mortality in Western societies. The major pathological process associated with CHD is atherosclerosis.

2 Atherosclerotic plaques develop slowly and are characterized by a gradual accumulation of cholesterol, triglycerides, connective tissue and smooth-muscle cells in the arterial intima.

3 Hyperlipidaemia, and particularly raised concentrations of LDL cholesterol, predispose to the development of atherosclerosis. Conversely, HDL cholesterol appears to confer some protection against the development of atherosclerosis.

4 Endothelial injury has been implicated in the development of atherosclerosis. Free radicals are thought to modify lipoproteins, enhancing their uptake into atherosclerotic lesions.

5 Activation of both the coagulation cascade and of platelets contributes to thrombosis, but may also promote the development of atherosclerosis. Release of platelet-derived growth factor by platelets causes migration of smooth-muscle cells to the arterial intima and also promotes their mitotic division.

6 Complications of atherosclerosis include necrosis and fissuring of the fibrous plaque, which may activate haemostatic mechanisms leading to thrombosis. Embolism occurs when a fragment of atheroma or thrombus breaks away and lodges elsewhere.

7 Strategies to prevent atherosclerosis include dietary modification, cessation of smoking, effective treatment of hypertension and control of diabetes.

Further reading

Ball & Mann (1988) *Lipids and Heart Disease: A Practical Approach.* Oxford Medical Publications, Oxford.

Durrington, P. (1989) *Hyperlipidaemia, Diagnosis and Management.* Butterworth, Kent.

Hypertension

Introduction

High blood pressure (*hypertension*) is one of the most common conditions that a doctor sees, affecting 10–15 percent of the adult population. The majority of people with hypertension do not have any symptoms, but if untreated for some years the condition may lead to heart attack (*myocardial infarction*), stroke (*cerebrovascular accident*), or renal failure. If detected early and treated effectively, these complications can be prevented.

This chapter considers the causes of hypertension, its clinical significance and its treatment.

Physiological control of blood pressure

The main determinants of arterial blood pressure are *cardiac output* and *peripheral resistance*. In addition, an increase in arterial blood volume increases blood pressure and a decrease in arterial blood volume lowers it.

Cardiac output

Cardiac output (CO) is determined by the volume of blood pumped out of the left ventricle (*stroke volume*) and heart rate.

CO = stroke volume × heart rate

It follows that an increase in heart rate tends to increase cardiac output and thereby increases arterial blood volume and blood pressure. Stroke volume is determined primarily by the strength of the heart beat, which is regulated mainly by the length of the myocardial fibres at the commencement of their contraction. The essence of *Starling's law* is that the more stretched the heart muscle fibres are at the start of their contraction, the longer is their contraction.

Peripheral resistance

Peripheral resistance is the resistance to blood flow imposed by friction between the blood and the vessel walls. Friction depends in part on *blood viscosity* and partly on the diameter of arterioles and capillaries. Blood viscosity depends on red cell count and plasma protein concentration. An increase in either increases viscosity and thereby tends to increase blood pressure.

However, under normal circumstances blood viscosity remains fairly constant. The major factor contributing to peripheral resistance is therefore *arteriole resistance*, which accounts for around half the resistance in the circulatory system and which is profoundly affected by *arteriole vasodilatation* or *vasoconstriction*.

The *vasomotor centres*, located in the medulla, can initiate vasoconstriction via sympathetic nerve fibres to maintain blood pressure and also to control the distribution of blood to areas of special need. In addition, a sudden fall in blood pressure causes aortic and carotid baroreceptors to stimulate vasoconstriction, and a sudden increase has the opposite effect.

Other control mechanisms include *vasomotor chemoreflexes* and a *medullary ischaemic reflex*, both of which are sensitive to severe hypoxia. Higher brain centres in the hypothalamus and cortex are also thought to influence the vasomotor centres in the medulla, explaining why anxiety often raises blood pressure.

Finally, when blood pressure in the afferent arterioles of the kidney falls substantially, cells of the *juxtaglomerular apparatus* secrete *renin*, a

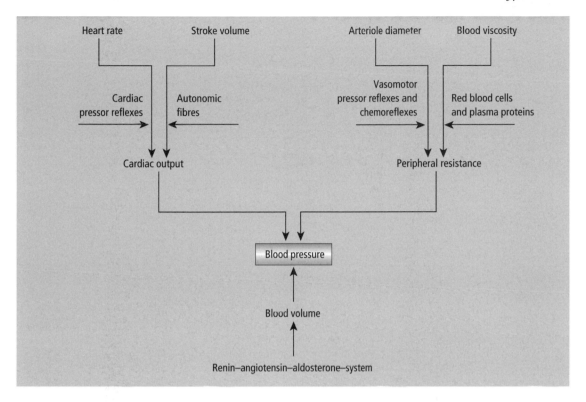

Fig. 23.1 Physiological control of blood pressure. Blood pressure is directly related to arterial blood volume which, in turn, is primarily dependent on cardiac output and peripheral resistance. Some of the many factors which regulate cardiac output and peripheral resistance are shown.

proteolytic enzyme which acts on a plasma substrate to release *angiotensin I*. Angiotensin I is inactive but is converted by *angiotensin-converting enzyme* (ACE) to angiotensin II which stimulates the release of aldosterone from the adrenal cortex. Aldosterone conserves sodium and increases reabsorption of water thereby increasing blood volume. Angiotensin II also has a direct *pressor* activity, thus increasing vasoconstriction. The renin–angiotensin–aldosterone system has important clinical implications in the regulation of blood pressure.

Thus, a series of complex homoeostatic mechanisms interact to regulate blood pressure when it falls or rises significantly. Some of these circulatory control mechanisms are shown in Figs. 23.1 and 23.2.

Definition and measurement of hypertension

Blood pressure is recorded as *systolic* and *diastolic* pressures in millimetres of mercury (mmHg). A blood pressure cuff (*sphygmomanometer*) is inflated around the upper arm until the pulse is occluded. The pressure is released until the pulse sounds are heard by a stethoscope over the brachial artery (systolic pressure). As the pressure is released further, the sounds disappear again (diastolic pressure). The two readings are recorded thus: e.g. 140/90 mmHg. Electronic sphygmomanometers are also available that give automatic digital readings.

A blood pressure persistently above 160/95 mmHg is considered by the World Health Organisation as hypertensive. However, blood pressure naturally rises with age. A normal blood pressure in a 20-year-old should be around 120/80, while in people above 70 years a blood pressure of 165/100 might be accepted as not

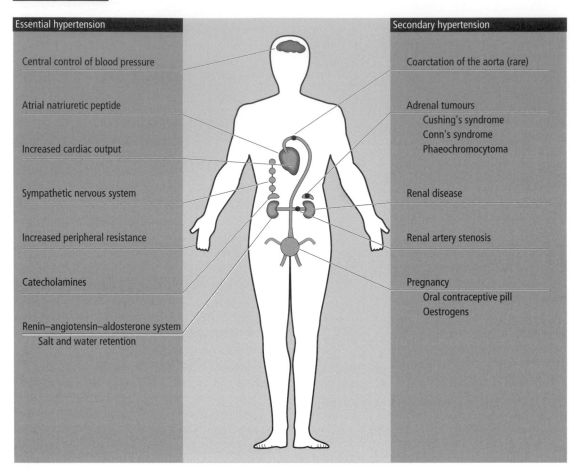

Fig. 23.2 Mechanisms of hypertension. The major factors known to cause hypertension are shown. Essential hypertension comprises 95 percent of all cases of hypertension and is probably multifactoral in origin. Five percent of hypertension is secondary to other disorders such as renal disease.

requiring treatment. The age of the patient will influence the decision as to what level of blood pressure needs treatment.

Blood pressure should be measured on several occasions over some weeks before a decision is made as to whether the patient is consistently hypertensive, and therefore requires treatment. This is important as blood pressure can vary from day to day and even minute to minute. Anxiety and stress, and particularly a first visit to a doctor ('white coat hypertension') can artificially elevate blood pressure.

There is a normal diurnal variation of blood pressure, with blood pressure being higher during the day and lowest during the night. Twenty-four-hour ambulatory blood pressure monitors may give a helpful indication of the 'normal' blood pressure. It may be worth, in some cases, waiting 3–6 months before deciding whether a person's blood pressure needs treating.

As even severely high blood pressure often causes no symptoms, family doctors in the UK should routinely measure blood pressure in all patients on their list.

Potential consequences of untreated blood pressure

Moderately raised blood pressure over many years leads to arterial wall muscle hypertrophy (thickening) and narrowing of the lumen, and also contributes to the development of atheroma, resulting in myocardial infarction, heart failure, and stroke (see also Chapter 22). Damage to the blood vessels in the kidneys can result in deterioration of renal function. Other risk factors, such as smoking or high cholesterol levels (*hypercholesterolaemia*) will accelerate this process. Risk of death increases progressively as diastolic blood pressure rises above 80 mmHg. A diastolic pressure of 100 mmHg increases risk of death from myocardial infarction by up to three times, and rising systolic pressure carries a similar increasing risk. All three risk factors, of hypertension, smoking, and hypercholesterolaemia, if present, together increase mortality by 16-fold or more.

Hypertension in diabetic patients markedly increases cardiovascular risk, and justifies a particularly active policy of blood pressure reduction in diabetics, 50 percent of whom will be hypertensive.

Severe hypertension (e.g. 240/140) can cause blindness, brain haemorrhage, or severe renal failure in only days or weeks. Large studies, particularly in the USA such as the Hypertension Detection and Follow-up Program (HDFP), have shown that treating blood pressure reduces the incidence of cardiovascular complications. The benefit of treating mild hypertension (diastolic pressures less than 100 mmHg) has been difficult to prove. However, most doctors would accept that the treatment of persistent mild hypertension is justified.

Causes and mechanisms of hypertension

Essential hypertension

Ninety five percent of hypertension is of unknown cause, and is termed *essential* or *idiopathic*.

The development of high blood pressure is often multifactorial, and commonly not clinically obvious (see Fig. 23.2). It can be related to imbalance of blood pressure control mechanisms in the nervous system (from brain and sympathetic nervous system, resulting in increased heart rate, cardiac stroke volume, and peripheral vascular resistance); and from hormonal control (renin–angiotensin-aldosterone system, aldosterone, and catecholamines).

Abnormalities in the several cell-membrane sodium-transport mechanisms have been demonstrated, resulting in increased intracellular sodium concentrations, which contributes to vascular smooth-muscle cell contraction and increasing peripheral vascular tone. Hypertension may also be inherited. Although the mechanism of inheritance is frequently unclear, sodium transport defects appear to run in families, and can be more prevalent in certain population groups, e.g. Afro-Caribbeans.

An increased dietary sodium intake increases blood pressure. Excess total body sodium results in water retention via *antidiuretic hormone* (ADH) secretion as a response to the rise of oncotic pressure. *Atrial natriuretic peptide* (ANP) is also involved in the control of sodium and water homeostasis. The rise in blood volume causing hypertension may be reduced by suppression of aldosterone, which results in reduced reabsorption of sodium in the renal tubules, and increased urinary sodium and water loss.

Cell membrane calcium channels also affect vascular tone. Vasoconstriction is mediated by *alpha-adrenergic receptors* in the vessel wall. Many anti-hypertensive agents act on vascular tone to induce vasodilatation and hence reduce blood pressure.

Secondary hypertension

The remaining five percent of hypertension is due to other medical conditions (see Fig. 23.2) and is termed *secondary hypertension*. Most secondary hypertension is the result of renal diseases such as immune-mediated glomerular injury (*glomerulonephritis*), previous infection causing inflammation and scarring (*chronic pyelonephritis*), hereditary renal disease (e.g. *polycystic kidneys*), *diabetic nephropathy* or *systemic immune-mediated diseases* (e.g. systemic lupus erythematosus (SLE) and polyarteritis). Narrowing of a renal artery can be due to atheroma or hyperplasia of the vascular muscle (*renal artery stenosis*). Here the reduced blood flow to the kidney results in release of renin from the juxtaglomerular cells, and raises blood pressure by sodium and water retention and increased peripheral vascular resistance via the renin–angiotensin–aldosterone system.

The remaining causes are rare. Benign tumours of the adrenal cortex secrete cortisol (*Cushing's syndrome*), or aldosterone (*Conn's syndrome*) and cause hypertension by salt and water retention. Catecholamines (e.g. adrenaline) can be produced from a benign adrenal medullary tumour (*phaeochromocytoma*). Narrowing of the aorta (*coarctation*) is a very rare cause of hypertension. Pregnancy, oestrogen therapy and oral contraceptives sometimes induce hypertension.

Examination

Routine examination of the patient will give some indication of the duration and severity of hypertension, whether there were pre-existing causes of high blood pressure (secondary hypertension); and whether any complications resulting from hypertension have developed.

In long-standing hypertension, the left ventricle of the heart may be enlarged (*left ventricular hypertrophy*) or dilated where the heart fails due to the strain of contraction against long-standing increased peripheral resistance. In heart failure the patient will be short of breath (dyspnoea) and fine crackles may be heard at the lung bases due to accumulation of fluid in the alveoli (pulmonary oedema) from left ventricular failure. If there is right ventricular failure, fluid will accumulate as leg oedema.

There may be evidence of atheroma as indicated by a 'rushing' sound (*bruits*) caused by blood flow through a narrowed artery, or more seriously, absent leg pulses from arterial occlusion. If atheroma affects the renal arteries (*renal artery stenosis*) hy-

pertension might be severe or resistant to treatment. An abdominal bruit from the renal arteries may be heard with a stethoscope.

Examination of the retinal vessels in the eye gives an indication of the duration and severity of hypertension. A moderate degree of hypertension over several years can result in relatively minor changes in the vessels including narrowing of the vessel or thickening of the vessel wall (*grade 1*). More severe hypertension causes *arterio-venous nipping*, where artery and vein cross (*grade 2*), or *haemorrhages* and *exudates* (*grade 3*), caused by areas of retinal infarction. In severe accelerated hypertension, swelling of the optic disc (*papilloedema, grade 4*) may result in the deterioration of vision, if not blindness, if left untreated.

Investigations

Hypertension should be investigated firstly to establish whether there is any pre-existing (secondary) cause of hypertension which might need specific treatment, and secondly to determine the extent of any end-organ damage. The complex investigations required to elucidate the possible mechanisms of essential hypertension are not usually performed in clinical practice.

Urine testing is carried out routinely at family doctor surgeries and in hospitals. If urinary tract infection is excluded, proteinuria (protein in the urine) and haematuria (blood-stained urine) suggest renal disease. *Glycosuria* (glucose in the urine) suggests diabetes mellitus.

Cardiac complications are shown by performing an electrocardiogram (ECG), which will show left ventricular hypertrophy from long-standing hypertension, or ischaemic heart disease from coronary atheroma. A chest radiograph will show cardiac enlargement associated with heart failure or hypertrophy.

Blood tests are carried out to determine plasma levels of electrolytes, urea and creatinine. Markers of renal function, urea and creatinine, rise in renal impairment from reduced excretion. If there is a suggestion of renal impairment, this can be more accurately determined by calculating the creatinine clearance from a 24 hour urine collection. Urinary protein excretion can be measured at the same time. Increased urinary protein loss suggests renal disease, and this can be further investigated by imaging the size and shape of the kidneys by ultrasound or *intravenous urogram* (IVU). In some cases, a renal biopsy is indicated to make a histological diagnosis of the renal disease.

Plasma sodium levels usually remain within the reference range, since excess total body sodium is balanced by water retention. However, low plasma potassium can indicate Cushing's and Conn's syndromes. If either is suspected, estimations of cortisol and aldosterone levels will be needed. If severe and episodic hypertension is found, urinary catecholamine estimation may suggest phaeochromocytoma.

The presence of arterial bruits raises the possibility of renal artery stenosis, particularly if there is severe or resistant hypertension, a small kidney and/or renal impairment. An *isotope renal scan* gives an indication of renal perfusion, and a *renal arteriogram* will show any narrowing of the renal artery. If found, the stenosis can be dilated at the same time by a *balloon angioplasty*. However, since 95 percent of hypertension is idiopathic, these more complex investigations will usually either be unnecessary or give negative results.

Treatment

The objective of treatment is to reduce blood pressure to normal levels and then to maintain blood pressure control with the minimum dose of anti-hypertensive drugs, without producing unnecessary side effects.

Non-pharmacological methods can be used with effect. Weight reduction, lowered salt intake, and regular moderate exercise will all help to reduce blood pressure, and may in many people remove the need for drug therapy. Other risk factors need to be addressed. Patients must stop smoking, and cholesterol levels, if elevated, need to be reduced by dietary modification, and, if necessary, by drug therapy. If there is a treatable secondary cause of hypertension, such as renal artery stenosis or adrenal tumour then this requires attention.

There are several groups of anti-hypertensive drugs with different pharmacological actions. In essential hypertension any of these drugs can potentially be used and it is not necessary in most cases to know the underlying cause of the hypertension. Treatment is commenced with a small dose of a single drug. If blood pressure control is not achieved then the dose can sometimes be increased or a drug from a different group added, or both administered in a 'step-care' approach (see Table 23.1). There are several alternative drugs within each group, each with slightly different pharmacological profiles, such as dose range, length of action, selectivity, and side-effect profile. Compliance with treatment will be optimized if the minimum number of tablets are prescribed, given once, or at most twice a day, and with as few side-effects as possible. Side-effects can occur in up to 20 percent of patients given a particular drug.

Treatment is usually commenced with a thiazide diuretic, a beta-blocker or a calcium antagonist. Thiazide diuretics (e.g. bendrofluazide, hydrochlorthiazide) increase salt and water excretion, but most of their hypotensive action

Table 23.1 Step-care approach to drug treatment of hypertension

---

Step 1
Beta-blocker or calcium antagonist or thiazide diuretic

If side-effects use ACE inhibitor or alpha-blocker

Step 2
Combination of beta-blocker + calcium antagonist

Alternative: replace with ACE inhibitor

Step 3
Combination of ACE inhibitor + calcium antagonist

Step 4
Add beta-blocker or alpha-blocker (triple therapy)

Step 5
Add frusemide
Followed by minoxidil

---

is probably by vasodilatation. They are effective, inexpensive, mild anti-hypertensive agents, but can sometimes precipitate diabetes, gout, impotence, and potassium depletion resulting in cardiac *extrasystoles* (premature heart beats). As Afro-Caribbeans often have increased intra-cellular sodium concentrations, thiazides may be the starting treatment of choice in this group.

Beta-blockers (e.g. propranolol, atenolol) are beta-adrenergic antagonists, and act by slowing heart rate, but have several other actions including effects on cerebral control of blood pressure. They are very commonly used, but can produce lethargy and cold peripheries and can exacerbate asthma. Labetolol has both alpha- and beta-blocker actions. A newer beta-blocker, celiprolol, acts predominantly by vasodilatation.

Calcium antagonists or calcium channel blockers (e.g. nifedipine, nicardipine, amlodipine, diltiazem) block calcium influx into cells, so causing smooth-muscle cell relaxation, and vasodilatation. They are effective and well tolerated. Side effects of this vasodilatation include headache and leg oedema.

Alpha-blockers (e.g. prazosin, terazosin, doxazosin) also induce vasodilatation, and postural hypotension (sudden fall in blood pressure on standing) which is less of a problem if these drugs are initially administered in small doses.

Angiotensin-converting enzyme inhibitors (ACE inhibitors, e.g. captopril, enalapril, lisinopril) block production of the vasoconstrictor angiotensin II. Aldosterone production will also be inhibited, so reducing sodium and water retention. These drugs are increasingly being used and are well tolerated, although an irritating cough may be produced. ACE inhibitors may protect against decline of renal function, particularly in diabetics. They should be used with close monitoring, since severe elevation of potassium levels may result in patients with renal impairment.

Drugs that act on the CNS are now rarely used to control hypertension. Methyl-dopa is given three times a day, and in higher doses can cause depression and red cell lysis (haemolysis).

Clonidine and reserpine are no longer used because of their potentially serious side-effects.

In severe hypertension, intravenous hydrallazine, labetolol and sodium nitroprusside can be used, but with caution, since a precipitous fall of blood pressure should be avoided.

Summary

The objectives of anti-hypertensive therapy are to identify all patients with hypertension, to effectively reduce blood pressure and to maintain its control. This should be achieved with the minimum amount of medication and avoidance of side-effects.

Changes in blood pressure medication may be needed in cases where blood pressure is difficult to control, or where side effects occur. Patients need to realize that anti-hypertensive medication will almost always have to be taken for life. Hypertension, although usually asymptomatic, may have potential life-threatening consequences in the long term, which can be prevented if blood pressure is satisfactorily controlled.

Key points

1 Physiological control of blood pressure is complex. The following all contribute to the maintenance of normal blood pressure: cardiac output; arterial blood volume and peripheral resistance.

2 It is important to screen for hypertension because the condition is often asymptomatic. Untreated prolonged hypertension can lead to myocardial infarction, stroke and renal failure.

3 The majority (95 percent) of hypertension is of unknown cause. This is essential (or idiopathic) hypertension. The remaining five percent of cases of hypertension are attributable to other disorders.

4 Active treatment of hypertension reduces the risk of cardiovascular disease.

5 Effective treatment of hypertension may sometimes be achieved without the use of drugs. When drug treatment is indicated, a step-care approach may be employed.

Further reading

Sever P. *et al.* (1993) Management guidelines in essential hypertension: report of the second working party of the British Hypertension Society. *BMJ* **306:** 983–7.

Swales J. *et al.* (1991) *Clinical Atlas of Hypertension*. Gower Medical Publishing, London, New York.

Case Studies

24.1 Chest pain radiating to the left arm

Clinical features

A 53-year-old Asian man was admitted to hospital with severe crushing central chest pain, coming on at rest, which radiated to the left arm. This was associated with sweating, nausea, vomiting and breathlessness. On questioning, he had experienced similar but less severe pain for the previous month whilst walking. He had not seen a doctor for many years. He smoked 20 cigarettes a day. His father was diabetic and died from 'heart trouble' aged 48 years.

On examination he was obese, pale and sweaty. His heart rate was 100 beats per minute and irregular. He was hypertensive (blood pressure: 170/100 mmHg).

Investigations

Investigations included those shown in Table 24.1.1.

Clinical investigations included an electrocardiogram (ECG) and a chest radiograph. The ECG showed atrial fibrillation, left ventricular hypertrophy and raised ST segments in anterior chest leads. The chest radiograph showed evidence of slight cardiac enlargement and mild pulmonary oedema.

Diagnosis

The clinical history and features are suggestive of myocardial infarction (MI) preceded by a short

Table 24.1.1 Initial investigations performed

Analyte	Value	Reference range
Blood		
Sodium	148 mmol/l	136–145
Potassium	4.3 mmol/l	3.4–5.2
Urea	5.7 mmol/l	2.5–6.7
Creatinine	98 μmol/l	70–150
Cholesterol	8.2 mmol/l	3.6–6.7
Fasting glucose	13.6 mmol/l	<7
Aspartate transaminase	235 U/l	5–40
Lactate dehydrogenase	2263 U/l	300–650
Urine (dipstick tests)		
Glucose	2⁺	0–trace
Protein	0	0–trace

A 2⁺ glucose reading approximates to a urinary glucose of at least 28 mmol/l

history of angina pectoris (see Chapter 21). The diagnosis is supported by the electrocardiogram ST segment elevation in the anterior region of the heart (i.e. the left ventricle) and the raised levels of the cardiac enzymes, aspartate transaminase (AST) and lactate dehydrogenase (LDH).

Diagnosis: acute myocardial infarction

Discussion

MI defines death of myocardial tissue. It is the result of inadequate blood flow to the myocardium (myocardial ischaemia) sufficient to produce lethal cell injury. Myocardial ischaemia is most often due to thrombosis in a coronary artery, usually at a site of a previous atheromatous plaque (see Chapter 22).

Following MI, some parts of the damaged heart

are unable to conduct impulses. These changes in impulse conduction can be detected on the ECG and are one basis for determining whether an infarct has occurred and its likely location. This can result in the development of abnormal heart rhythms (dysrhythmias) some of which may be life-threatening.

Myocardial cell death also results in the release of intracellular enzymes into the extracellular fluid. Monitoring the serum levels of these enzymes can be useful indicators of the presence and extent of an MI. The substantial rise in the levels of the cardiac iso-enzymes LDH and AST, observed in this patient suggests significant myocardial damage.

The previous history of angina pectoris, due to transient myocardial ischaemia, suggests that blood flow to the myocardium may have been compromised for some time in this patient. This has produced an overall reduction in cardiac function resulting in mild cardiac failure. Cardiac failure is indicated. This is supported by enlargement of the heart and the accumulation of fluid in the lungs (*pulmonary oedema*).

Treatment and prognosis

The management of a patient with an MI is in three stages, as follows. Firstly, the patient is treated with bed rest, analgesia using diamorphine, and oxygen to try to reduce the myocardial ischaemia. Thrombolytic therapy (for example, using intravenous streptokinase to promote fibrinolysis) is also given and can reduce the size of the infarction if given early enough. In this patient the myocardial ischaemia produced an irregular rhythm and atrial fibrillation. Digoxin can revert the heart to its normal rhythm and will also improve cardiac contractility. After 48 hours in bed the patient should commence mobilization and provided there are no further complications, may be discharged after 5–7 days. Rehabilitation continues over the following 6 weeks.

Secondly, it is important to identify any risk factors for MI. The patient is a smoker, has *hypercholesterolaemia* (raised blood cholesterol

levels) and left ventricular hypertrophy suggesting long standing previously undiagnosed hypertension. The elevated blood glucose level suggests mild, maturity onset diabetes mellitus (non-insulin dependent diabetes mellitus, Type II diabetes). Mild diabetes is frequently asymptomatic and may be present for a number of years before it is detected. The normal blood urea, sodium and potassium and absence of proteinuria (protein in the urine) suggests that the patient has not yet developed diabetic renal disease. The early death of his father from heart disease suggests an inherited risk of MI which may be the result of genetically determined hypercholesterolaemia, hypertension or diabetes. There is increasing interest in the role of high insulin levels as a risk factor for MI. In the UK Asian patients, in particular, have an increased risk of death from MI which is 40 percent above that of the British caucasian population. They also have a four times greater risk of developing diabetes.

Finally, additional investigations and treatment may be necessary to prevent further MI. Most importantly, the patient must stop smoking as this is an important risk factor. An exercise test on a treadmill is also generally performed 6 weeks after MI. If further ischaemic changes develop on ECG then coronary angiography needs to be performed. If there is significant stenosis or occlusion of the coronary arteries then coronary artery bypass-graft or percutaneous coronary artery angioplasty should be considered.

The progress of most patients is monitored in an out-patient clinic. In this case, the patient had been clearly overweight at the time of his MI. Since then, he had seen a dietitian who had given him advice on healthy eating and suggested a reduction of his fat intake to less than 30 percent of his total energy intake. The patient was noted to have *corneal arcus* (deposition of lipids in the periphery of the cornea), which is often, though not always, indicative of hyperlipidaemia. A full profile of his blood lipids was performed, the results are shown in Table 24.1.2.

In order to prevent further accumulation of cholesterol in his arteries the patient was prescribed a drug to lower his cholesterol levels. This drug acts

Table 24.1.2 Blood lipid profile

Analyte	Value	Optimal value
Blood		
Triglyceride	1.4 mmol/l	<2.3 mmol/l
Cholesterol	7.7 mmol/l	<5.2 mmol/l
High density lipoprotein cholesterol	1.2 mmol/l	>1.0 mmol/l
Lipoprotein(a)	811 mmol/l	<300 mmol/l

as an inhibitor of a key enzyme involved in the synthesis of cholesterol by the liver. The patient was again advised to stop smoking and to take more exercise. His diabetes was successfully controlled by the administration of oral hypoglycaemic agents (sulphonylureas, see Case Study 24.3). Low dose aspirin as an anti-platelet agent (see Chapter 21) and beta-blockers (see Chapter 23) were also prescribed. Both of these agents have been shown to reduce the incidence of re-infarction.

Questions

1 What is the physiological basis of left ventricular hypertrophy in long-standing hypertension?

Answer: the increased work of the heart in pumping against prolonged resistance in the form of high blood pressure causes thickening of the walls of the left ventricle (left ventricular hypertrophy).

2 How do you account for the pulmonary oedema observed in this patient?

Answer: a reduction in efficiency of the left side of the heart (left ventricular failure) increases the venous pressure in the pulmonary circulation. Hydrostatic pressure in the pulmonary capillary bed rises, forcing excess fluid into the interstitial spaces where it interferes with gaseous exchange. Eventually some fluid may pass into the alveoli causing marked *dyspnoea* (shortness of breath).

24.2 Protein in the urine and hypertension

Clinical features

A 45-year-old man was found to have protein in his urine on dipstick testing at an employment medical. He was also hypertensive (blood pressure: 180/100). On questioning he admitted to having had some swelling of his ankles at the end of the day for the last 6 months, but otherwise had no symptoms.

Investigations

Laboratory investigations included those shown in Table 24.2.1.

Anti-nuclear antibodies were not detectable. Renal ultrasound showed normal size and appearance of kidneys.

A renal biopsy was performed. Histological analysis of the renal biopsy showed glomerulonephritis (inflammation of the renal glomeruli) of membranous type, characterized by thickening of the glomerular basement membrane and sclerosis (scarring) of individual glomeruli. Immunofluorescent analysis showed granular deposition of immunoglobulin G (IgG) within the

Table 24.2.1 Investigations performed

Analyte	Value	Reference range
Blood		
Albumin	27 g/l	34–48
Sodium	138 mmol/l	136–145
Potassium	3.8 mmol/l	3.4–5.2
Urea	11.2 mmol/l	2.5–6.7
Creatinine	155 µmol/l	70–150
Creatinine clearance	64 ml/min	75–140
Fasting glucose	4.6 mmol/l	<7
Cholesterol	9.2 mmol/l	3.6–6.7
Urine		
24 hour urinary protein	6.3 grams/24 hours	<0.1

glomerular basement membranes. On electron microscopy there were electron-dense deposits within glomerular basement membranes.

Diagnosis

The moderately large amount of protein in the urine (proteinuria) is consistent with chronic glomerulonephritis. Other forms of renal disease such as chronic pyelonephritis and chronic interstitial nephritis produce much less severe proteinuria. The absence of anti-nuclear antibodies rules out systemic lupus erythematosus (see Chapter 13) as a cause of the renal disease. Other forms of glomerulonephritis, for example proliferative glomerulonephritis, are excluded as are other causes of heavy proteinuria such as diabetic nephropathy (fasting blood glucose levels were within the reference range).

Diagnosis: membranous glomerulonephritis

Discussion

Membranous glomerulonephritis is due to the deposition of antigen–antibody complexes (immune complexes) within the glomerular basement membranes. These immune complexes can be detected by immunofluorescence analysis or as electron-dense deposits on electron microscopy.

The precise stimulus for the formation of these immune complexes cannot always be clearly identified. Rarely, in some cases exogenous antigens (e.g. hepatitis B virus, *Treponema pallidum* antigens) and endogenous antigens (e.g. thyroglobulin) have been implicated. The deposition of immune complexes within glomeruli leads to glomerular inflammation, glomerular damage, including the deposition of collagen within glomeruli (glomerular sclerosis), and subsequent impairment of renal function. In membranous glomerulonephritis the changes in the basement membrane are manifested as the leakage of protein through the damaged glomerulus and into the urine. This patient has moderately severe proteinuria sufficient to reduce the blood albumin levels below normal (hypoalbuminaemia). The hypoalbuminaemia has in turn caused a reduction in the oncotic pressure of the blood, with leakage of fluid into the tissues resulting in the accumulation of fluid (oedema) in the legs. The triad of proteinuria, hypoalbuminaemia and oedema is termed *nephrotic syndrome*. The patient shows evidence of impaired renal function with a slight elevation of blood urea and creatinine and reduction in creatinine clearance. The history of oedema for 6 months suggests the condition is not of recent origin. Hypertension has developed secondary to renal disease (see Chapter 23).

Treatment and prognosis

Diuretics, either orally or intravenously, can be used to increase water excretion and reduce oedema. Where oedema is resistant then intravenous albumin infusions can be used to raise plasma oncotic pressure and facilitate diuresis. In some forms of glomerulonephritis corticosteroids can be used to suppress the glomerular inflammation. There are two possible outcomes of patients with membranous glomerulonephritis. In some patients there will be a partial resolution of proteinuria with stabilization of renal function. Alternatively, renal function may decline progressively over the course of between 5 and 20 years, eventually requiring dialysis. In the latter group of patients, corticosteroids have been shown to have no effect. Hypertension will accelerate the decline of renal function and treatment of hypertension is therefore indicated.

Questions

1 Hypercholesterolaemia (raised blood cholesterol level) is frequently encountered in patients with the nephrotic syndrome. Why is it important to administer lipid-lowering drugs to this group of patients?

Answer: hypercholesterolaemia is associated with the development of atherosclerosis (see Chapter 22). In addition, the development of vascular damage associated with atherosclerosis is accelerated by hypertension (see Chapter 23).

2 Why is plasma creatinine a useful marker of renal function? Are there more accurate methods for the measurement of renal function?

Answer: creatinine is released from skeletal muscle at a fairly constant rate and excreted in the urine. In renal disease, creatinine may accumulate in the blood as a result of impaired excretion. The rate of creatinine clearance from the blood may therefore be a useful measure of renal function.

The relationship between plasma creatinine concentration and creatinine clearance rate is not linear. In some people, creatinine clearance may fall to 50 mls/min before plasma creatinine levels rise above the reference range. Glomerular filtration rate may be more accurately measured by intravenous injection of radioactive chromium-labelled EDTA followed by the measurement of its clearance over several hours. Alternatively, inulin clearance may be measured under certain experimental conditions.

24.3 Fever and leg ulcer

Clinical features

A 54-year-old man presented to an Accident and Emergency Department with fever and a large ulcer on the sole of his right foot. This had been present and gradually enlarging over 2 weeks. Earlier action had not been taken because the ulcer was painless. He claimed to be otherwise fit and well, although on direct questioning he had noticed increased thirst and urination over 18 months, a 10 kg weight loss over 2 years and non-specific lethargy of longer duration which had been attributed to 'old age'. On examination he was thin, somewhat dehydrated and febrile (temperature; 39°C). Examination of his retina revealed capillary haemorrhages. He was unable to

detect vibration sensation below his knees and had lost soft touch sensation below his ankles. There was a large deep malodorous ulcer under his great toe that was surrounded by spreading skin infection. Exploration of this ulcer revealed a cavity full of pus tracking deep along the sole of his foot. His dipstick urine analysis showed 3$^+$ glucose, 2$^+$ protein and 3$^+$ ketones.

Investigations

The results of laboratory investigations are shown in Table 24.3.1.

Table 24.3.1 Investigations performed

Analyte	Value	Reference range
Blood		
Random glucose	24.7 mmol/l	3.5–8.9
Urea	19.4 mmol/l	2.5–6.7
Creatinine	157 µmol/l	70–150
Bicarbonate	23 mmol/l	20–30

No islet cell or insulin autoantibodies were detected.
A radiograph of the patient's right foot showed destruction of the bone in the great toe.
Microbiological analysis of the pus from the ulcer showed the presence of both aerobic (including *Staphylococcus aureus*) and anaerobic bacteria.

Diagnosis

The patient has *hyperglycaemia* (raised blood glucose levels) confirming diabetes mellitus. The raised blood urea and creatinine indicate poor renal function, almost certainly due to diabetic renal disease (diabetic nephropathy). This is further supported by the proteinuria (protein in the urine) which is the result of protein leaking through a damaged renal glomerular capillary basement membrane. The dehydration is the result of the osmotic loss of water induced by glycosuria (glucose in the urine) resulting in increased urination and stimulation of thirst. His bicarbonate levels were normal so the blood accumulation of ketone bodies (i.e. aceto-acetate and 3-hydroxybutyrate which are the breakdown products of non-esterified fatty acid metabolism) was not sufficient to cause acidosis (lowered blood pH).

The failure to detect islet and insulin autoantibodies is against a diagnosis of Type I diabetes mellitus which has an autoimmune basis (see Chapter 13). Clearly he has had diabetes for a long time. Microvascular complications involving the eyes (diabetic retinopathy, manifested by the presence of retinal capillary haemorrhages) and kidneys, and peripheral nerve damage (diabetic neuropathy) relate to a long exposure to high blood glucose levels. His onset of diabetes was insidious, possibly developing 10 years or so before presentation, and so this is probably Type II diabetes mellitus. The mean pre-diagnosis duration of unrecognized hyperglycaemia is estimated at 4 years. Ten percent of patients with Type II diabetes have complications at diagnosis.

Diagnosis: Type II diabetes mellitus with diabetic nephropathy, diabetic neuropathy and infected neuropathic foot ulcer.

Discussion

Diabetes mellitus is a metabolic disorder in which blood glucose concentrations are elevated. Conventionally, two major forms of diabetes mellitus are recognized. Type I diabetes (juvenile onset, insulin-dependent diabetes mellitus) usually presents acutely in young patients and is the result of an autoimmune response to pancreatic beta-cells. This leads to destruction of the beta-cells with consequent lack of secretion of insulin. There is a genetic predisposition to Type I diabetes which is explained in part by an association with specific HLA types (see Chapter 13).

Insulin lowers blood glucose levels, increases protein synthesis, and inhibits lipolysis (fat breakdown) including inhibition of the release of fatty acids from adipose cells. In the absence of insulin these fatty acids are released from adipose cells and converted to ketones in the liver resulting in the accumulation of ketones in the blood and their

excretion in the urine (ketonuria). The excess keto-acids in the blood require buffering by the bicarbonate ion; this leads to a marked decrease in serum bicarbonate levels and acidosis. Patients with Type I diabetes mellitus, therefore, have a mandatory requirement for insulin injection therapy to prevent acidosis-induced coma and inevitable death.

In contrast, patients with Type II diabetes (maturity onset, non-insulin dependent diabetes mellitus) are usually older, often obese, and there is usually an insidious or gradual onset of symptoms. Genetic factors are even more important than in Type I diabetes and among identical twins there is a concordance rate of 90 percent. However, Type II diabetes is not linked to any HLA haplotype and there is no evidence that autoimmune mechanisms are involved in its pathogenesis.

The following two metabolic defects characterize Type II diabetes.

1 A relative but not absolute *insulin deficiency*. The cause of this insulin deficiency is not known but may be related to a progressive loss of beta-cell function and beta-cell mass.

2 An inability of peripheral tissues to respond to insulin, termed *insulin resistance*, due to a number of abnormalities of post-receptor transport of glucose.

In clinical practice, the distinction between Type I and Type II diabetes mellitus is not always clear cut and an appreciation of the underlying biochemical abnormalities often aids therapeutic decision making.

Treatment and prognosis

Insulin resistance can be reduced by weight loss and by exercise, but insulin deficiency is of greater significance. After altering diet by reducing the content of simple, refined carbohydrates and increasing complex carbohydrate and fibre, the diminished insulin secretion in Type II diabetes may more easily cope with the consequent reduced rate of entry of glucose into the circulation. If still insufficient to achieve good glucose control, then oral hypoglycaemic drugs (e.g. sulphonylureas) can be used. These act by stimulating insulin secretion from the beta-cell and by enhancing the effect of insulin at the post-receptor level in peripheral tissues. However, if insulin deficiency and beta-cell loss are marked then these drugs become ineffective in the treatment of Type II diabetes. Obviously these drugs are not used in Type I diabetes where insulin deficiency is absolute. On average, because of the slow progression of Type II diabetes, a patient responding initially to diet alone will require oral hypoglycaemic agents after a period of approximately 3 years and insulin treatment some 7 years later.

The patient was started on twice daily insulin injection therapy with rapid disappearance of urinary ketones and correction of blood glucose. Despite antibiotic therapy he required surgical removal of the infected tissue losing his first two toes and part of his forefoot. With healing his mobility remained impaired and he never returned to employment. His retinopathy was stabilized using retinal laser photocoagulation to prevent blindness. Normal kidney function was not restored. Slow but progressive decline of renal function would be expected and he will eventually require dialysis. Six months after commencing therapy he was given a trial of oral hypoglycaemic tablets but had a brisk recurrence of symptomatic hyperglycaemia and ketonuria and was restarted on insulin therapy for life.

Questions

1 Given that a number of patients with Type II diabetes respond well to dietary restriction and/or oral hypoglycaemic agents, why was the patient started on insulin therapy?

Answer: the patient was thin and losing weight, had marked hyperglycaemia and ketonuria. This pointed to severe insulin deficiency requiring insulin replacement therapy and predicted his subsequent failure to respond to oral hypoglycaemic agents.

2 How can you explain the development of the leg ulcer in this patient?

Answer: this man's foot had diminished sensation due to peripheral nerve damage (neuropathy) secondary to his diabetes. A further consequence of neurological damage is an abnormal gait leading to very high pressures in localized areas of the foot during walking. The consequent trauma very rapidly leads to ulcer formation which is often unrecognized by the patients. Once the skin is damaged, infection may ensue causing further inflammation and necrosis. The patient's ability to respond to infection is impaired because of circulatory disturbance due to microvascular disease together with other factors such as impaired leucocyte function which render patients with diabetes more susceptible to a number of forms of infection.

Part 7
Genetic Disorders

Inherited Single Gene Disorders

Introduction

Over the last decade there have been major advances in the diagnosis of genetic diseases. This has been brought about in part by the increased awareness of the role of a genetic component in the pathogenesis of many diseases and partly by the increased application of molecular techniques. Together these factors have resulted in genetics being one of the fastest moving fields in medicine today.

This chapter examines the different types of mutations which occur in the genes leading to some of the major inherited single gene disorders and shows how the genotypic changes lead to expression of a specific disease phenotype.

The nature of mutations

A mutation is a change in the genetic make-up (*genotype*) of a cell. If mutations occur in the cells that form the *gametes*, that is the germ cells, then the mutation may be transmitted to the offspring where it will be present in every cell of an affected individual. These heritable mutations may arise as *de novo* (new) mutations in the germ cells of one or both parents or may have been inherited by the parents from previous generations.

Alternatively, mutations occuring in other body cells, termed *somatic mutations*, will not be inherited by subsequent generations but will result in genetic differences between the cells of the same organism. Somatic mutations may have consequences for the individual, since particular types of these mutations are thought to contribute to the development of cancer (see Chapter 28).

Mutations range from rearrangements or deletions involving large sections of whole chromo-somes through to single base changes. Large deletions or rearrangements of entire sections of a chromosome can be detected by the examination of chromosome morphology and are the subject of Chapter 26. Mutations involving single genes are usually the result of either the substitution of a single base with another (known as a *point mutation*), or the deletion or insertion of bases. These mutations may arise within the regions of a gene which code for protein (*exons*), within the non-coding regions (*introns*), or within nearby control elements.

Mutations arising in the exons of a gene often affect the nature of the protein product. For example, the insertion or deletion of one or two base pairs will lead to alterations in the reading frame of the DNA. Mutations arising in this way are known as *frameshift mutations*. A point mutation may alter the code in a triplet of bases (*codon*) and lead to the replacement of one amino acid by another in the protein product. This is referred to as a *mis-sense mutation* and if it occurs in a critical region can dramatically change the function of the encoded protein. A point mutation can also change an amino acid codon to a stop codon resulting in premature termination of protein synthesis and a truncated protein product. Such a mutation is called a *non-sense mutation*.

Mutations within gene control regions can lead to a marked reduction or total lack of transcription, as seen in several forms of haemolytic anaemia (see Chapter 20). Point mutations within introns can result in defective splicing of intervening sequences. This in turn affects normal processing of messenger RNA (mRNA) and hence formation of the mature mRNA necessary for protein synthesis.

It is important to recognize that for some inherited single gene disorders (e.g. sickle cell anaemia) all affected individuals will carry an identical mutation. However, for many diseases there is often more than one type of mutation which can produce the same phenotype. Beta-thalassaemia, for example, may result from many different mutations in the beta-globin gene.

Testing for inherited single gene disorders

The identification of specific disease-causing genes has a number of implications. Firstly, for a severe disorder, such as Duchenne muscular dystrophy or cystic fibrosis, it is possible to offer parents the option of pre-natal testing and termination of an affected fetus at an early stage in pregnancy. Secondly, in diseases where pre-symptomatic diagnosis is possible, for example in inherited cancer syndromes, early treatment can lead to a substantial improvement in survival and the quality of life. Thirdly, population screening has become possible for diseases which are common in the population, for example cystic fibrosis. This can reduce the incidence of the disease in the population and at the same time reduce the health burden from these disorders.

Patterns of inheritance

The majority of single gene disorders show clear patterns of Mendelian inheritance. Diseases can either be *X-linked* (i.e. the affected gene is on the X chromosome), or *autosomal* (the affected gene is on one of chromosomes 1–22). In addition, they may be *dominant*, requiring a mutation in only one copy of the gene, or *recessive*, where mutations in both copies are needed for expression of the phenotype. Examples of these different patterns of inheritance are shown in Fig. 25.1.

Methods of diagnosis of single gene disorders

Pre-natal and pre-symptomatic diagnosis of genetic diseases can be indirect or direct. If the chro-

mosomal location of a gene is known but the gene itself has not yet been isolated, indirect analysis, termed *linkage analysis*, is possible. This depends on the tracking of a disease gene through a family by the use of polymorphic markers, that is, markers which vary from one individual to the next, to 'tag' the chromosome carrying the disease mutation. The principle of this approach for family analysis is illustrated in Fig. 25.2. Direct analysis is possible by the detection of specific mutations in the affected gene(s) and is the subject of the following sections.

Molecular basis of the single gene disorders

Deletions

Large *deletions* are a major cause of *Duchenne muscular dystrophy* (DMD). This is an X-linked recessive condition seen primarily in boys which causes muscle degeneration and eventually death. 50–60 percent of affected boys show deletions of one or more exons of the very large dystrophin gene (Fig. 25.3). These deletions occur with particularly high frequency at certain points ('hot spots') throughout the gene. The deletions cause an alteration in the reading frame of the dystrophin gene so that a premature stop codon is introduced and hence a truncated and unstable protein is produced. If muscle tissue from affected boys is examined it can be seen that dystrophin protein is virtually absent.

In contrast, in *Becker muscular dystrophy* (BMD), a milder disease also caused by abnormalities in the dystrophin gene, muscle sections show the presence of dystrophin. The dystrophin gene in BMD patients also shows large deletions but because they occur in triplets they leave the reading frame intact. Therefore, although part of the protein is missing it is still able to function at a lower level and the phenotype of the disease is consequently milder than that of DMD.

Cystic fibrosis (CF) is one of the most common autosomal recessive conditions. It is characterized by abnormally thick mucus secretions in the lungs and by pancreatic enzyme insufficiency.

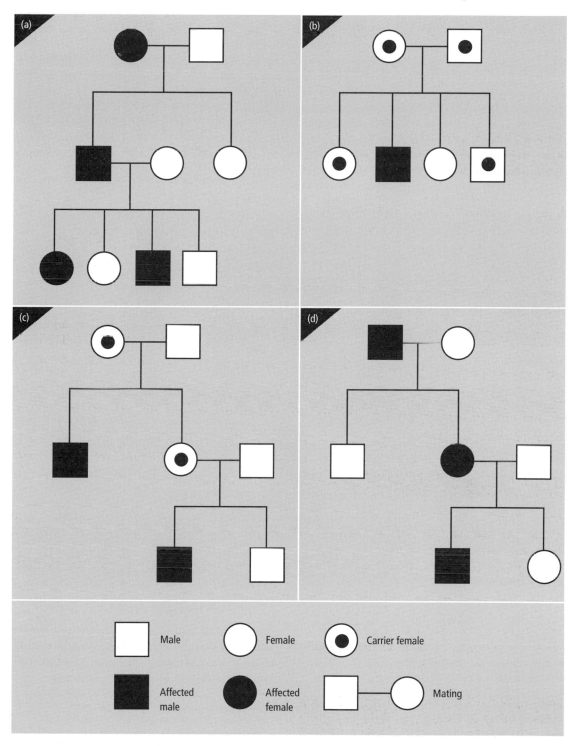

Fig. 25.1 Mendelian patterns of inheritance: (a) autosomal dominant inheritance; (b) autosomal recessive inheritance; (c) X-linked recessive inheritance; and (d) X-linked dominant inheritance.

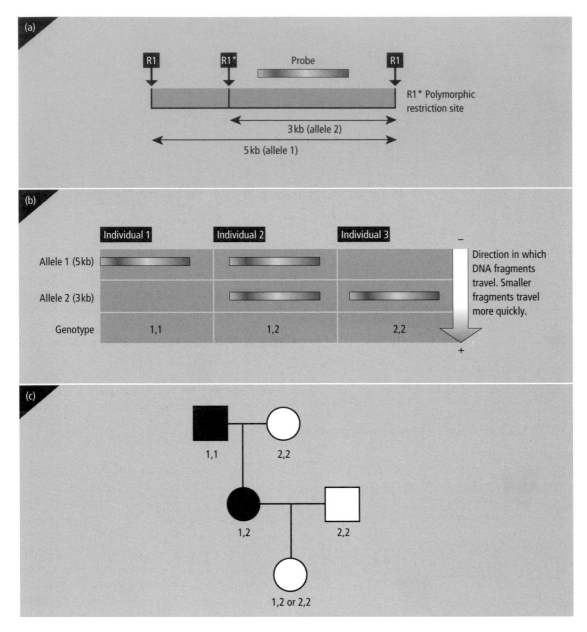

Fig. 25.2 Linkage analysis using *restriction fragment length polymorphisms* (RFLPs). This approach relies on the ability to cleave DNA at specific sites (*restriction sites*) using restriction enzymes. Restriction enzyme digestion of DNA yields a number of fragments (*restriction fragments*) of different sizes depending on the number of restriction sites and their position within the DNA. (a) Two different restriction fragment length polymorphisms known to be located on a specific chromosome near the gene of interest. If restriction site, R1* is present then restriction enzyme digestion will yield two fragments and the probe will recognize a 3 kilobase (kb) sized fragment. If R1* is absent then the probe will recognize a single 5 kb fragment.

(b) Gel electrophoresis separates the restriction fragments on the basis of their size, and below the genotype results of three individuals with the three possible outcomes using the RFLP in (a). (c) Results of an RFLP entered into the pedigree. By looking at the affected individual in the first generation, it can be seen that he has allele 1 on both chromosomes, one of which carries the mutated gene. He has passed the disease to his daughter along with allele 1. If she in turn passes on the chromosome with allele 1 to her 'at risk' daughter, the daughter will be affected. If she passes on the chromosome with allele 2 the daughter will not be affected.

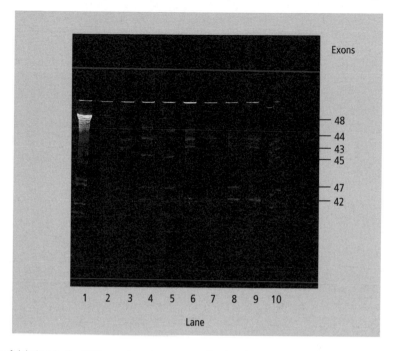

Exons

48
44
43
45

47
42

1 2 3 4 5 6 7 8 9 10

Lane

Fig. 25.3 Detection of deletions in the DMD gene by gel electrophoresis of amplified DNA. A normal female in lane 8 shows 6 bands corresponding to 6 exons of the DMD gene. Other lanes from affected boys show absence of some of the bands indicating that DNA from these exons of the gene has been deleted. Lane 1 is a molecular weight marker. (Photograph courtesy of Dr Sarah Bullock, DNA laboratory, Regional Genetics Service, Birmingham Maternity Hospital.)

The observation of elevated sweat electrolytes suggested that the causative abnormality might be a defect in the regulation of chloride ion conductance. When the cystic fibrosis gene was isolated in 1989, it was shown to encode a transmembrane protein which functions as a chloride ion channel. The gene is now referred to as the *cystic fibrosis transmembrane regulator* (CFTR) gene. The CFTR protein produced by the gene has five functional domains as shown in Fig. 25.4.

Over 300 different CF mutations have so far been identified (see Fig. 25.4). These include nonsense mutations, frameshift mutations, or splice site mutations. Unlike DMD, large deletions are rare. The majority of mutations occur at low frequency, but one, known as ΔF508, has been found on approximately 75 percent of CF chromosomes in the UK population. This mutation is a 3-basepair (bp) deletion in exon 10 which causes the deletion of the amino acid phenylalanine from the ATP-binding domain of the protein.

CFTR gene mutations fall into three functional groups. Group one mutations, which include the ΔF508 mutation, prevent correct folding and maturation of the protein. CF proteins with the second group of mutations are processed correctly but the chloride ion channel fails to open on stimulation. Group 3 mutations are likely to produce chloride channels with slightly altered properties but have not yet been fully characterized.

An analysis of genotype/phenotype correlations has been made in CF but many of the correlations are not clear cut. However, one group of patients, comprising between 10 and 15 percent of cases, have some preservation of pancreatic enzyme levels. These patients tend to have 'milder' mutations such as mis-sense mutations and rarely have the ΔF508 mutation.

Point mutations

Single base changes (point mutations) are a

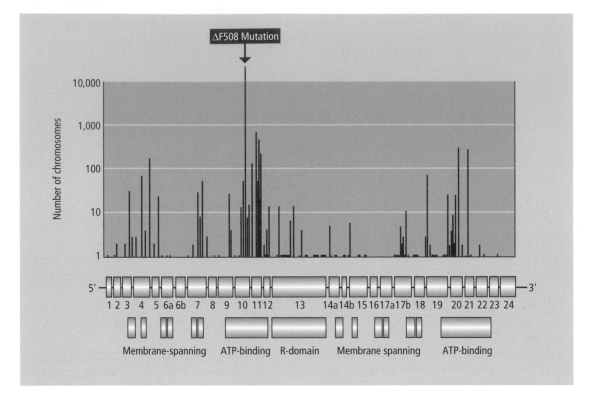

Fig. 25.4 Distribution and frequency of cystic fibrosis mutations in each of the 5 domains of the CFTR gene. Exons are numbered 1–24 (From Lap-Chee Tsui, 1992).

common disease-causing mechanism. For some diseases all affected individuals carry the same point mutation, whereas for other disorders the nature of the point mutation may vary between affected individuals.

An example of a disease in which all affected individuals have the same single point mutation is sickle cell anaemia (see also Chapter 20). This autosomal recessive disease has an incidence of about 1 in 500 in the black population and carries significant morbidity and mortality. It is caused by a point mutation in the beta-globin gene, changing codon 6 from CTC, which codes for glutamic acid, to CAC, encoding valine. The alteration in this single amino acid results in the production of insoluble haemoglobin. As soon as haemoglobin formed from mutant beta-globin becomes de-oxygenated, it aggregates and forms crystalline deposits in the red cell causing the cells to assume the characteristic sickle shape. Re-

peated sickling and unsickling damages the red cell membrane and shortens its lifespan. This leads to haemolytic anaemia, blockage of the microcirculation and associated tissue death.

Other diseases have a more complicated pattern of point mutations. One such disease is a form of inherited colon cancer called *familial adenomatous polyposis* (FAP). In this autosomal dominant disease, affected individuals develop polyps throughout their colon and rectum. By the third or fourth decade of life, at least one of these polyps will become malignant, and if left untreated, the patient will die. The ability to diagnose the disease early, means that preventative surgery can be carried out (see Case Study 27.1).

When the gene for this disease (the APC gene, sometimes referred to as the FAP gene) was identified it became apparent that the majority of patients had different mutations and that most of these were either point mutations or very small insertions or deletions of a few bases. The mutations are scattered throughout the 5′ end of the gene. Over 95 percent of mutations result in the introduction of a premature stop codon and a truncated protein is produced. In FAP, a mutation in only one allele of the FAP gene is necessary for disease. This is thought to be because the normal protein produced by the unaffected allele is inactivated by its interaction with the abnormal protein. In order to detect the mutation in a particular FAP family, it is necessary to scan each exon in turn until an abnormality is found (Fig. 25.5). Once the location of a mutation is pinpointed to a particular exon, the mutation can be confirmed by sequencing of the DNA in that region.

As the phenotype of patients with FAP can be variable, for example with regard to the age of onset, it was initially believed that this would be explained by the position and nature of the mutations. On the whole this has not been the case although there are some exceptions. An attenuated form of the disease with fewer polyps and a delayed age of onset is caused by mutations in exon 3. The protein made from this mutated gene is very short and rapidly degraded. Only low levels of normal-sized protein (produced by the unaffected allele) are present and the subsequent effect is a milder phenotype.

Duplications

Charcot–Marie–Tooth (CMT) syndrome is the most common inherited disorder of the peripheral nervous system affecting one in 2500 people and is characterized by wasting of the distal muscles of the limbs. It is subdivided into a number of types based on pathology and electrophysiology, the most common of which is Type 1A. The gene for the disease has been mapped to chromosome 17 and a surprising mechanism of mutation was identified. In this disorder the phenotype is associated with a large duplication of DNA. The most likely explanation for the phenotype is over-expression of a gene within the duplicated region, probably the gene encoding peripheral myelin protein (PMP). Interestingly, the CMT Type 1A phenotype is also seen if point mutations occur in this gene—yet another example of the same disease occurring via a number of different mechanisms.

Expansion of trinucleotide repeats

In recent years a completely different mechanism has been identified as the cause of genetic disease. This involves the expansion of trinucleotide repeat sequences (either CAG, CTG or CGG) and has been recognized as causing seven different single gene disorders to date (Table 25.1). Each of these diseases share some features in common, particularly the increasing severity of the disease with successive generations (termed *anticipation*) and a parental bias in the transmission of the severe forms of the disorder. There is, however, some variation in the way in which these repeats function at the DNA or mRNA level.

The first of these diseases to be recognized was *Fragile X mental retardation*, the most common inherited form of mental retardation, affecting 1 in 1000 males and 1 in 2000 females. The pattern of inheritance in Fragile X is unusual for an X-linked dominant disease in that there are both carrier males and carrier females. In addition, a proportion of carrier females are affected and these affected females always inherit the disease from their mothers.

The gene causing the disease is known as the *FMR1 gene* and when it was identified, an unstable region was noted in the 5' end of the gene. This region contains a repeat of the trinucleotide, CGG. In normal individuals, the number of these repeats varies between 10 and 50. Carriers of the repeat have between 50 and 200 copies (the so-called *premutation* for Fragile X), whereas affected individuals have over 200 copies. The clinical phenotype is only seen if there are over 200 copies of the repeat.

Now that the gene has been identified the patterns of inheritance can be explained. A male carrier will transmit the premutation to all his daughters. The number of CGG repeats varies only slightly during this process but remains within the premutation range so that all of his daughters are carriers of the disease and clinically unaffected. It is only when the premutation is transmitted by a female that there is a significant increase in the number of repeats leading to expression of the full mutation. If a carrier female

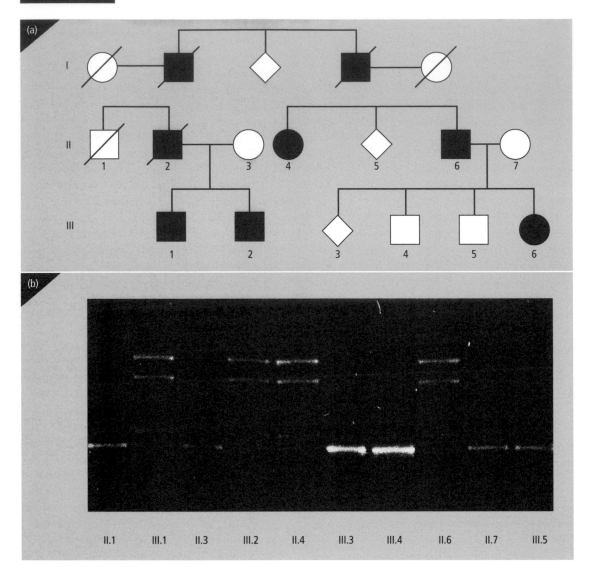

Fig. 25.5 Mutation analysis of a family with familial adenomatous polyposis. (a) Family pedigree (note that symbols with a diagonal line through them indicate that the patient is deceased). (b) Gel electrophoresis of amplified DNA from the FAP gene. Lanes II.1, II.3, III.3, III.4, III.5 and II.7 show only a single normal band indicating that no mutation is present. The other lanes show four bands indicating the presence of mutant DNA fragments.

transmits the mutation to her son the number of repeats will increase significantly to the full mutation range and he will be clinically affected. The premutation can also be transmitted to a daughter with a similar increase in repeat number but in this case only about 50 percent of females who inherit the full mutation will be mentally retarded. At the molecular level, expansion of the CGG repeat above 200 copies, results in abnormal methylation of DNA sequences at the 5' end of the gene and complete shut down of transcription of the FMR-1 gene.

Following identification of the FMR-1 gene, other diseases were identified where trinucleotide repeat expansion was shown to be the cause of the disorder. *Myotonic dystrophy* is a progressive wast-

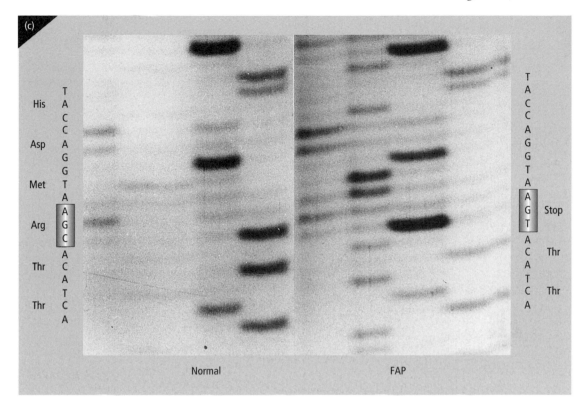

Fig. 25.5(c) DNA sequence of part of the FAP gene from a normal and an affected individual. There is a C to T transition which changes the codon for the amino acid arginine to a stop codon. (From Walker M.R. & Rapley R. © John Wiley & Sons, Ltd.)

ing disease of the muscles. When the responsible gene (the *DM* gene) was identified, an unstable CTG repeat was found in the 3' untranslated region. Normal individuals have 5–37 repeats. Affected patients have between 50 and several thousand repeats (Fig. 25.6).

There are many similarities to Fragile X. In general, the greater the number of repeats the more severe the disease. Again the disease increases in severity with successive generations but can be transmitted by both males and females. There is also a sex bias in transmission of the disease. There is a congenital form of myotonic dystrophy which results in the birth of a severely affected child and this only arises if the mother transmits the mutation. Unlike Fragile X, expansion of the

CTG repeats does not result in the shut down of transcription of the gene. Instead the mechanism of action may be an abnormal gain in function of the product of the DM gene.

Huntington's disease is one of the most serious genetic diseases affecting the CNS. It was one of the first single gene disorders to be localized to a specific chromosome (chromosome 4) but it has taken longer to isolate the gene. Recently an unstable CAG repeat sequence has been identified in the 5' coding sequence of a gene now known as 'huntingtin'. As with Fragile X and myotonic dystrophy there is a variation in repeat number in the normal population and an unstable expansion of the repeat number in affected individuals. Again there is evidence of anticipation—those with early onset disease have the highest number of repeats. There is also a sex bias with juvenile onset disease seen this time with transmission from the father. The precise effect of the trinucleotide repeat in Huntington's disease remains unclear, although it is more likely to be a

Table 25.1 Diseases associated with expansion of trinucleotide repeats

Disease	Inheritance	Sex bias for transmission	Gene function	Location of repeat	Disease causing mutation	Size of repeat in normal individuals	Size of repeat in disease
Fragile X	X-Linked dominant (partially penetrant i.e. not all individuals with the mutation will show the disease phenotype)	Full mutation only if transmitted by female	Unknown	5' Untranslated region	Transcription shut down	10–50	50–200 (premutation) >200 (full mutation)
Myotonic dystrophy	Autosomal dominant	Congenital form transmitted by female	Possible protein kinase	3' Untranslated region	Altered level of mRNA	5–37	50–2000
Huntington's disease	Autosomal dominant	Early onset transmitted primarily by male	Unknown	Protein-coding	? Gain of function	9–34	38–100
Spinobulbar muscular atrophy	X-Linked, recessive	Not yet known	Androgen receptor	Protein-coding	? Gain of function	11–31	40–62
FraxE	X-Linked dominant	Not yet known	Unknown	? Untranslated region	? Gain of function	6–25	? 25–200 (premutation) ? >200 (full mutation)
Spinocerebellar ataxia	Autosomal dominant	Possible paternal	Unknown	Protein-coding	Not yet known	25–36	43–81
Dentatorubral and Pallidoluysian atrophy	Autosomal dominant	Mainly paternal	Unknown	Protein-coding	? Gain of function	8–25	49–75

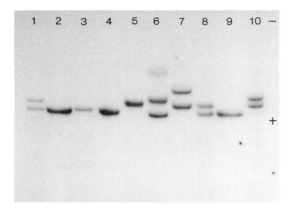

Fig. 25.6 Molecular analysis of the DM gene followed by gel electrophoresis. Normal individuals have either two 9 kb-sized DM alleles, two 10 kb-sized alleles, or are heterozygous. (This pattern in normals is due to an insertion of 1 kb in the gene which is not directly related to the disease.) Affected individuals have amplification of the CTG repeat which can be seen as an increase in size of the 10 kb allele. Lanes 1 and 8 show normal individuals heterozygous for the 9 and 10 kb alleles. Lanes 2–4 and 9 show normals homozygous for the 9 kb allele. Lane 5 shows a normal individual homozygous for the 10 kb allele. Affected individuals are in lanes 6, 7 and 10 and show an increase in the fragment size (bands do not travel as far to the anode) due to amplification of the CTG repeat (Photograph courtesy of Andrea Mitchell, DNA laboratory, Regional Genetics Service, Birmingham Heartlands Hospital).

gain in function of the abnormal protein as with myotonic dystrophy, rather than a shut down in transcription of the gene as with Fragile X. As with the other diseases, molecular diagnosis of Huntington's disease is now possible.

The features of other diseases associated with expansions in trinucleotide repeats are summarized in Table 25.1. It is likely that over the next few years a number of other single gene disorders will be associated with this novel disease-causing mechanism.

Summary

Genetic diseases are a significant cause of illness and death. It is estimated that 10 percent of all adult admissions and up to 50 percent of paediatric admissions to hospital are due to a genetic cause. Molecular techniques can now be used to diagnose the more common of these diseases. In some cases it is possible to show that a fetus is affected with a disease and also to give some idea about the severity of the disease. Pre-symptomatic diagnosis of some genetic diseases is also possible in selected cases.

Currently, new genes are being identified at the rate of about one a month. The next few years are therefore likely to be a very exciting time, enabling geneticists not only to understand more about the basic functions of cells but also to benefit individuals who are carriers of a genetic defect or are themselves affected by a genetic disease.

Key points

1 Mutations are changes in the genetic make-up of cells.

2 If a mutation is present in the cells that form the gametes, then the mutation may be transmitted to the offspring where it will be present in every cell of an affected individual. This mutation may arise as a new mutation in the germ cells of one or both parents, or it may have been inherited by the parents from previous generations.

3 The inherited single gene disorders are characterized by the presence of mutations involving only a single gene. These mutations may be deletions or insertions of bases, or involve the substitution of one base for another (point mutation).

4 Single gene disorders show clear patterns of Mendelian inheritance. They may be either X-linked (mutation is present in a gene on the X-chromosome, or autosomal (mutation is present in a gene present on one of chromosomes 1–22). In addition, they may be dominant, requiring a mutation in only one copy of the gene, or recessive, when a mutation in both copies of the gene is required.

Further reading

Gelehrter T.D. & Collins F.S. (1990) *Principles of Medical Genetics*. Williams & Wilkins, Baltimore.

Grompe M. (1993) The rapid detection of unknown mutations in nucleic acids. *Nature Genetics*, **5**: 111–117.

Lap-Chee Tsui. (1992) The spectrum of cystic fibrosis mutations. *Trends in Genetics*, **8**: 392–398.

Walker M.R. & Rapley R. (eds.) (1994) *Molecular and Antibody Probes in Diagnosis*. Wiley, Chichester.

Chromosome Abnormalities

Introduction

The previous chapter described a group of mutations which disrupt the expression of single genes. These mutations give rise to various single gene disorders (e.g. muscular dystrophy) that can now be defined using molecular techniques. This chapter describes the other clinically important group of mutations which involve changes in chromosome number or structure.

A point worth emphasizing is the difference in scale between the two groups of mutations. Single gene mutations may involve as little as a single base substitution ranging up to deletions of tens of kilobases of DNA. In contrast, the gain or loss of entire chromosomes, or the presence of microscopically visible deletions, involves relatively huge amounts of DNA, inevitably involving a large number of genes. The smallest chromosomal deletion, visible by light microscopy of suitably prepared and stained chromosomes, will remove a minimum of several megabases of DNA.

Constitutional and acquired chromosome abnormalities

Chromosome abnormalities may be broadly subdivided into two types: *constitutional* and *acquired*.

Constitutional chromosome abnormalities

Constitutional chromosome abnormalities are those that are either inherited from one or other parent, or arise as *de novo* (new) mutations during gamete development (*gametogenesis*) or during early embryogenesis. The mutation is usually found in all cells of an affected individual and since it is present in the germ cells can be transmitted to the next generation.

Acquired chromosome abnormalities

Acquired chromosome abnormalities may arise either during fetal growth, or later in cells retaining the ability to undergo cell division. Such acquired chromosomal mutations are confined to the cell in which they arise and its progeny. Nonrandom acquired chromosome abnormalities have now been described in a variety of leukaemias and solid tumours and are believed to contribute to the development of these lesions. This area is dealt with in more detail in Chapter 29.

Mitotic errors, resulting in gain or loss of single chromosomes at cell division, also occur at a very low rate in all individuals. Most of these errors are lethal for the cell progeny but a few are benign and may accumulate with age. Examples are the loss of the Y chromosome which occurs in a proportion of lymphocytes in elderly men and the addition of an extra X chromosome which occurs in a proportion of lymphocytes in elderly women.

The structure of chromosomes

Chromosomes are complex macromolecular structures which are a fundamental unit of genome organization. In order to appreciate the potential phenotypic effect of chromosome abnormalities it is helpful to have some idea of the relationship between the size of a chromosome and the DNA base-pair sequence from which genes are transcribed. Human somatic cells each contain about 6000 million base pairs of DNA organized in 46 chromosomes (known as the *diploid set*) consisting of 22 pairs of autosomes and two sex chromosomes, (XX in females and XY in males). At a conservative estimate there are 10 000 genes per *haploid set* (i.e. 23 chromosomes), this implies that each chromosome contains on average about 400 genes.

Chromosomes are highly organized structures consisting of a single, linear, double-stranded DNA molecule which interacts with various DNA-binding proteins in a complex manner (Fig. 26.1). The overall packing ratio from DNA strand to a chromosome at metaphase is about 8000:1. Chromosome 1 is the largest and contains approximately 300 megabases (i.e. 300 million base-pairs) of DNA, whereas chromosome 21 contains only 50 megabases of DNA.

Chromosome examination

'Banding' and other techniques allow unequivocal identification of chromosome pairs and detection

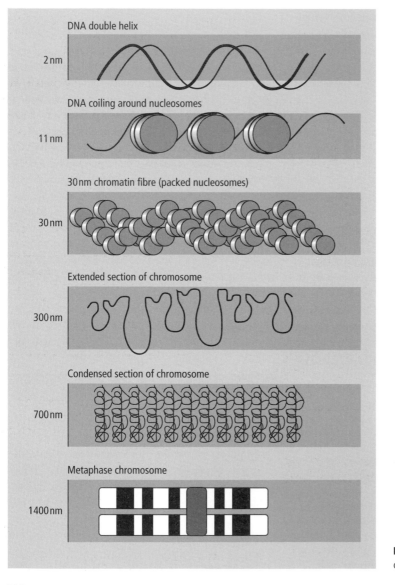

DNA double helix

2 nm

DNA coiling around nucleosomes

11 nm

30 nm chromatin fibre (packed nucleosomes)

30 nm

Extended section of chromosome

300 nm

Condensed section of chromosome

700 nm

Metaphase chromosome

1400 nm

Fig. 26.1 The organization of the chromosome.

of chromosome abnormalities. The simplest starting material for the examination of chromosomes is a small volume of blood (usually as little as 0.2 ml). This is cultured for 72 hours in medium containing *phytohaemagglutinin* (PHA). PHA stimulates the lymphocytes present in the blood to divide. Addition of colchicine arrests the lymphocytes at metaphase by inhibiting the polymerization of tubulin in the formation of spindle fibres. Preparations of the lymphocytes in metaphase (so called *metaphase spreads*) are then made on microscope slides, stained and examined.

Various stains may be employed which enable bands within each chromosome to be identified. This technique, known as *banding*, allows unequivocal identification of chromosome pairs, enabling delineation of many types of chromosome abnormality. Typically a combination of the protease *trypsin*, and Leishman's stain reveals 550 chromosome bands per haploid set. This approximates to about 6 megabases of DNA per chromosome band.

Newer molecular cytogenetic techniques exploit the fact that single-stranded DNA, tagged with a fluorescent label, will hybridize with its complementary strand on pretreated metaphase chromosomes. This technique, known as *fluorescence in situ hybridization* (FISH), allows the detection of submicrosopic deletions at critical points in the genome known to be associated with genetic disease (see Case Study 27.2). This approach underlines the fact that disruption of genetic material at the chromosomal level is part of a size continuum of mutation from a single base-pair alteration to the gain or loss of whole chromosomes involving tens of thousands of kilobases of DNA.

Types of chromosome abnormalities

Chromosome abnormalities are relatively more common than is generally supposed (Tables 26.1 and 26.2). They generally involve either a change in chromosome number, a change in chromosome structure, or abnormalities in the way chromosomes are inherited.

Numerical abnormalities

Numerical abnormalities may involve either the gain or loss of individual chromosomes (known as *aneuploidy*) or more rarely the gain of entire haploid sets of chromosomes resulting in *triploidy* ($n = 69$) or *tetraploidy* ($n = 92$). Aneuploidy may take the form an extra chromosome, known as *trisomy* (three copies present) or loss of a chromosome, referred to as *monosomy* (one copy present). Monosomy or trisomy involving the sex chromosomes are compatible with life and are usually associated with varying degrees of phenotypic abnormalities. This is because X inactivation normally ensures that only one X chromosome is actively transcribed in each cell and the Y chromosome contains a large amount of inert, highly repetitive, DNA. Clinically, the best defined sex chromosome abnormalities are *Klinefelter's syndrome* and *Turner's syndrome*.

Table 26.1 Frequency of chromosome abnormalities in various groups

Group	Frequency %
Clinically recognized pregnancies	8
Spontaneous abortions	50
Stillbirths	5
Livebirths (overall)	0.5

Table 26.2 Frequency of specific chromosome abnormalities

Chromosome abnormality	Frequency (live conceptuses)
Trisomy 21	1:700
Trisomy 18	1:3000
Trisomy 13	1:5000
47,XXY	1:1000 males
47,XXX	1:1000 males
45,X	1:10 000 females
Balanced translocations	1:500
Unbalanced translocations	1:2000

Klinefelter's syndrome (frequency 1 in 1000 males) occurs when two X chromosomes and one Y chromosome are present (47, XXY). The clinical features may include *hypogonadism* (small reproductive organs), *gynecomastia* (enlargement of male breasts). Individuals are invariably infertile. Verbal IQ may be lower compared to that of normal siblings.

Turner's syndrome (frequency 1 in 10 000 females) results from complete or partial monosomy of the X chromosome and is characterized primarily by short stature and sterility in affected females. Intelligence is normal. In just over one half of all cases there is complete monosomy of the X chromosome (i.e. 45, X). The remainder of patients show only partial monosomy, involving various structural rearrangements (e.g. deletions, rings or iso-chromosomes) of one X chromosome.

In contrast, monosomy or trisomy involving autosomes generally results in the loss or gain of too much important genetic information to be compatible with live birth. However, a number of autosomal trisomies may survive to birth. Trisomy 21 or Down's syndrome (see Fig. 26.2), Trisomy 18 (Edward's syndrome) and Trisomy 13 (Patau's syndrome) are the most common, in descending order of frequency.

Structural abnormalities

Structural abnormalities can take many forms in-

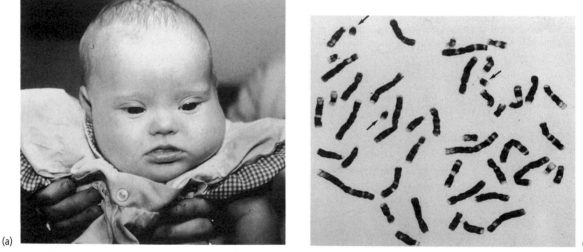

Fig. 26.2 (a) A child showing the typical facial chacteristics of Down's syndrome (see Table 26.4), (b) a chromosomal metaphase spread from a case of Down's syndrome showing 3 copies of chromosome 21 (arrowed). (c) Chromosomes from the same spread organized into groups (a karyotype) to show trisomy 21 more clearly.

cluding large deletions or insertions of genetic material, duplication of segments of a chromosome, inversions or translocations. The features of some of these structural abnormalities are illustrated in Fig. 26.3.

Many structural abnormalities produce chromosome imbalance as a result of gain or loss of genetic material. This usually results in profound physical and mental disability. Imbalance can be expressed as a percentage of the ratio of the length of the missing or additional segment over the total length of the haploid chromosome complement (percent HAL). This crude measurement, takes no account of gene content. Excess material, if less than 1 percent of HAL, in the form of partial trisomy, may result in a viable pregnancy with frequent livebirth. An excess of between 1–2 percent HAL increases the risk of a severely compromised phenotype resulting in non-viability *in utero* and therefore abortion. Partial monosomy

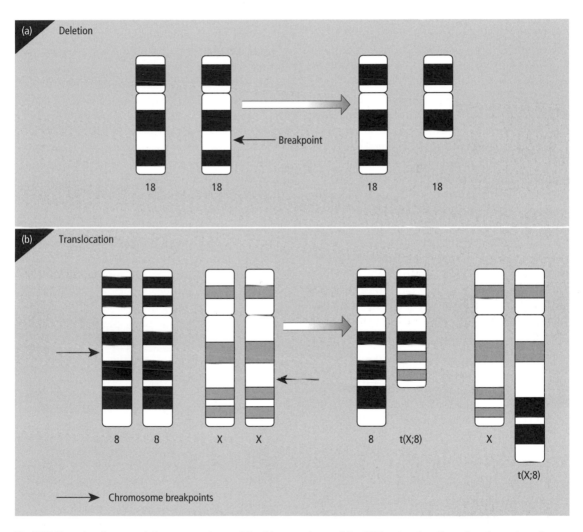

Fig. 26.3 Examples of structural chromosome abnormalities. (a) Deletion. Loss of chromosomal material, in this case from one of the chromosome 18 pair. Losses of segments of a chromosome may remove many important genes leading to severe phenotypic abnormalities. (b) Translocation. Shown here is a reciprocal translocation. Part of one chromosome 8 has been transferred to one X chromosome, and part of the X chromosome has been transferred to chromosome 8.

(i.e. a HAL deficit of 1–2 percent) is much less well tolerated than partial trisomy.

Translocation or inversion of chromosomal material may have no phenotypic effect on the individual because the rearrangement results in no gain or loss of material. However, such rearrangement of genetic material may give rise, through recombination or through segregation of translocated chromosomes during meiosis, to the production of unbalanced gametes with profound reproductive consequences for the carrier individual resulting in infertility, miscarriage or disabled offspring.

Structural abnormalities occur with high frequency in certain conditions associated with an increased sensitivity to chromosome breakage. These diseases include Fanconi's anaemia, Bloom's syndrome and ataxia telangiectasia (see also Chapter 28). The type of breakage, which is not generally site-specific, is characteristic for each disease and reflects the underlying DNA repair defect in each case.

Site-specific fragility may also occur both spontaneously and in the presence of various inducing agents. Only one site appears to be clinically important, and that is a site towards the end of the long arm of the X chromosome at Xq27.3. Expression of this fragile site is seen in the Fragile X syndrome which in affected males results in mild to moderate mental retardation, large ears, prominent forehead, macro-orchidism (enlarged testes), hyperflexibility of joints and perserverative speech. The underlying molecular basis for this chromosome fragility is now known to be an expansion beyond a critical threshold of the number of copies of a trinucleotide (CGG) repeat sequence (see Chapter 25).

Uniparental disomy

A third class of abnormality results when both chromosomes of a pair are inherited from one or other parent resulting in *uniparental disomy*. Such a finding implies that the parental origin of a chromosome may determine gene expression on that chromosome. This phenomenon is called *imprinting*. The best example of imprinting is the relationship between the pattern of inheritance of chromosome 15 in *Prader–Willi* and *Angelman* syndromes.

Prader–Willi syndrome (PWS) is characterized by infantile *hypotonia* (poor muscle tone), short stature, small hands and feet, almond shaped eyes, hypogonadism, psychomotor retardation, *hypopigmentation* (pale skin) and early onset of childhood *hyperphagia* (over eating) with consequent obesity.

Angelman's syndrome (AS) is characterized by severe mental retardation, seizures, inappropriate laughter, *ataxic gait* (unsteady posture, lurching walk), puppet-like upper-limb movements, lack of speech and a large jaw.

In PWS, deletions within the long arm of chromosome 15 (q11–q13) are always found on the paternally derived chromosome. Non-deletion cases can display uniparental disomy and in these cases two copies of the maternal chromosome 15 are present. These findings imply that the absence of a sequence on the paternally derived chromosome 15 at q11–q13 gives rise to the PWS phenotype.

In contrast in AS, deletions are always on the maternally derived chromosome and uniparental disomy, although much less frequent than in PWS, manifests itself in the presence of two paternal copies of chromosome 15. Another example of imprinting is seen in triploidy ($n = 69$). The phenotypic outcomes of triploid chromosome complements are listed in Table 26.3.

Table 26.3 Phenotypic consequences of triploid chromosome complements. The phenotypic effects depend upon the parental origin of the extra chromosome set

Syndrome	Genotype	Phenotype
Triploid conceptus	Two maternal sets, one paternal set	Small and fibrotic placenta, embryo retarded
Partial mole	One maternal set, two paternal sets	Trophoblast hyperplasia, embryo retarded and/or malformed

Chromosome abnormality and clinical syndrome

Variation is the hallmark of the relationship between a chromosome abnormality and a clinical syndrome. Using the example of Down's syndrome (trisomy 21) it can be seen (Table 26.4) that there is considerable variability in the phenotype of such individuals. Indeed no single feature is considered to be *pathognomic* (i.e. unique) for Down's syndrome. Such variation may well partly reflect the different genetic background, consisting of the other chromosomes that make up the diploid set, in each individual. It should also be noted that a 'critical region' within chromosome 21 is required to be trisomic to express the Down's syndrome phenotype (Fig. 26.4).

Another general consideration is that the influence of a gene or set of genes acts through a myriad of developmental pathways. Chromosome abnormalities therefore increase the probability of particular developmental anomalies without predetermining them.

How do chromosome abnormalities arise?

It is now possible to determine both the parental

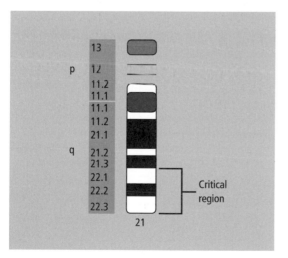

Fig. 26.4 A critical region within chromosome 21 is required to be trisomic for the Down's syndrome phenotype to be expressed.

origin of chromosomal abnormalities and in some cases the mechanisms by which they arise. In general, maternal errors account for most aneuploidy states, whereas point mutations and structural rearrangements are more likely to result from paternal errors.

Maternal errors

By the time of birth the average human ovary contains about 2 million oöcytes in the diplotene stage of the first meiotic division. Here they remain in a resting phase until further maturation through the meiotic cycle occurs prior to ovulation.

Many trisomies arise as a result of errors in segregation at the first maternal meiotic division (M1) in oöcytes. *Non-disjunction* is the most common segregation defect. Non-disjunction occurs when an homologous pair of chromosomes fail to disjoin at M1, resulting in two aneuploid cells. The oöcytes formed will therefore have either an extra chromosome ($n + 1$), or one less chromosome ($n - 1$). Fertilization of such oöcytes with normal spermatocytes will result in either

Table 26.4 Frequency of phenotypic abnormalities seen in Down's syndrome patients

Phenotypic feature	Frequency in Down's syndrome patients (%)
Oblique (up-slanting) palpebral fissures	82
Loose skin on nape of neck	81
Brachycephaly (short antero-posterior skull length)	75
Hyperflexibility	73
Flat nasal bridge	68
Short, broad hands	64
Epicanthic folds (skin folds over inner canthi)	59
Short fifth finger	58
Brushfield spots (speckled iris ring)	56
Furrowed tongue	55
Transverse palmar crease	53
Folded or dysplastic ear	50
Protruding tongue	47
Congenital cardiac defects	40

trisomic ($2n + 1$), or monosomic ($2n - 1$) zygotes. The underlying mechanism(s) leading to non-disjunction at MI are not known but alterations in the level of recombination between chromosomes are associated with non-disjunction. Trisomy 21, 47, XXY and 47, XXX, but not trisomy 16 and 18, have been associated with a significant reduction in recombination.

Paternal errors

'*De novo*' structural rearrangements and point mutations giving rise to a variety of inherited conditions, such as familial retinoblastoma and Type-1 neurofibromatosis (see also Chapter 28), show a strong bias towards a paternal origin. In contrast to oögenesis, spermatogenesis is a continuous process of production of spermatozoa from puberty onwards.

Studies in mice and *Drosophila* which closely resemble humans with respect to spermatogenesis, indicate that point mutations arise and accumulate in spermatogonia which are pre-meiotic cells capable of mitotic division. In contrast, in mice and *Drosophila* and by extrapolation in humans, structural rearrangements fatally disrupt meiosis and therefore must arise during post-meiotic maturation (i.e. during spermatid and spermatozoon stages).

Summary

The ability to recognize and define chromosome abnormalities has contributed to our understanding of the nature and origin of much congenital abnormality and in many cases allows the possibility of prenatal diagnosis in subsequent pregnancies. The nature of the fundamental causes of chromosome abnormalities are still not clear.

Key points

1 Chromosome abnormalities may be defined as microscopically visible changes in chromosome morphology and represent mutations involving a large number of genes. The smallest detectable chromosomal deletions remove a minimum of several megabases of DNA.

2 Chromosome abnormalities may be either constitutional, if they are inherited from one or other parent, or acquired, if the mutation arises during fetal growth or later in cells retaining the ability to undergo cell division.

3 Chromosome abnormalities may involve either a change in chromosome number, structure or pattern of inheritance.

4 Changes in chromosome number may involve either the gain or loss of individual chromosomes (aneuploidy) or the gain of entire haploid sets (triploidy or tetraploidy). Aneuploidy of the germ cells can give rise to either trisomic or monosomic zygotes.

5 Structural abnormalities include large deletions or insertions of genetic material, duplication of segments of a chromosome, inversions or translocations.

6 A third class of abnormality arises when both chromosomes of a pair are inherited from one or other parent. This is known as uniparental disomy and implies that the parental origin of a chromosome may determine gene expression on that chromosome.

Further reading

Connor J.M. & Ferguson-Smith M.A. (1993) *Essential Medical Genetics*, 4th edn. Blackwell Scientific Publications, Oxford.

Strachan T. (1992) In Read A.P. & Brown T. (Eds.) *The Human Genome*. Bios Scientific Publishers, Oxford.

Therman E. & Susman M. (1993) *Human Chromosomes: Structure, Behaviour and Effects*. Springer–Verlag, New York.

Case Studies

27.1 Rectal bleeding with diarrhoea

Clinical features

A 17-year-old girl was referred to the gastro-enterology department with a 6-month history of rectal bleeding and diarrhoea. When asked about the delay in seeing a doctor she replied that her father had died when she was 6-years old from what her mother called 'bowel problems' and that she had been afraid she might have the same problem.

Details of her father's medical history showed that he had died from a metastatic colonic adenocarcinoma when only 35-years-old. The post mortem report revealed that he also had multiple polypoid adenomas situated throughout the entire length of his colon.

Previous family history revealed that the patient's brother had died from a rare form of liver cell cancer, known as *hepatoblastoma*, when only 5-years old.

Investigations

The results of laboratory investigations performed are shown in Table 27.1.1.

The total white cell count is towards the upper limit of normal. The differential white cell count is normal.

Erythrocyte morphology showed microcytic (cells reduced in size) and hypochromic (staining intensity reduced) red blood cells. Normal erythrocytes would appear normocytic and normochromic (see Chapter 20).

Table 27.1.1 Laboratory investigations

Analyte	Value	Reference range (female)
Total white cell count	$10.6 \times 10^9/l$	4.0–11.0
Red cell count	$3.46 \times 10^{12}/l$	3.8–5.8
Haemoglobin	7.6 g/dl	11.5–15.5
Haematocrit	0.244	0.37–0.47
Mean cell volume	70.5 fl	82–92
Mean cell haemoglobin	21.96 pg	27.0–32.0
Platelet count	$460 \times 10^9/l$	150–400

Blood film
White blood cell differential

Neutrophils	70%
Lymphocytes	22%
Monocytes	6%
Eosinophils	2%
Basophils	0%

The blood count results indicate iron deficiency anaemia. Iron deficiency can arise due to dietary deficiency, malabsorption or chronic blood loss (see Chapter 20). In this case, in view of the clinical history and presentation, the most likely cause is chronic rectal blood loss.

Chronic rectal bleeding and diarrhoea may be due to a number of inflammatory conditions of the colon, including ulcerative colitis and Crohn's disease (see Chapter 18), or may have an infective cause. Examination of the colon and rectum by sigmoidoscopy is therefore indicated. On sigmoidoscopy, multiple polyps were observed throughout the patient's colon and rectum, some of which were biopsied. Histological examination of these polyps revealed that they were benign tumours of colonic epithelial cells (*adenomas*). Microbiological culture of the stools was negative.

Diagnosis

The presence of multiple polypoid adenomas in the colon indicates a diagnosis of *familial adenomatous polyposis* (FAP). This is consistent with the early onset of colonic adenocarcinoma in the patient's father which had presumably arisen in at least one of the mutiple adenomas situated throughout his colon.

Diagnosis: familial adenomatous polyposis.

Discussion

FAP is an autosomal dominant condition, therefore any offspring of an affected parent have a 50 percent risk of developing the disease. Hepatoblastoma is a relatively rare childhood tumour but is often found in association with FAP. A diagnosis of FAP in the deceased boy is therefore highly likely. The genetic basis of FAP is discussed in detail in Chapter 25.

Screening of children in FAP families begins at the age when polyps start to develop (i.e. usually in the mid-teens). The three ways in which screening can be carried out are outlined below.

1 Annual clinical investigations from mid-teens until mid-40s. This involves inspection of the colon by sigmoidoscopy and eye examination. Approximately 90 percent of FAP patients have lesions in their eye known as *congenital hypertrophy of the pigment epithelium* (CHRPE). These lesions, if present in affected members of a family, are good markers of gene carriers. Patients generally accept eye examination better than sigmoidoscopy (although sigmoidoscopy is still necessary once a patient is identified by eye examination).

2 Linkage analysis using restriction fragment length polymorphisms (RFLPs, see Chapter 25) around the FAP gene locus can be carried out in suitable families. This can be used to identify those at highest risk, who can then be screened annually as above. Those individuals identified to be at low risk by RFLP analysis may still need to be screened occasionally by sigmoidoscopy as the technique can produce false negative results.

3 Finally, it may be possible to identify the specific mutation in an affected family member. At-risk family members can then be screened for the presence of this mutation. The detection of mutations in this way is more accurate than RFLP analysis.

A mutation in exon 15 of the FAP gene at codon 1309 was identified in the patient described above. This mutation is the most common in FAP families, occuring in about 10 percent of families worldwide and would be the first to be tested for in any new family.

A full pedigree of the case family revealed that there were two younger male siblings, aged 14 and 11, both of whom would be expected to have a 50 percent risk of developing the disease. The mutation was not found in the 14-year-old sibling so further screening was not necessary in his case. The 11-year-old brother was too young to be screened since there was no evidence of a particularly early onset of the disease in this family. Testing would be offered to the younger boy in two to three years time unless requested earlier by the family, or if symptoms appeared.

Treatment and prognosis

Since it is certain that one of the adenomas in affected individuals will become malignant, treatment is by removal of the colon. The prognosis for patients who have had this type of surgery at an early stage is relatively good. However, regular investigations to check for the presence of any further polyps developing in the remains of the rectal tissue or in the upper gastrointestinal tract are essential.

Questions

1 What is the likely diagnosis in a family showing a history of colonic cancer in which affected members develop right-sided tumours at around 40–50 years of age without any prior evidence of adenomas.

Answer: FAP is only one of several inherited colon cancer syndromes. The later age of onset, in conjunction with tumours of the right side of the colon and a lack of adenomas suggests a diagnosis of *hereditary non-polyposis colon cancer* (HNPCC). This disease accounts for 10–15 percent of all colon cancer cases and is therefore more common than FAP. Four causative genes have so far been identified. Two are DNA repair genes, one is situated on chromosome 2, and is responsible for approximately 60 percent of cases. The other, on chromosome 3, accounts for a further 30 percent. Detection of mutations in HNPCC families is now possible.

2 Can you explain the basis of the iron deficiency anaemia observed in this patient?

The total iron content of the human body is typically 3–5 grams, two-thirds of which is contained within erythrocytes. At the end of the erythrocyte life span, haemoglobin is catabolized and iron is released. The majority of this is conserved, being transported to iron stores or to the bone marrow for reincorporation into new erythrocytes. To compensate for the small amounts of iron which are lost normally, around 2 mg of iron are absorbed daily from dietary sources. Each millilitre of erythrocytes contains approximately 1 mg of iron, so in chronic blood loss there can be a substantial loss of iron from the iron pool, which must be replaced from other sources. Iron for haemopoiesis is drawn from iron stores and absorption increases to compensate for this. However, if blood loss is great, losses of iron invariably exceed iron available from iron stores and from dietary sources. Iron deficiency anaemia is the usual outcome. For this reason, patients presenting with unexplained iron deficiency anaemia must always be investigated for possible occult (hidden) blood loss.

27.2 Heart murmur and cleft palate

Clinical features

A 10-day-old baby boy with cleft palate and a cardiac murmur required assisted ventilation. Several hours later he developed twitching, neuromuscular irritability, and convulsions.

Investigations

Laboratory investigations revealed a plasma calcium level of 1.6 mmol/l (reference range: 2.2–2.6). Values for all other analytes measured were within normal reference ranges.

Investigation at a regional paediatric cardiothoracic centre by echocardiography revealed obstructive lesions of the left (pulmonary) outflow tract together with a ventral septal defect (VSD).

A clinical geneticist reviewing the case noted that the facial features were slightly *dysmorphic* (mis-shapen). Inner canthi were slightly displaced and the palpebral fissures were short. The root and bridge of the nose were noted to be wide and prominent. The mouth was relatively small. The ears were low-set and posteriorly rotated. Deficient upper helices together with an increase in anterior–posterior diameter gave a relatively circular shape to the ear. Previous family history revealed that a half-sibling from the father's previous marriage had died from cardiac failure within five weeks of birth. A post mortem examination had revealed the presence of congenital heart defects together with *hypoplastic* (underdeveloped) thymus and parathyroid glands. Further questioning of the family also revealed that the patient's father had learning problems at school and a repaired cleft palate.

Blood samples were taken from the patient and his parents for chromosome analysis. No abnormalities were detected on conventional cyto-

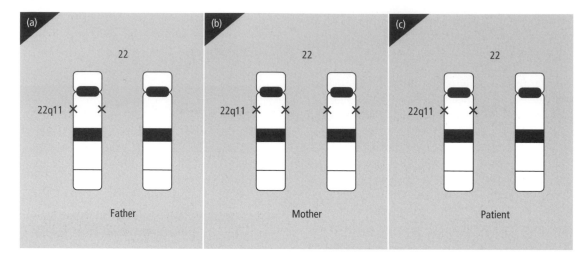

Fig. 27.2.1 Fluorescence *in situ* hybridization analysis of chromosomes from the case family. (a) Father's chromosome 22 pair. Fluorescent dye-labelled probe to a region within the DiGeorge critical region (DGCR) hybridizes (shown as star) to one chromosome 22 only. (b) Mother's chromosome 22 pair. Hybridization of probe to both chromosomes. (c) Patient's chromosome 22 pair. The probe only hybridizes to one chromosome 22. These results suggest that the patient and his father have a deletion of the DGCR on one copy of chromosome 22. The mother is deletion-negative.

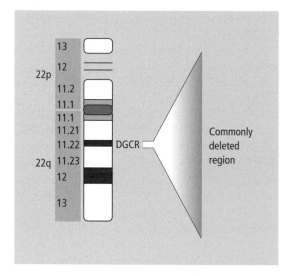

Fig. 27.2.2 DiGeorge's syndrome is characterized by deletions within chromosome 22 encompassing the 'DiGeorge critical region' (DGCR). This region occupies approximately 2 megabases of DNA.

genetic analysis using banding techniques (see Chapter 26).

Fluorescence *in situ* hybridization (FISH) analysis of the patient's chromosomes (Fig. 27.2.1) re-vealed a sub-microscopic deletion on one copy of chromosome 22 at q11. This region encompasses the so called *DiGeorge critical region* (Fig. 27.2.2). The same abnormality was also present in the father's case, but the mother's chromosomes were normal.

Further laboratory investigations revealed reduced numbers of circulating T lymphocytes. A chest radiograph failed to show any conclusive evidence of thymus gland hypoplasia.

Diagnosis

The association of congenital cardiac defect, dysmorphic facies, thymus gland hypoplasia, cleft palate and *hypocalcaemia* (reduced serum calcium levels), together with a microdeletion of chromosome 22 at q11 suggests a diagnosis of Di George's syndrome. The FISH results show that the patient has inherited the chromosome abnormality from his father (Fig. 27.2.3).

Diagnosis: DiGeorge's syndrome.

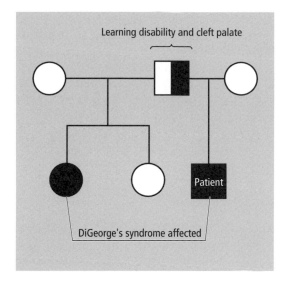

Learning disability and cleft palate

Patient

DiGeorge's syndrome affected

Fig. 27.2.3 Family pedigree of case family.

Discussion

DiGeorge's syndrome comprises thymus and parathyroid gland hypoplasia, hypocalcaemia, cardiac outflow tract defects, and dysmorphic facies. It is almost invariably associated with an interstitial microdeletion of chromosome 22 encompassing the DiGeorge critical region (DGCR) comprising about 2 megabases of DNA. The hypocalcaemia seen in DiGeorge's syndrome is due to an underdeveloped parathyroid gland which produces less than normal levels of parathyroid hormone (parathyroid hormone increases serum calcium levels). Clinically, hypocalcaemia manifests as neuromuscular irritability and convulsions.

DiGeorge's syndrome is now thought to be at the severe end of a spectrum of overlapping clinical disorders associated with the same deletion. *Conotruncal anomaly face syndrome* (dysmorphic facial appearance and cardiac outflow defects) and *velocardiofacial syndrome* (VCFS) (cleft palate, cardiac anomalies, and characteristic facial appearance) show a deletion within 22q11 in most cases. All three syndromes show considerable phenotypic overlap and variability even within a single family. The acronym CATCH-22: Cardiac defects; Abnormal facies; Thymic hypoplasia; Cleft palate; Hypocalcaemia, has been coined as an umbrella term for this overlapping group of syndromes.

A great deal of effort is currently being expended to unravel the molecular basis of these conditions and to identify the relevant gene or genes. A better understanding of the molecular basis of the disease will allow more accurate diagnosis and prognosis and ultimately pave the way for gene therapy.

Treatment and prognosis

Convulsions are controlled by administering 2.5 percent calcium gluconate in a 5 percent glucose solution which is given intravenously until the convulsions cease. It is important to monitor heart rate during treatment since *bradycardia* (a decreased heart rate, usually defined as less than 60 beats/minute) may develop. From then on, calcium gluconate is added to feeds until the serum calcium concentration rises to normal. Any congenital heart defects will require surgery in an appropriate unit.

In one recent study, 24 children with DiGeorge's syndrome were assessed during the first few weeks after diagnosis. All the patients studied had a cardiac defect. Thirteen of the 24 children died during the period of study, 11 as a consequence of their cardiac defect and two as a result of infection secondary to severe immunodeficiency. It should be noted that thymus gland hypoplasia in DiGeorge's syndrome, whilst resulting in underproduction of T lymphocytes, does not normally produce a life-threatening immunodeficiency (see also Chapter 14). However, common infections may occur frequently up to 2–3 years of age which is then often followed by a spontaneous improvement.

Moderate to severe developmental delay may be expected to occur in approximately half of all patients with DiGeorge's syndrome who survive beyond infancy. Symptoms of deafness may be present in older children and this should be confirmed by formal testing.

Genetic counselling of parents of children with DiGeorge's syndrome depends on whether a parent has the deletion. When one parent has the deletion the risk of any offspring being affected is 50 percent.

The value of FISH in the diagnosis of chromosome abnormalities is well illustrated in this case. FISH may also be useful in the prenatal diagnosis of DiGeorge's syndrome. Screening for microdeletions of 22q11 using FISH has been successfully accomplished on cells from chorionic villus samples at 11–12 weeks of pregnancy. Counselling for this approach may still present clinical and ethical dilemmas because of the phenotypic variability that is seen in affected individuals.

Questions

1 Why do you think the patient is more severely affected than his father?

Answer: unlike other inherited disorders (e.g. myotonic dystrophy) DiGeorge's syndrome shows no evidence of increasing severity from one generation to the next. The most likely explanation in this case is that only mildly affected individuals (i.e. the father) will survive to adulthood and therefore reproduce.

2 Does the risk of having affected offspring increase or decrease in a man or woman who is a known deletion carrier who has two 'normal' (i.e. deletion-negative) offspring?

Answer: if one or other parent is a known carrier of the deletion, the chance that any individual offspring will inherit that deletion is 50 percent irrespective of the number of deletion-negative offspring.

Part 8
Neoplasia

Principles of Neoplasia

Introduction

Neoplasia, literally meaning 'new growth', is a disorder characterized by the abnormal and continuous growth of cells which are no longer subject to the homeostatic controls which maintain the appropriate number of cells in normal tissues. In most cases these cells form a solid mass of tissue which is referred to as a *tumour* (literally 'swelling') or *neoplasm*. An exception to this is leukaemia in which the abnormal cells arise from precursor cells in the bone marrow and pass into the bloodstream in the same way as normal blood cells.

This chapter introduces the basic principles of neoplasia. The cellular basis of neoplasia is outlined and benign and malignant forms of this disorder are described. The role of causative influences, including both environmental and genetic factors, are considered in relation to the development and progression of neoplasia. Finally, host responses to neoplasia are reviewed.

Growth characteristics of neoplasms

Under normal circumstances the number of cells in a given tissue is subject to variation. Thus, when an increased workload demand is placed upon a particular tissue, the tissue may respond by increasing cell number, a process known as *hyperplasia*. In some settings hyperplasia may be abnormal. Cells which no longer have the capacity to divide respond to increases in workload demand by increasing cell size. This is known as *hypertrophy*. Examples of hypertrophy include the increase in skeletal muscle size in training athletes and the 'pathological' hypertrophy of the muscle cells of the left ventricle (left ventricular hypertrophy) that occurs in long-standing hypertension (see Case Study 24.1).

In contrast to the processes of hyperplasia and hypertrophy which are essentially reversible once the provoking stimulus has been removed, neoplastic growth is usually not reversible. Neoplastic cells are no longer responsive to the controlling mechanisms that maintain cell number in normal tissues and therefore continue to divide under circumstances in which normal cells cease proliferation. The net result is the progressive accumulation of neoplastic cells and the formation of a tumour mass. The differences in growth regulation between normal and neoplastic cells may be summarized under the following five headings.

Growth factor dependency

Stimulation of a normal cell into a proliferative state often depends upon an external signal in the form of a growth factor. *Platelet-derived growth factor* (PDGF) is an example of a growth factor. Following tissue damage, PDGF is released by platelets and stimulates adjacent fibroblasts to divide and form a fibrous scar. Many growth factors bind to receptors situated on the surface of target cells. Binding of growth factor to a receptor initiates a series of biochemical changes within the cell which ultimately leads to cell division.

Tumour cells are not as dependent on growth factors as normal cells and are able to proliferate when concentrations of growth factors are much lower than those required by normal cells. These differences in growth factor requirements can be explained by several possible mechanisms. Tumour cells may secrete growth factors which are able to stimulate their own proliferation (*autocrine stimulation*), or they may respond more vigorously to growth factors produced by other cells. Alternatively, the tumour cells may proliferate in the absence of the usual growth factors required by normal cells. These mechanisms are outlined in Fig. 28.1.

Density-dependent inhibition of growth

Once normal dividing cells reach a finite density they stop proliferating. In contrast, neoplastic cells do not cease proliferation but continue to

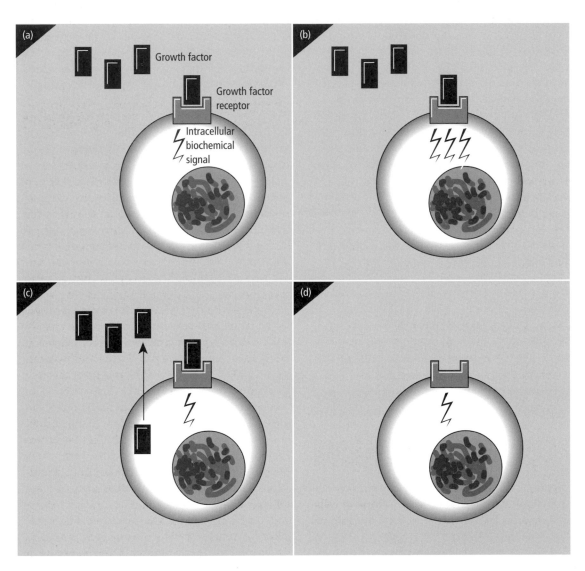

Fig. 28.1 Possible mechanisms leading to reduced growth factor dependency by neoplastic cells. (a) Normal cell. Ligation of a growth factor to a receptor on the cell membrane leads to intracellular biochemical signalling which will eventually produce cell division. (b) Neoplastic cells may respond more vigorously to growth factor ligation, or (c) they may secrete growth factors which stimulate their own proliferation. Alternatively, (d) a defective receptor may transmit intracellular growth signals in the absence of an extracellular growth factor.

replicate to much higher densities than normal cells.

Anchorage dependence

Most normal cells need contact with a substratum in the extracellular environment to reproduce. Neoplastic cells, on the other hand, are able to grow without attachment to a substratum. This is well illustrated *in vitro* by the ability of tumour cells to form colonies when suspended as single cells in agar.

Contact inhibition of movement

When normal cells are placed in culture, they have the ability to respond to the presence of other cells. Thus, when two cells come into contact, one or both will change direction ensuring that the cells do not overlay each other. This characteristic is referred to as *contact inhibition of movement*. Neoplastic cells lack contact inhibition of movement and often grow over or under each other.

Adhesiveness

Tumour cells are less adhesive than normal cells and are less firmly attached to neighbouring cells or the extracellular matrix. Loss of adhesiveness contributes to the invasive and metastatic properties of some neoplasms (see Chapter 30).

Tumour growth rate

Tumour growth rate is determined by various factors, including the rate at which new tumour cells are generated by cell division, and the rate at which cells are lost from the dividing cell pool, either by cell death or by differentiation. Factors other than cell kinetics can modify the rate of growth of neoplasms. An adequate blood supply, for example, is necessary for tumour growth. In experimental systems, tumours can only grow to several millimetres in diameter without provision of a blood supply. Although tumours often rely upon the host for their blood supply, tumour cells can secrete *angiogenic* (blood vessel-forming) factors, which result in the proliferation of blood vessels within the tumour.

Hormones can also influence the growth rate of tumours arising in hormone-responsive cells. Some breast tumours, for example, grow very rapidly during pregnancy in response to the high oestrogen levels. Some of these oestrogen-dependent breast tumours have been successfully treated with the use of anti-oestrogen drugs (e.g. tamoxifen).

The cellular basis of neoplasia

Neoplasms are believed to arise from a single *target cell* which has undergone a series of genetic changes (*mutations*) that ultimately result in its ability to escape the normal proliferative controls imposed upon normal cells. Mutations may occur spontaneously within cells or they may be induced following exposure to chemicals or radiation. Most mutations impair cell survival and ultimately result in cell death. However, in some cases a mutation may provide a cell with a growth advantage when compared to its normal counterparts. Mutations that enhance cell growth usually arise either in genes that stimulate cell division (*oncogenes*), or in those that inhibit cell division (*tumour suppressor genes*). The functions of these genes are discussed in detail in Chapter 29.

A cell bearing a beneficial mutation may continue to divide until a collection of genetically identical cells or *clone* is formed. Cells from this clone may in turn acquire new mutations which further enhance their growth potential. Eventually a point may be reached when some of these cells are able to grow in an uncontrolled fashion and a tumour results. Once a tumour is established, mutations within tumour cells may give rise to multiple subclones within the tumour, each with differing properties. This is referred to as *tumour heterogeneity* and is an important concept in relation to tumour progression (see Chapter 30).

Benign and malignant neoplasms

Neoplasms are broadly divisible into *benign* and *malignant* subgroups. *Cancer* is a term which is commonly used to describe the disease which results from the presence of a malignant neoplasm. Benign and malignant neoplasms differ in a number of important ways as outlined in the following sections.

Invasion and metastasis

Malignant neoplasms are characterized by their capacity to invade surrounding normal tissue and to spread to distant parts of the body to generate secondary growths. This latter property is known as *metastasis* and is described in detail in Chapter 30. In general, benign tumours do not invade adjacent tissues and do not metastasize.

Degree of differentiation

The tumour cells of benign neoplasms closely resemble the cell of origin and are therefore described as being *well differentiated*. Although malignant neoplasms may also be well differentiated, many are either *poorly differentiated* (cells of the tumour do not closely resemble cell of origin) or *undifferentiated* (the origin of the tumour cells cannot be determined). In general, undifferentiated tumours have higher growth rates than their well differentiated counterparts.

Clinical outcome

Malignant neoplasms are often fatal to their host. This is primarily due to their ability to metastasize and to develop resistance to various forms of therapy (see Chapter 30). In contrast, benign neoplasms are life-threatening only in the following exceptional circumstances.

If the tumour is present within, or impinges upon, a vital structure. Certain benign tumours of the atrium (*atrial myxomas*) may cause valve obstruc-tion, cardiac insufficiency and sudden death in some cases.

If the tumour produces a physiologically active substance in increased amounts. Some benign tumours of the adrenal medulla (*phaeochromocytomas*) secrete excessive amounts of adrenaline leading to hypertension which can precipitate myocardial infarction or cerebral haemorrhage. Likewise, beta-cell adenomas of the pancreas can secrete enough insulin to produce fatal hypoglycaemia (low blood glucose levels).

If the tumour is present within the central nervous system (CNS). Because the CNS is an enclosed system, expanding lesions can cause pressure damage to surrounding nervous tissue or produce more serious complications as a result of associated rises in intracranial pressure.

Classification of neoplasia

Neoplasms are usually classified on the basis of the presumed cell or tissue of origin irrespective of the site at which the tumour is found. Thus, squamous cell carcinomas are malignant neoplasms derived from squamous epithelial cells. Since this type of epithelial cell is found in many locations within the body, squamous cell carcinoma can arise in many sites which include skin, oesophagus and cervix.

Some neoplasms, for example *chronic myeloid leukaemia* (CML, see also Case Study 31.1), arise in *stem cells*. Stem cells are present in small numbers in cell populations and have two critical functions: to generate descendants which will become differentiated and perform the function of the tissue; and to renew themselves so that a stable number of stem cells remain. CML is characterized by the accumulation of neoplastic cells of differing myeloid lineages which have all descended from a common neoplastic myeloid stem cell. Table 28.1 gives a brief classification of some neoplasms.

Table 28.1 Some neoplasms and their cell or tissue of origin

Tissue or cell of origin	Benign neoplasm	Malignant neoplasm
Epithelium		
Squamous epithelium	Squamous cell papilloma	Squamous cell carcinoma
Glandular epithelium includes glandular epithelium of solid organs	Adenoma	Adenocarcinoma
Mesothelium	Mesothelioma	Malignant mesothelioma
Connective tissue		
Cartilage	Chondroma	Chondrosarcoma
Bone	Osteoma	Osteosarcoma
Smooth muscle	Leiomyoma	Leiomyosarcoma
Striated muscle	Rhabdomyoma	Rhabdomyosarcoma
Lymphocytes	–	Lymphoma
Haemopoietic cells	–	Leukaemia
Melanocytes	Melanoma	Malignant melanoma

Note that there are no well defined benign counterparts of the lymphomas and leukaemias.

Causal factors in the development of cancer

Analysis of the incidence of cancer in different human populations throughout the world has lead to the identification of groups of causal factors. These are broadly divided into environmental and genetic subgroups.

Environmental factors

Chemical agents

The classic example of cancer following exposure to chemicals was described in 1775 by Percival Pott who noted that chimney sweeps had a high incidence of cancer of the scrotum which he attributed to exposure to soot. Subsequently, many hundreds of chemical carcinogens have been implicated in the causation of cancer. Examples of these are listed in Table 28.2.

Most chemical carcinogens are *electrophilic* (electron-seeking) and chemically modify the DNA of exposed cells, thereby inducing mutations. Some chemical agents are not themselves carcinogenic but are converted to carcinogenic derivatives by metabolic enzymes of the body (Fig. 28.2). These are called *indirect carcinogens*. Carcinogens which do not require chemical modification for their cancer-causing properties are known as *direct carcinogens*.

The process of chemical carcinogenesis can be observed experimentally by monitoring the effect

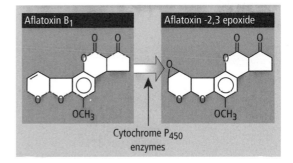

Fig. 28.2 Aflatoxin B_1 is an indirect carcinogen requiring conversion to aflatoxin-2,3 epoxide by the action of the cytochrome P_{450} enzymes in the liver. This compound then reacts with guanine residues in DNA.

Table 28.2 Examples of chemical carcinogens

Chemical agent	Nature of exposure	Resultant cancer
Beta-naphthylamine	Chemical used in rubber industry	Bladder cancer in exposed workers
Benzo(a)pyrene	Constituent of cigarette smoke	Lung cancer
Asbestos	Inhalation of asbestos fibres	Malignant mesothelioma of pleural cavity
Aflatoxin B_1	Produced by mould *Aspergillus flavus* found on groundnuts	Hepatocellular adenocarcinoma in populations whose diet includes affected nuts
Cyclophosphamide	Drug used in the treatment of cancer	Lymphomas and leukaemias

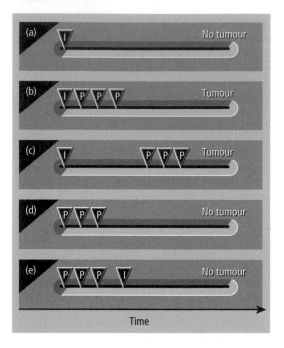

Fig. 28.3 Experiments demonstrating the initiation and promotion stages of chemical-induced skin cancer in mice. (a) application of an initiating agent (I) alone does not result in tumour formation. (b) Initiating agent followed by promoter (P) results in tumour formation. (c) Application of promoter delayed for several months after initiation also results in tumour formation indicating that initiation has 'memory'. (d) Promotion alone and (e) promotion followed by initiation do not produce tumours.

of chemical carcinogens on experimental animals. This has led to the concepts of *initiation* and *promotion* (Fig. 28.3).

Initiation is the acquisition of a mutation (or mutations) by a cell following exposure to a carcinogen. Initiation is rapid and irreversible but alone is not usually sufficient for tumour formation. If the initiated cell is then exposed to a second agent known as a *promoter* then a tumour may be formed. Application of a promoter without prior initiation will not lead to tumour formation. Promoters include substances such as phorbol esters and unlike *initiators* are not mutagenic but are potent mitogens. The role of promoters, therefore, is to induce clonal proliferation of initiated cells which will ultimately lead to tumour formation. It should be noted that some chemicals possess the

capability of both initiation and promotion, as evidenced by their ability to induce tumours without any added factors. These chemicals are known as *complete carcinogens* to distinguish them from *incomplete carcinogens* which are only capable of initiation. Although these concepts are based on animal studies there is evidence that these stages are also discernible in some human cancers. Fig. 28.4 gives an overview of events in chemical carcinogenesis.

Radiation

The increased risk of cancer in individuals exposed to *ionizing radiations* is well documented. Uranium miners, for example, have a 10-fold increase in the incidence of lung cancer, and mortality rates from leukaemia and other cancers are increased in survivors of the Hiroshima and Nagasaki atom bombs. Ionizing radiations are carcinogenic because they can interact with DNA and induce mutations.

Particulate radiation (e.g. alpha and beta particles) can react with DNA directly, whereas *electromagnetic radiation* (X-rays, gamma rays) are indirectly ionizing by releasing energetic electrons when these rays are absorbed. These rays can either be absorbed directly by DNA or by other molecules such as water. The release of electrons from water generates *free radical species* such as the hydroxyl ion which then react with DNA. The resulting disruption of chemical bonds leads to a variety of lesions in DNA including base damage, intermolecular cross-linking, and strand breaks.

Epidemiological studies have shown an increased incidence of various skin cancers following exposure to *ultraviolet radiation*. In contrast to ionizing radiation, ultraviolet rays deposit energy which is insufficient to ionize molecules but is enough to temporarily excite them and make them chemically active. Ultraviolet rays, for example, excite pyrimidine bases of DNA which then react with each other forming *pyrimidine dimers*.

DNA damage caused by exposure to chemical carcinogens or radiation is not necessarily perma-

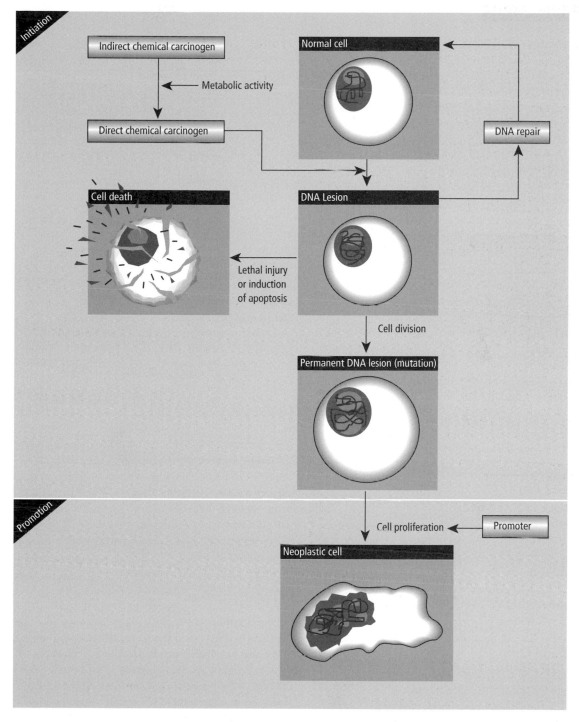

Fig. 28.4 An overview of events in chemical carcinogenesis. DNA damage following exposure of a normal cell to a chemical carcinogen may either be repaired or result in cell death. Alternatively, if the cell divides, the genetic change may be transmitted to daughter cells. Clonal expansion of mutated cells can lead to the development of a neoplasm.

nent because cells have the capacity to repair DNA. *DNA repair* must take place prior to cell division to prevent the transmission of a potentially harmful mutation to the daughter cells. Cells can delay their progression through the cell cycle to allow sufficient time for DNA repair to take place prior to cell division. Many cells carrying damaged DNA have the additional option of activating apoptosis (see Chapter 3) to precipitate their self-destruction.

A key strategy used by mammalian cells to remove damaged DNA caused by ultraviolet light or other mutagens is *excision repair* (Fig. 28.5). During this process a multiprotein system locates a lesion in DNA and removes the damaged nucleotides. DNA synthesis proceeds using the remaining normal strand as a template. Finally, the newly synthesized DNA is joined to the two ends of the undamaged strand by a *DNA ligase* enzyme.

The importance of DNA repair in preventing the transmission of potentially carcinogenic mutations is highlighted by the increased cancer risk observed in patients with defects in DNA repair (Table 28.3).

Table 28.3 Examples of inherited defects in DNA repair associated with an increased cancer risk. All are autosomal recessive disorders

Disorder	Defect	Common neoplasms
Xeroderma pigmentosum	Variable, but many patients have defect in excision repair pathway (see Fig. 28.5)	Various skin cancers, including basal cell carcinoma and malignant melanoma
Bloom's syndrome	Defect in DNA ligase leading to increased sister chromatid exchange	Various, characterized by early onset
Fanconi's anaemia	Increased susceptibility to DNA cross-linking agents	Leukaemia, particularly myelomonocytic type
Ataxia telangiectasia	Increased sensitivity to radiation and spontaneous chromosome translocations, impaired ability to delay cell cycle progression	Leukaemias and lymphomas particularly of T cell type, some epithelial tumours e.g. ovaries and stomach

Oncogenic viruses

A large number of viruses including both DNA and RNA viruses have proved to be cancer-causing in a wide variety of animals. There is increasing evidence that viruses are also important in the development of some human cancers. The contribution of viruses as oncogenic agents is discussed in Chapter 29.

Genetic factors

Evidence indicates that for a large number of cancers there exist not only environmental influences but also hereditary predispositions. The classical example here is *retinoblastoma*, a tumour of the retina, which is inherited in some families as an autosomal dominant disorder. Affected individuals inherit a mutation in one allele of the *retinoblastoma gene*, a known tumour suppressor gene, so that only a single somatic mutation in the second allele is required for the development of a tumour.

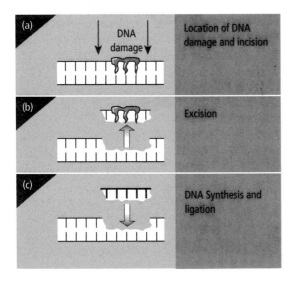

Fig. 28.5 Excision repair of DNA. During this process, DNA damage is located (a) and removed by a series of enzymes (b). New DNA is synthesized and joined to the two ends of the undamaged strand (c).

A defect in a tumour suppressor gene (NF-1) has also been shown to be responsible for the increased risk of tumours in Type 1 neurofibromatosis. This autosomal dominant condition is characterized by the development of multiple benign tumours derived from Schwann's cells (*neurofibromas*), some of which may become malignant in later life. *Familial adenomatous polyposis* (FAP) is another autosomal dominant condition in which affected people develop multiple adenomas of the large bowel. In adulthood there is a high risk of one or more adenomas developing a focus of carcinoma. Many of the gene defects responsible for FAP have now been identified (see Chapter 25 and Case Study 27.1). Other inherited conditions that predispose individuals to cancer include some DNA repair disorders (see Table 28.3) and immunodeficiency syndromes.

Clustering of cancers within families in the absence of any recognizable underlying inherited condition also occurs. Some of these familial cancers may be due to common environmental factors within the families or may have occurred by chance. However, in other families the pattern of inheritance, specific associations of certain malignancies within the familial clusters and an unusually early age at diagnosis suggest a genetic aetiology.

Of particular interest is the *Li-Fraumeni cancer family syndrome*. The principal features of this syndrome are soft tissue sarcomas in children and young adults, and the early onset of breast cancer in their mothers and other close female relatives. Osteosarcoma and leukaemia also occur to excess. An autosomal dominant pattern of inheritance is seen and there is a high incidence of multiple primary malignancies. The Li-Fraumeni cancer family syndrome is the result of the genetic transmission of mutations within the p53 tumour suppressor gene (see Chapter 29).

Host responses to neoplasia

The concept of *immune surveillance* suggests that the immune system is able to eradicate potential cancer cells and that cancer arises because of a defect in this surveillance process. This is supported by the observation that cancer is more common in immunosuppressed individuals. However, only certain cancers occur with increased frequency in immunosuppression, particularly lymphomas and leukaemias, and the incidence of the more common cancers, such as lung and breast, is not significantly increased.

Host defence systems include both *adaptive* and *innate* systems. The adaptive arm of the immune system includes antigen-specific T and B lymphocytes which have the capacity of distinguishing self from non-self. It follows that if tumours are to be recognized by T or B lymphocytes they must express non-self antigens. Non-self antigens found on tumour cells are referred to as *tumour antigens*. Experimental cancers induced in laboratory animals either by chemicals, radiation or viruses frequently express antigens which are not found on normal cells and which are often unique to individual tumours. These tumour antigens are known as *tumour-specific antigens*. In contrast, spontaneous tumours in animals are weakly, if at all, immunogenic.

The majority of antigens present on human cancers are not unique to tumour cells but are also present on normal cells and are called *tumour-associated antigens*. These antigens may be normally expressed only on fetal cells and not on adult cells, or they may be expressed at low levels on normal adult cells but at increased levels on tumour cells. An example of a tumour-associated antigen is a protein designated p97 which is found at high levels on melanoma cells. A vaccine has been developed against this protein which has been shown to protect mice from developing malignant melanoma. Results such as this highlight the potential use of tumour-associated antigens as targets for therapeutic intervention in some forms of cancer. Immune responses to tumour antigens may be mediated by a number of integrated and interdependent cell systems as described in the following sections.

B cells

For antibodies to have an anti-tumour effect, the

tumour must express an antigen recognizable to B cells. In most cases the antigen must also be recognized by T helper cells that are capable of secreting lymphokines including the interleukins IL-4, IL-5, and IL-6 which are necessary for B cell proliferation and differentiation. Once antibody has bound to the target cell it may induce *antibody-dependent cellular cytotoxicity* (ADCC), or *complement-mediated lysis* (see Chapter 4).

T cells

Cytotoxic T cells recognize antigen in association with MHC Class I molecules and are important in the recognition and elimination of virus-infected tumour cells. T cell secretion of interferon-gamma (IFN-γ) activates macrophages and increases expression of MHC molecules on tumour cells. The precise role of T cells, however, is unclear since some T cell depletion syndromes, for example athymic mice and Di George's syndrome in humans, (see Case Study 27.2) do not show a significant increase in spontaneous malignancies.

Natural killer cells

Natural killer (NK) cells are a distinct lymphocytic lineage as illustrated by patients with *severe combined immunodeficiency* (SCID) who have no B or T cells but do have NK cells, The importance of NK cells in tumour immunity is highlighted in the beige mouse strain and in *Chèdiak–Higashi syndrome* in humans. In both cases there is a marked impairment of NK function and an increase in the incidence of certain types of cancer. Although it is not known how NK cells recognize tumour cells, recognition does not require processing or presentation and is not MHC-restricted. NK cells possess neither surface immunoglobulin nor T cell receptors. However, NK cells do have Fc receptors and can participate in ADCC.

Macrophages

Activated macrophages also have Fc receptors and can participate in ADCC. They can also induce tumour cell lysis by the release of a variety

extracellular factors which include tumour necrosis factor-alpha (TNFα).

Summary

Neoplastic cells differ from normal cells because they do not respond to normal growth control mechanisms. In most cases this subversion of growth control is the result of mutations in important growth control genes. These mutations may be the result of a variety of environmental insults (including exposure to carcinogenic chemicals or radiation), or they may be inherited. Other inherited conditions, such as disorders of DNA repair and some immunodeficiency states, may predispose individuals to cancer.

Key points

1 Neoplasia, literally meaning 'new growth' is a disorder characterized by the accumulation of cells which are no longer responsive to the controlling mechanisms that maintain cell number in normal tissues.

2 Neoplasms or tumours are the tissue masses which result from the accumulation of these abnormal cells. Neoplasms may be either benign or malignant. Malignant neoplasms are almost always life-threatening, whereas benign neoplasms rarely are.

3 Neoplasms are usually classified on the basis of the presumed cell of origin, irrespective of where they are found.

4 Neoplasms are believed to arise from a single target cell which has undergone a series of mutations. These mutations enable the cell to escape the normal proliferative constraints imposed upon normal cells.

5 These mutations may arise spontaneously, as a result of exposure to a variety of environmental agents including chemicals and radiant energy, or they may be inherited.

6 The incidence of some forms of cancer is increased in a number of immunodeficiency states. This suggests that the immune system is important in preventing the development of some forms of cancer.

Further reading

Higginson J. (1993) Environmental carcinogenesis. *Cancer*, **72**, 971–977.

Kaufmann W.K. & Kaufmann D.G. (1993) Cell cycle control, DNA repair and initiation of carcinogenesis. *FASEB*, **7**, 1188–91.

Lynch S.A. & Houghton A.N. (1993) Cancer immunology. *Curr. Op. Oncol.* **5**, 145–50.

Oncogenes, Tumour Viruses and the Molecular Basis of Cancer

Introduction

A fundamental characteristic of malignant cells is that they continue to divide under circumstances in which normal cells cease proliferation. It is now clear that this is due to the aberrant expression of genes that regulate cell proliferation. There are two kinds of regulatory genes: those that promote growth, called *oncogenes*; and those that suppress growth, termed *anti-oncogenes* or *tumour suppressor genes*. This chapter examines how changes in the expression of these genes can lead to the development of cancer.

Oncogenes and viruses

The concept that there are genes capable of causing cancer (oncogenes) is based largely on studies carried out on tumours arising in animals. In 1911, P. Rous described a transmissible sarcoma in chickens. The original tumour found in an adult bird could be transmitted to other chickens by injection of a cell-free filtrate of the tumour. Later, similar observations were made for tumours arising in other animals.

The causative agents for these transmissible tumours were found to be *retroviruses*. When a retrovirus infects a cell it employs the enzyme reverse transcriptase to generate a double-stranded DNA copy of its RNA genome (see Chapter 8). This DNA copy, known as the *provirus*, integrates into the host cell DNA. The structure of a typical retrovirus genome is shown in Fig. 29.1a.

Retroviruses are responsible for a variety of diseases in humans and other animals although not all of them are able to cause cancer. The cancer-causing (oncogenic) retroviruses may be divided into those that are able to induce tumours in infected animals after very short latency periods, generally days or weeks (*acutely transforming*) and those which induce tumours over a much longer period of time, often many months or even years (*slowly transforming*). The mechanisms of tumour formation in both groups are different, and are discussed later.

Acutely transforming retroviruses

Dissection of the genome of acutely transforming retroviruses revealed that they possessed genes that were responsible for their transforming properties (Fig. 29.1b). These genes were therefore called oncogenes (*onc*). Approximately 20 different oncogenes were identified and each was given a three-letter name derived from the virus in which the oncogene was identified (Table 29.1). Most acutely transforming retroviruses contain only one oncogene, although some (for example, the *Avian erythroblastosis virus-ES4*) contain two.

Later, studies showed that these viral oncogene sequences were almost identical to endogenous sequences in the DNA of the animal species in which the virus was isolated. These cellular sequences were designated *cellular oncogenes* (c-*onc*) or *proto-oncogenes* to distinguish them from their viral counterparts (v-*onc*). It is now generally accepted that the v-*onc* were created when a retrovirus captured genetic information from the host cell in the form of whole or part of the cellular oncogene sequence (Fig. 29.2). In most cases, the incorporation of the oncogene into the virus resulted in the deletion of important viral sequences, thus rendering the virus defective for replication. Such viruses require co-infection with a *helper* virus, which provides the structural

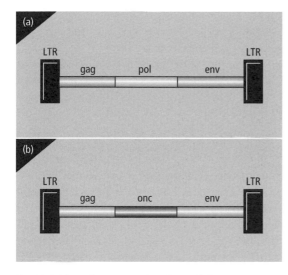

Fig. 29.1 Schematic representation of retroviral genomes. (a) Typical retrovirus. The genome is split into three regions. The *gag* encodes the structural proteins of the viral nucleocapsid; *pol* encodes reverse transcriptase; and *env* encodes the envelope proteins. The long terminal repeats (LTRs) are able to bind host factors and initiate transcription of viral genes. (b) Acutely transforming retrovirus. The virus contains an oncogene which is responsible for its transforming nature. Incorporation of the oncogene resulted in disruption of the viral genome and the virus in this case is replication defective.

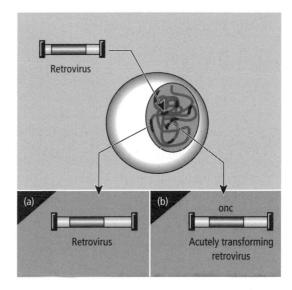

Fig. 29.2 Proposed evolution of acutely transforming retroviruses. A retrovirus infects a cell and its complementary provirus integrates into the host cell DNA. (a) Normal life cycle; new virus is produced which contains intact genome. (b) Viral sequences are lost and replaced by sequences derived from a cellular oncogene. The new genome is packaged into viral particles. The new virus released henceforth is an acutely transforming variant of the original infecting virus.

Table 29.1 Examples of acutely transforming retroviruses

Acutely transforming retrovirus	Species affected	Tumour type	Oncogene present in viral genome
Rous sarcoma virus	Chicken	Sarcoma	*src*
Avian myelocytomatosis virus MC29	Chicken	Sarcoma	*myc*
Simian sarcoma virus	Monkey	Sarcoma	*sis*
Avian erythroblastosis virus – ES4	Chicken	Erythroblastosis, sarcoma	*erbA* and *erbB*

proteins and enzymes necessary for the propagation of the acutely transforming virus. The single exception to this is the *Rous sarcoma virus*. Incorporation of *src*, the oncogene present within this virus, did not disrupt the viral genome, and the virus is therefore able to replicate without the need for a helper virus.

Although acutely transforming retroviruses are responsible for many neoplasms in animals, to date no members of this group have been shown to cause cancer in humans.

The function of oncogenes in normal cells

The identification of cellular oncogenes has prompted investigation of the function of these genes in normal cells. What is now clear is that the protein products of cellular oncogenes are involved in pathways controlling cell division. To understand the function of cellular oncogenes it is firstly important to be familiar with the transduction of growth signals within cells.

Control of cellular growth

Stimulation of a cell into a proliferative state often depends upon an external signal in the form of a growth factor. In order for a growth factor to alter cell function, it must transmit its message through the cell membrane. Some growth factors, for example the steroid hormones, are lipid soluble and readily pass through the cell membrane. Once inside the cell they bind to intracellular receptors. These receptors then bind to DNA and regulate the transcription of important cellular genes.

Many growth factors do not enter the cell but bind instead to receptors situated on the cell membrane. These membrane bound receptors have a cytoplasmic domain which becomes activated once the growth factor has bound. Activation of the receptor in this way allows the signal to be transferred to other molecules, usually proteins, situated within the cytoplasm. There are a number of ways in which this may be achieved. The receptor may be able to attach phosphate ions to specific amino acids, either tyrosine or serine and threonine, on the target protein. Molecules which are able to phosphorylate other proteins in this way are known as *protein kinases*. Those that phosphorylate serine and threonine amino acids are referred to as *serine—threonine kinases* and those that phosphorylate tyrosine are known as *tyrosine kinases*. Epidermal growth factor (EGF) receptor and platelet-derived growth factor (PDGF) receptor are examples of receptors that are tyrosine kinases.

Receptors may transmit extracellular signals via activation of *guanine nucleotide-binding proteins (G proteins)*. G proteins can stimulate enzyme systems (e.g. adenylate cyclase) located on the cytoplasmic side of the plasma membrane. These enzyme systems may in turn stimulate cytoplasmic protein kinases. The purpose of these complex interactions among proteins is to substantially amplify the initially small growth factor signal as it is transduced through the cytoplasm.

From the cytoplasm and by mechanisms which are poorly understood the growth signal is ultimately transferred to the nucleus, whereupon a number of nuclear proteins are activated. Many of these are able to bind to gene regulatory sequences (promoters or enhancers) and initiate the expression of genes necessary for cell division. Proteins which bind to DNA to regulate gene expression are known as *transcription factors*.

Role of oncogenes in cell growth

Cellular oncogene products have been identified that function at each step of the pathway outlined above. Thus, several oncogenes are related to growth factors, including the *sis* oncogene which codes for the beta chain of PDGF. Oncogenes coding for growth factor receptors with tyrosine kinase activity include c-*erb*B which codes for the EGF receptor, and c-*fms* which codes for colony-stimulating factor-1 (CSF-1) receptor. Oncogenes coding for cytoplasmic protein kinases include c-*src* and c-*abl*, which have tyrosine kinase activity and c-*raf* and c-*mos*, which have serine–threonine kinase activity.

Oncogenes of the *ras* family exhibit many characteristics similar to G proteins involved in adenylate cyclase activation. Several oncogenes represent transcription factors. These include the *myc* family. Two other oncogenes, c-*fos* and c-*jun*, are components of the transcription factor complex known as AP-1.

Altered oncogene expression in malignant cells

Oncogenes clearly play a fundamental role in the transduction of growth signals within cells, and in normal cells, as we might expect, their expression is tightly regulated. In malignant cells, however, this is not so and the expression of one or more oncogenes is either quantitatively or qualitatively different from that seen in normal cells. It is these changes in oncogene expression which are primarily responsible for the subversion of growth control which is so characteristic of malignant cells.

The mechanisms responsible for these changes

in oncogene expression may be broadly subdivided into the following two categories.

Activation of cellular oncogenes

Most changes in oncogene expression are the result of either amplification of an oncogene, point mutation within an oncogene, or a chromosome translocation. In these circumstances the cellular oncogene is said to be activated.

Gene amplification

Increase in the number of copies (*amplification*) of a cellular oncogene often results in its overexpression. Examples in human tumours include amplification of N-*myc* in neuroblastomas, and c-*neu* in breast cancer. In both cases high levels of amplification correlate with poor prognosis. The amplified genes may be seen on cytogenetic analysis where they are represented by *homogeneously staining regions* (HSRs) or *double minutes* (Fig. 29.3).

Point mutation

Single base changes (*point mutations*) in an onco-

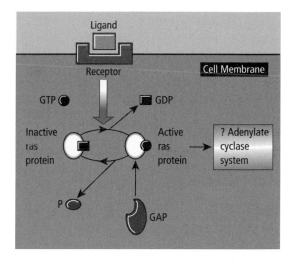

Fig. 29.4 Schematic illustration of the proposed role of *ras* protein in signal transduction. On binding of an unidentified ligand inactive *ras* protein binds GTP and becomes activated, and signal is transmitted to effector molecules. The *ras* protein has GTPase activity which brings about its own inactivation. The GTPase activity of *ras* protein appears to result from its interaction with a cytoplasmic protein, GTPase-activating protein (GAP). Point mutations in *ras* are associated with reduced GTPase activity and may be due to the inability of GAP to stimulate GTPase activity of mutant *ras* protein. In such circumstances, signals to effector molecules would be expected to be prolonged.

gene can often dramatically affect the function of the encoded protein. For example, *ras* genes frequently undergo point mutations which reduce their GTPase activity. Activation signals to effector molecules are therefore prolonged (Fig. 29.4). Many point mutations in oncogenes are the result of the activity of chemical carcinogens or radiation (see Chapter 28).

Chromosome translocation

Transfer of part of one chromosome to another (*chromosome translocation* see Chapter 26) is a common finding in many neoplasms. Translocations are commonly seen in lymphomas and are thought to be the result of mistakes in the process of gene rearrangement which occurs during normal lymphocyte development (see Chapter 5). In *Burkitt's lymphoma*, a neoplasm of B lymphocytes,

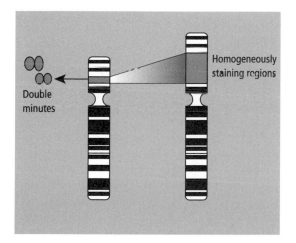

Fig. 29.3 Morphological manifestations of gene amplification in neuroblastoma. N-*myc* gene is amplified in neuroblastoma cells and is seen cytogenetically as either homogeneously staining regions (HSRs) or extra chromosomal fragments, known as double minutes.

there is typically a reciprocal exchange of chromosomal material between chromosomes 8 and 14. In this translocation the c-*myc* gene, normally located on chromosome 8, moves to the immunoglobulin heavy chain (IgH) locus on chromosome 14, and part of the IgH locus migrates to chromosome 8. The effect is constitutive expression of the c-*myc* gene and continuous cell proliferation. In some cases the change in c-*myc* regulation is due to the presence of potent transcriptional enhancer elements of the IgH locus which are now located next to the c-*myc* gene, whereas in others it is the result of the loss of c-*myc* regulatory sequences which remain on chromosome 8.

The follicular B cell lymphomas are characterized by a translocation in which the *bcl*-2 gene moves from its normal position on chromosome 18 to the IgH locus on chromosome 14. The result of this translocation is an increase in *bcl*-2 expression. Expression of the *bcl*-2 gene has been shown to protect cells from apoptosis (see Chapter 3). Consequently, follicular lymphomas are characterized by an accumulation of B lymphocytes which are resistant to apoptosis and are therefore long lived. Another example of chromosome translocation is seen in chronic myeloid leukaemia (see Case Study 31.1) This translocation involves chromosomes 9 and 22 and generates the so-called 'Philadelphia chromosome'.

Retroviral oncogenesis

Although retroviruses are a rare cause of human cancer their study has been indispensable in the discovery and analysis of oncogenes. The oncogenic retroviruses are divided into the following two groups.

Acutely transforming retroviruses

These retroviruses transform cells by virtue of the fact their genomes contain oncogenes. Once they infect a cell, expression of the v-*onc* is initiated. In contrast to its normal cellular partner, the v-*onc* is expressed constitutively and at relatively higher levels since its transcription is under the control of the viral LTRs. In addition, the v-*onc* often represent modified forms of their cellular progenitors that have been truncated, mutated, or fused to viral coding sequences, and as a result the encoded proteins are often more active than their normal counterparts. For example, the v-*erb*B oncogene encodes a defective EGF receptor in which the ligand-binding domain and part of the regulatory domain are deleted, and which therefore exhibits constitutive tyrosine kinase activity (Fig. 29.5).

Slowly transforming retroviruses

Unlike their acutely transforming counterparts, the slowly transforming retroviruses do not possess oncogenes, but induce tumours by other means. A common mechanism is *insertional mutagenesis*. This involves integration of the retrovirus into close proximity of a cellular oncogene. In this position the retrovirus can alter the expression of the cellular oncogene. A good example is provided by the *avian leukosis viruses* (ALVs), which are responsible for B cell lymphomas in chickens. In most tumours the ALV provirus is integrated within or near to the normal

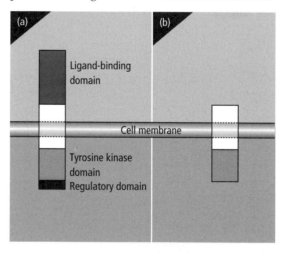

Fig. 29.5 Structure of the EGF receptor. (a) Normal receptor encoded by c-*erb*B showing ligand-binding, tyrosine kinase, and regulatory domains. The regulatory domain exerts a negative influence on tyrosine kinase activity. (b) Truncated receptor encoded by v-*erb*B. Ligand-binding and regulatory domains are absent and the receptor has constitutive tyrosine kinase activity.

250

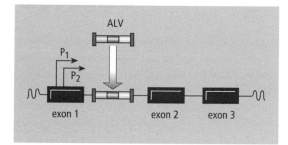

Fig. 29.6 Structure of the c-*myc* gene showing a typical insertion point for ALV provirus. The c-*myc* gene is composed of three coding regions (exons). Normal promoters are shown (P₁ and P₂). ALV commonly inserts between the promoters and exon 2 of c-*myc*, effectively divorcing c-*myc* from its normal transcriptional control. Transcription of c-*myc* is now controlled by the viral LTRs.

c-*myc* gene, usually between the normal promoters for c-*myc* and exon 2 (Fig. 29.6). This divorces the body of the c-*myc* gene from its promoters, and hence its normal transcriptional control. Expression of c-*myc* is now initiated from the viral LTRs resulting in a considerable increase (20–100-fold) in the levels of c-*myc* mRNA.

The human T lymphotropic virus-1 (HTLV-1) is a slowly transforming retrovirus which is responsible for adult T cell leukaemia and lymphoma (ATLL) in humans. In contrast to the majority of slowly transforming retroviruses, HTLV-1 does not induce tumour formation by insertional mutagenesis. The initiating event in this disease is immortalization of T helper lymphocytes by HTLV-1, which is achieved by expression of an additional coding region present within the viral genome known as *tax*-1. The *tax*-1 protein increases the expression of the cellular interleukin-2 (IL-2) receptor gene making the cell more responsive to IL-2, which is a potent growth factor for T lymphocytes. As a result infected cells are stimulated to proliferate, and the subsequent accumulation of mutations by the proliferating cell may lead to the development of ATLL.

Tumour suppressor genes

Oncogenes code for protein which when present in abnormal form or amount may induce malignant growth by upregulating or turning on cell division. Genes with the opposite function are called *anti-oncogenes* or *tumour suppressor genes*. The proteins of tumour suppressor genes downregulate cell proliferation, and their inactivation may produce a neoplastic cell in which the effect of a growth-promoting factor goes unopposed. Many tumour suppressor genes are said to act recessively since abnormalities in both alleles are often necessary for loss of function. Inactivation of one allele alone is usually insufficient since the normal allele continues to produce protein which can suppress cell proliferation. Tumour suppressor genes include those briefly outlined in the following sections.

The retinoblastoma gene

Abnormalities in the retinoblastoma (Rb-1) gene were first detected in retinoblastoma, a neoplasm of the retinal precursor cells (*retinoblasts*), and subsequently in other tumours, notably osteosarcomas. Normal Rb-1 product binds to a number of transcription factors including c-*myc* protein and inhibits their activity. When a normal cell is required to divide, Rb-1 product is phosphorylated and is unable to interact with the transcription factors. The free transcription factors then bind to DNA and initiate gene expression leading to cell division.

In retinoblastoma, both alleles of the Rb-1 gene on chromosome 13 are inactivated, either by deletion or point mutation. This results in neoplastic growth since Rb-1 product can no longer suppress cell division. The majority of cases of retinoblastoma arise in a sporadic fashion in the population. In these cases, defects in both alleles of the Rb-1 gene occur *somatically* (i.e. post-conception) in the same retinoblast. However, as many as one-third of retinoblastomas arise from a genetic predisposition. In these cases a mutation is already present in one allele at conception (and consequently present in all cells of the developing retina), whereas the second occurs as a somatic event. This model explains the observed single focus of tumour formation in sporadic cases, since the tumour arises following the convergence of two rare genetic events on a single target retinoblast.

Multiple tumour foci in both eyes are usually seen in heritable retinoblastoma. This can be explained by the fact that one of the two mutations is already present in the retinal cells and only a single mutation is required to complete the triggering process.

The p53 gene

One of the most common defects in human cancer involves the tumour suppressor gene p53. Abnormalities in this gene have been detected in many common cancers including those of the colon, breast and lung. The p53 protein exists as a complex composed of four molecules (*tetramer*) of p53 and normally stimulates the expression of genes that suppress cell growth. Following cell injury p53 expression is increased, resulting either in cell cycle arrest until the damage is repaired, or cell death by apoptosis. Tumour cells are frequently exposed to conditions which may result in cell injury, for example, they are often deprived of oxygen. In such circumstances, inactivation of p53 would be advantageous to these cells since they would be able to escape the proliferative constraints imposed on cells having normal p53 function. There are a number of ways in which normal expression of p53 can be lost.

1 Deletion of one or both p53 alleles which reduces the concentration of p53 tetramers below that required for normal function.

2 Mutation in the p53 gene, resulting in the production of a truncated p53 product which is unable to form tetramers.

3 Mutation in the p53 gene, producing a protein which forms inactive tetramers. In tumours in which one allele remains normal, activity of the normal protein may be inhibited due to its participation in inactive tetramer formation. In some cases therefore, abnormalities in only one allele are sufficient for inhibition of normal p53 function.

The neurofibromatosis-1 gene

Abnormalities in the neurofibromatosis (NF-1) gene have been detected in neurofibromatosis type-1 which is characterized by the development of multiple benign neurofibromas some of which may become malignant in later life. The NF-1 gene codes for a GTPase-activating protein (GAP) called *neurofibromin* which negatively regulates *ras* protein (see Fig. 29.4). Most neurofibromatosis type-1 sufferers have loss of function mutations in the NF-1 gene.

There is evidence that in some cases, mutations in tumour suppressor genes are due to the activity of carcinogenic agents. For example, when exposed to aflatoxin B_1, cells show specific p53 mutations (at codon 249). These same mutations are seen in aflatoxin-induced hepatocellular carcinoma. Both p53 and Rb-1 proteins are bound to and inactivated by the transforming proteins of a number of oncogenic DNA viruses. This represents a further mechanism by which tumour suppressor gene function may be inhibited.

Oncogenesis by DNA viruses

The oncogenic DNA viruses are a diverse group which are responsible for many cancers in humans and other animals (Table 29.2). Following infection of a host cell, oncogenic DNA viruses produce proteins that are responsible for their transforming nature. There are four important groups of oncogenic DNA viruses.

The adenoviruses

The *adenoviruses* are widespread in nature. In humans they account for relatively minor infections (see Chapter 8), but do not cause cancer. Human adenoviruses, however, are able to induce tumours in newborn hamsters and rats. Two proteins produced by these adenoviruses, designated E1A and E1B, are responsible for their cancer-inducing properties. Both bind to and inactivate the protein products of known tumour suppressor genes. E1A binds to Rb-1 protein and E1B to p53

Table 29.2 Some oncogenic DNA viruses

Virus family	Virus	Natural host	Host in which virus is oncogenic	Tumour produced	Oncogenic protein
Adenovirus	Human Adenoviruses A, B, D	Humans	Hamster, Rat	Various	E1A, E1B
Papovavirus	Polyoma	Mouse	Mouse	Various	Middle T antigen, Large T antigen
	SV40	Monkey	Hamster, Rat	Various	Large T antigen
	HPV 16, 18	Humans	Humans	Cervical cancer	E6, E7
Herpesviruses	EBV	Humans	Humans	Burkitt's lymphoma, Nasopharyngeal carcinoma, Hodgkin's lymphoma	EBNA-2, LMP-1
Hepadnaviruses	Hepatitis-B virus	Humans	Humans	Hepatocellular carcinoma	Hepatitis-B x-antigen

protein. In this way the normal anti-proliferative effects of these two genes are inhibited.

E1A is also able to decrease the expression of MHC Class I molecules on infected cells. Since expression of MHC Class I molecules is important in the elimination of virus-infected cells (see Chapters 5 and 8), their downregulation by E1A contributes to the survival of adenovirus-infected cells.

The papovaviruses

The *papovavirus* family comprise the *polyoma* and *papillomaviruses*. The polyoma group include the polyoma virus, simian virus 40 (SV40), and the human polyoma viruses, BK and JC. With the exception of the polyoma virus, these viruses do not cause cancer in their natural hosts but do induce tumours in newborn animals, including hamsters and rats. Proteins produced by each of these viruses interact with host-derived proteins to bring about transformation. The so called large T antigen (*tumour antigen*), a protein produced by SV40, is able to bind to and inactivate Rb-1 and p53 proteins. The large T antigen produced by polyoma virus can bind Rb-1 protein, but not p53.

Most of the oncogenic effects of the polyoma virus are attributable to a second protein, known as the middle T antigen. This protein complexes with the product of the cellular oncogene c-*src*.

As discussed earlier, *src* protein transmits intracellular growth signals by virtue of its ability to activate other proteins by phosphorylating their tyrosine component (*tyrosine kinase activity*). By complexing to *src* protein, polyoma middle T antigen enhances this tyrosine kinase activity.

In humans the most important papillomaviruses are the human papilloma viruses (HPV) types 16 and 18 which are implicated in the development of cervical cancer. Their transforming potential is partly due to the viral proteins, E6 and E7, which are able to bind p53 and Rb-1 proteins respectively.

The herpesviruses

The herpesvirus family includes the Epstein–Barr virus (EBV) which is important in the development of a number of malignancies in humans including Burkitt's lymphoma, nasopharyngeal carcinoma, lymphomas in immunosuppressed individuals, and more recently Hodgkin's lymphoma.

EBV infects approximately 90 percent of the world's adult population and in the majority of individuals is carried as a clinically silent infection. EBV is able to infect and immortalize B lymphocytes. In the normal host there is a balance between the growth of B lymphocytes immortalized by EBV and their destruction by the immune system. In immunosuppressed individuals these

EBV-infected lymphocytes are able to proliferate unchecked and often develop into a tumour (see Case Study 31.2). The viral genes responsible for B-lymphocyte immortalization include the EBV nuclear antigen-2 (EBNA-2) and latent membrane protein-1 (LMP-1) genes. LMP-1 has been shown to transform cells in culture.

EBV is thought to contribute to the development of Burkitt's lymphoma by immortalizing the progenitor B lymphocytes thereby increasing the likelihood of the 8;14 translocation occurring.

The hepadnaviruses

Of this group probably the most important is the *hepatitis-B virus* (HBV), which is implicated in the development of *hepatocellular carcinoma* (HCC) in humans. In certain parts of the world (e.g. Taiwan) where HBV is endemic, HCC is very common, particularly among males. In addition to HBV infection, several independent risk factors of HCC have also been documented, including aflatoxin B_1 exposure, *hepatitis C virus* infection and alcoholism.

There are a number of putative transforming proteins encoded by HBV. These include the hepatitis B x-antigen (HBxAg), which has been shown to transform hepatocyte cell lines and fibroblasts in culture.

Multistep transformation

Much experimental and epidemiological evidence argues that malignant change is a process which results from multiple genetic alterations involving both oncogenes and tumour suppressor genes. Experiments with mice, for example, show that the activation of a single oncogene is usually not sufficient to cause a tumour, and that changes in at least two oncogenes or tumour suppressor genes are required.

If tumours arise as a result of multiple events then an important question is: at which stage of malignant transformation is a particular oncogene or tumour suppressor gene involved? From studies on the experimental activation of c-*ras* in car-cinogen-treated animals, it has been shown that *ras* gene activation is an early initiating event in carcinogenesis. Likewise, mutations in the p53 gene constitute an intermediate or late step in tumour development. For example, mutations in p53 usually occur around or during the transition of benign tumours of the colonic epithelial cells (*adenomas*) to their malignant counterparts (*adenocarcinomas*). Similarly they are found in *blast crisis* of chronic myeloid leukaemia, but not in the earlier chronic phase.

Summary

At the beginning of this chapter, oncogenes were described as the genetic material carried by acutely transforming retroviruses that results in malignant transformation of infected cells. It is now clear that oncogenes represent normal cellular genes that function at key points in the transduction of growth signals within cells. They may contribute to the development of a malignant cell if their expression is altered through mutation, amplification or some other mechanism. In contrast, tumour suppressor genes inhibit cell growth and their inactivation can also lead to neoplastic growth. It appears that the development of cancer is a multistep phenomenon and that at least two or more changes in oncogenes or tumour suppressor genes are necessary.

Further reading

Hunter T. (ed.) (1993) Oncogenes and cell proliferation. *Curr. Opin. Gen. Dev.* **3**, 1–70.

Pitot H.C. (1993) The molecular biology of carcinogenesis. *Cancer*, **72**, 962–970

Smith M.R., Matthews N.T., Jones K.A. & Kung H.F. (1993) Biological actions of oncogenes. *Pharmacol. Ther.* **58**, 211–236.

Key points

1 Oncogenes were first identified as the genetic material carried by acutely transforming retroviruses that were responsible for their ability to induce tumours in animals.

2 Subsequently, similar genes were identified in the DNA of normal mammalian cells—these were termed cellular oncogenes (*c-onc*) to distinguish them from viral oncogenes (*v-onc*).

3 In normal cells, cellular oncogenes function to promote cell growth and division. Oncogenes that function at each step of the transduction of growth signals within cells have been identified. In normal cells, the expression of cellular oncogenes is tightly controlled.

4 Malignant cells show changes in oncogene expression. These changes are primarily responsible for the subversion of cell growth and division which is characteristic of neoplasia. These changes may involve amplification of the oncogene, a point mutation within an oncogene, or a chromosome translocation which involves an oncogene.

5 Virus infection can also affect oncogene expression.

Acutely transforming retroviruses carry v-oncogenes which are often abnormal forms of their cellular counterparts. Once infection occurs, v-*onc* expression by the host cell can lead to the development of malignancy.

6 Slowly transforming retroviruses do not possess oncogenes. They are able to induce tumours by integrating near to cellular oncogenes (insertional mutagenesis). In this position they can upregulate the expression of the cellular oncogene.

7 DNA viruses display a variety of different cancer-inducing mechanisms. In many cases, proteins produced by DNA viruses bind to and inactivate another group of cellular genes, known as tumour suppressor genes. In normal cells, the protein products of tumour suppressor genes inhibit cell growth and division. Inactivation of tumour suppressor proteins can lead to the development of malignancy.

8 The development of a tumour is a multistep process and alterations in the expression of two or more oncogenes or tumour suppressor genes is required.

Cancer: Invasion, Metastasis and Treatment

Introduction

In previous chapters, neoplasia was defined as the process of abnormal growth which gives rise to tumours or neoplasms. Two types of neoplasm are recognized. Benign neoplasms which are rarely life-threatening, grow within a well-defined capsule with size limitation, and only cause damage by mass effect or when causing compression within the confines of a closed environment such as the skull; and malignant neoplasms (cancers) which are defined by their ability to invade surrounding tissues (*invasion*) and spread to distant parts of the body to generate secondary growths (*metastasis*). This chapter describes the processes of invasion and metastasis and considers approaches for the treatment of malignant disease.

Invasion and metastasis

The most life-threatening aspect of cancer is not always growth of the primary tumour, but the consequences of tumour invasion and metastasis—the processes by which tumour cells grow out from the initial tumour site, invading into the local tissues and disseminating via the bloodstream and lymphatic vessels to form satellite lesions (*metastases*) throughout the body. Examples of invasion and metastasis are illustrated in Fig. 30.1.

The majority of human cancers are derived from epithelial cells and it is these *carcinomas* which are notorious for their ability to invade surrounding tissue and metastasize to distant sites. At this stage, the disease can no longer be treated by local therapy and the patient readily succumbs to direct anatomic compromise caused by disease spread and increasing tumour burden.

Around 60 percent of patients with cancer have microscopic or clinically evident metastases at the time when their primary tumour is diagnosed. Many of these patients will have multiple metastases, the distribution of which follows a remarkably reproducible pattern. Whilst this is often explained by the anatomical location of the primary tumour, a degree of *organ tropism* is exhibited by certain tumours. Thus, cancers of the bowel, by virtue of the portal venous system, metastasize early to the liver, whereas carcinoma of the kidney frequently metastasizes to the thyroid gland.

Tumours of comparable size have different metastatic potential, depending on their intrinsic aggressiveness. The ability of tumour cells to invade and metastasize appears to occur very soon after the primary tumour develops a blood supply (*angiogenesis*). Subpopulations of highly metastatic tumour cells pre-exist at a very early stage in the development of the primary tumour and, in the complex multistep pathogenesis of cancer, these more aggressive tumour cells are selected out because of their ability to successfully produce a metastatic colony.

Tumour cells and proteinases

The metastatic process begins when a tumour cell or group of cells leave the primary tumour, invade the local tissue, and survive to proliferate at another site. This complex process requires the tumour cells to enter the circulation, settle at a distant vascular bed, leave (*extravasate*) the blood vessels to enter a particular organ, and proliferate as a secondary colony of metastatic tumour cells

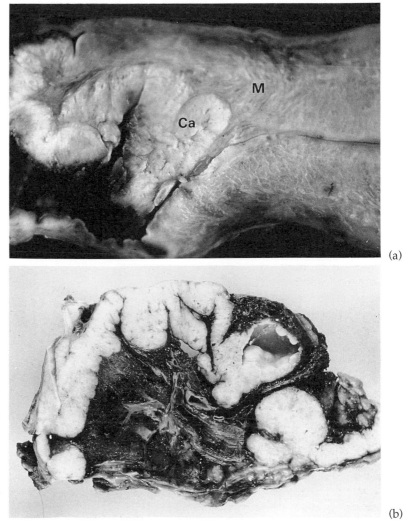

(a)

(b)

Fig. 30.1 Examples of cancer invasion and metastasis: (a) local invasion of cervical carcinoma (Ca) upwards from the cervix into the deep tissues of the myometrium (M); (b) local invasion of malignant mesothelioma from pleural cavity into the lungs, much of the normal lung tissue is replaced by pale tumour.

(Fig. 30.2). Only the fittest and most aggressive tumour cells can successfully survive all these stages and thus it is estimated that less than 0.01 percent of circulating tumour cells ultimately initiate metastatic tumour colonies.

An essential component of the invasive process is the degradation of extracellular matrix proteins that constitute the basement membranes. This proteolysis is mediated by degradative enzymes secreted by tumour cells. The best characterized of these enzymes are the *matrix metalloproteinases* which are categorized on the basis of their substrate specificities. Thus, interstitial *collagenases* preferentially degrade collagens Type I, II and III whereas *gelatinases* and *stromelysins* degrade Type IV collagen. The levels of Type IV collagenase activity correlate with the invasive potential of tumour cells and inhibition of this enzyme activity has been shown to block tumour cell invasion *in vitro*. The activity of metalloproteinases is controlled by natural inhibitors which are produced by normal tissue or

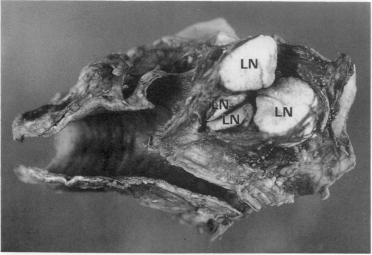

Fig. 30.1(c) Two bisected lymph nodes (LN) beneath the bronchi. Both lymph nodes have been replaced by pale tumour from a nearby bronchogenic carcinoma. This is an example of metastatic spread to lymph nodes.

(c)

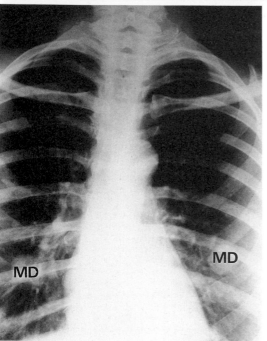

(d)

Fig. 30.1(d) Chest radiograph showing at least two well defined metastatic deposits within the lungs (MD), the original primary tumour was a malignant smooth-muscle tumour (leiomyosarcoma) of the uterus.

by the tumour cells. These *tissue inhibitors of metalloproteinases* (TIMPs) are a family of glyco-proteins which function as metastasis suppressor proteins, inhibiting the ability of tumour cells to invade the extracellular matrix.

Cell adhesion and movement

E-cadherin

The processes of invasion and metastasis are de-pendent on the modified behaviour of tumour

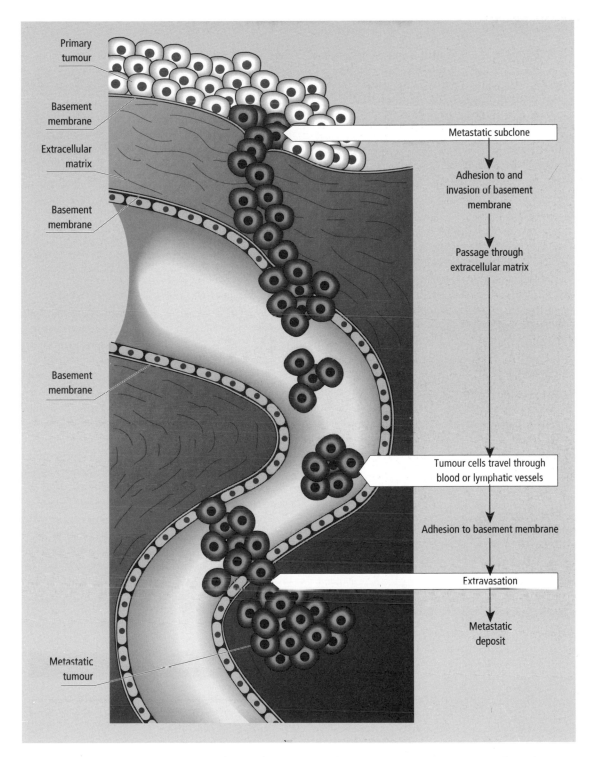

Fig. 30.2 The metastasis of a typical epithelial cancer. A metastatic subclone develops within the primary tumour mass and its cells eventually breach the underlying basement membrane and enter connective tissues. To complete the metastatic process they must move through connective tissue, enter blood/lymphatic vessels, leave the vessel and grow in a distant tissue. Redrawn, from Robbins, S. L. et al. (1990) *Pathologic Basis of Disease*, W. B. Saunders, Philadelphia.

cells with regard to cell–cell and cell–matrix inter-actions. A reduced ability of malignant cells to adhere to each other may facilitate the detach-ment of cells from the primary tumour and their subsequent invasion of local tissue. An epithelial cell–cell adhesion molecule called *E-cadherin* (also known as uvomorulin, L-CAM, or Arc-1) has been implicated in the invasive process. E-cadherin is a cell surface glycoprotein which mediates the Ca^{2+}-dependent adhesion of epithe-lial cells.

Experiments with cell lines and animal tumours suggest that down-regulation of E-cadherin ex-pression is associated with loss of differentiation and a more invasive phenotype. Analysis of tu-mour cell lines has established an association be-tween loss of E-cadherin expression, acquisition of a fibroblast-like morphology and ability to in-vade collagen gels.

A number of studies on human carcinomas have demonstrated an inverse correlation be-tween E-cadherin expression and both differen-tiation status and invasiveness (e.g. in breast carcinoma, head and neck squamous cell carci-noma). Thus, the down-regulation of E-cadherin expression appears to correlate with the grade and histological type of a tumour and may have prognostic significance.

Integrins and CD44

Other aspects of cell adhesion may also influence the invasion and metastasis of tumour cells. Integrins (see Chapter 4) have a central role in mediating the interaction of cells with the extra-cellular matrix. *In vitro* evidence suggests that increased expression of certain integrins can facili-tate metastasis presumably by enhancing the abil-ity of tumour cells to adhere to certain substrates. Whilst upregulation of integrins is not an inevita-ble consequence of tumour progression, increased levels of certain integrins have been observed in some tumours (e.g. melanoma). Many aspects of tumour metastasis resemble the normal trafficking and migration of lymphocytes (see Chapter 5). Thus, molecules involved in the adhesion of lymphocytes to endothelial cells

may have a role in tumour cell adhesion and also in the organ-specific patterns of metastasis.

CD44 is a lymphocyte-homing molecule that mediates binding to specialized lymph node endothelium. Work on rodent tumours originally identified a variant form of CD44, generated by differential mRNA splicing, which appeared to be associated with the capacity to metastasize. The expression of variant CD44 isoforms by human tumours, such as breast and colon carcinomas, may increase the metastatic potential of these malignancies.

Scatter factor

The movement of cells can be stimulated by a variety of factors which may also influence the invasion and spread of tumours. These factors include the so called *motogenic cytokines* such as *autocrine motility factor*, *migration-stimulating factor* and *scatter factor*. Scatter factor (SF) is of particular interest as it induces de-differentiation and increased motility of epithelial cells. SF has been shown to be identical to *hepatocyte growth factor* which is a potent mitogen for many normal cells including keratinocytes, melanocytes and endothelial cells. *In vitro* experiments have shown that SF can induce the progression of epithelial cells to a more motile and invasive phenotype. SF is produced by fibroblasts and ex-erts its effects on target cells by interacting with a specific receptor which has been identified as a transmembrane tyrosine kinase encoded by the c-MET oncogene. Thus the process of cell move-ment in tumour cells is linked with a known oncogene.

The genetic basis of metastasis

Most tumours are not homogenous cell populations but are composed of subpopulations of cells with differing properties. This phenemonen is referred to as *tumour heterogeneity* and is the result of somatic mutations occurring within tumour cells (see Chapter 28). Thus, a given tumour will contain subpopulations of cells which vary in their level of antigen expression, their degree of differentiation or some other characteristic. Likewise, tumours contain clones of cells with varying propensities for metastatic spread. Experiments also show that there are subpopulations of tumour cells within a primary tumour that have tissue-specific metastatic potential (Fig. 30.3).

That metastatic potential is derived and enhanced by progressive somatic mutations occurring within tumour cells has prompted the search for gene products involved in metastasis. Much of this work has relied on comparisons of metastatic variants derived from primary tumour cells. In

this way the *nm23 gene*, a potential metastasis suppressor gene, was discovered.

The nm23 gene was identified on the basis of its reduced expression at the mRNA level in highly metastatic variants of a single murine melanoma. Loss of nm23 expression correlates with poor survival in breast cancer while good prognosis is associated with increased expression. The nm23 gene product is homologous to the *abnormal wing disc (awd) gene* of the fruitfly *Drosophila* that is involved in the postmetamorphosis development and differentiation of multiple tissues. A role for nm23 in the signal transduction pathways responsible for cell–cell communication has been

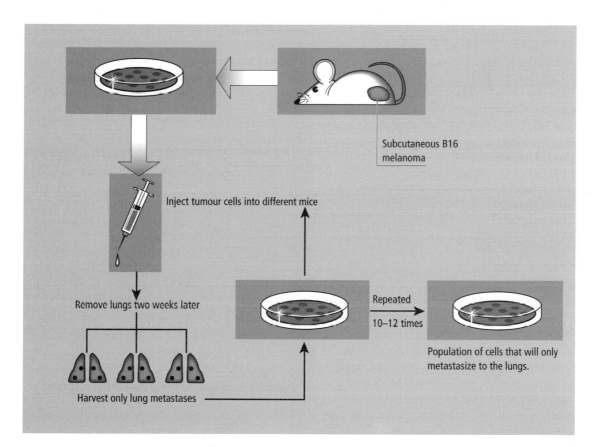

Fig. 30.3 Experiments showing that there are site-specific metastatic subclones within tumours. Subcutaneous B16 melanoma cells harvested from a single tumour will generate further tumours in mice after injection. These tumours will produce metastatic deposits in a variety of tissues, including the lungs. Only the lung metastases are harvested and re-injected into further mice. If this is repeated a number of times, a population of cells will be obtained that will only metastasize to the lungs.

suggested and may explain why loss of nm23 expression is associated with aberrant development or tumour progression.

Clues as to the precise function of nm23 came from the demonstration that cDNAs for nucleoside diphosphate (NDP) kinases, isolated from different species, encoded proteins that were highly homologous to the nm23/*awd* genes. Indeed, the *awd* gene product can function as an NDP kinase. The role of NDP kinases in microtubule assembly/disassembly and in G-protein-coupled signal transduction may explain the function of nm23 in metastasis. In particular, it is likely that aberrant NDP kinase activity may affect the cell adhesion and motility pathways which are critically important in the metastatic process.

Biological basis of cancer therapy

Most patients, in the course of being diagnosed with cancer, will have undergone surgery, either as a diagnostic procedure, or for removal of their primary tumour. However, many patients will have evidence of metastatic disease at the time of initial diagnosis, or are likely to experience disease recurrence during their lifetime. One of the first questions many patients then ask is, 'Can't you just cut it out, doctor?' In only a few cases is this actually possible, with surgery being limited by tumour accessibility, the requirement to preserve vital organ function, and (most often) the multifocal nature of metastatic spread. Management of metastatic cancer requires systemic therapy, aimed at eradicating widely disseminated macro- and microscopic disease from the whole body. In this context, most patients will receive treatment with conventional cytotoxic chemotherapy drugs.

Basic principles of modern chemotherapy

In theory, treatment specific for malignant disease should exploit some property of cancer cells not shared by normal cells. Unfortunately, while much cancer research is aimed at discovering such properties, none have been clearly defined, and most chemotherapeutic agents are essentially non-specific in their action. Most drugs interfere with one or more of the cellular processes involved in cell division, common to both normal and cancer cells, so that both cell populations are damaged. However, for reasons not entirely understood, normal growing cells vary in their susceptibility to cytotoxic drugs and are less sensitive than cancer cells. Secondly, the ability of normal cells to recover and repopulate after cytotoxic injury is greater than for cancer cells. For these reasons, chemotherapy has a degree of selectivity which can be exploited therapeutically.

The strategy for chemotherapy is therefore based on the necessity to achieve a balance between maximum tumour cell kill and an acceptable amount of toxicity to normal tissues. The narrow *therapeutic index*—the relationship between the desired and unwanted effects (Fig. 30.4)—of most cancer chemotherapy drugs is a major limitation to their clinical application. Some of the most sensitive tissues of the body are the rapidly dividing cells of the bone marrow and gastrointestinal mucosa. Drug-induced damage to these tissues can be life-threatening.

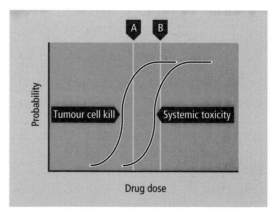

Fig. 30.4 Dose–response curves indicating probability of tumour cell and normal cell killing by a chemotherapy drug. (A) represents a dose achieving tumour control with minimum complications, (B) represents a dose achieving maximum tumour cell kill, but with significant systemic side effects.

The following two assumptions, based primarily on experimental work and not fully established in human malignant disease, underly the practice of chemotherapy.

1 Tumour cell growth proceeds exponentially, being largely independent of the homeostatic controls that regulate the growth of normal cells.

2 At a given dose, a chemotherapy drug will destroy the same proportion of cells, whatever the population at risk. Thus, the same dose that reduces a population of 10 million cells to 1 million would be required to reduce a population of 10 cells to 1 cell. This is known as the *fraction cell kill hypothesis* (Fig. 30.5).

However, tumour cells are a heterogeneous population, with different proliferation capacities. Some cells are likely to be slowly growing or non-dividing and therefore not susceptible to the cytotoxicity of a drug. Treatment will destroy the drug-sensitive cells, leaving behind a resistant cell population. In addition, tumour behaviour varies with size. Tumours are most susceptible to chemotherapy at their earliest stages of development. The increased sensitivity of small tumours is based on a higher growth fraction, shorter cell cycle time, and decreased time in which to enable drug-resistant mutations to arise. As a tumour enlarges, the growth fraction decreases, cell cycle time increases and drug-induced mutations leading to drug-resistance are more likely to occur.

The mechanism of action of chemotherapy agents can be defined either according to the phase of the cell cycle in which they are most active, or according to their pharmacological effect on the cell. Knowledge of the mechanism of action of a drug is important in designing drug combination regimens and scheduling, in order to maximize potential cell killing and minimize the side effects of treatment. Table 30.1 summarizes the major categories of chemotherapy agents currently being used in the clinic and the mechanisms by which they are thought to act.

The first effective drugs for treating cancer were introduced in the mid–late 1940s. Nitrogen mustard, antifolates, prednisolone and vinca alkaloids, in particular, were used to successfully treat lymphoblastic leukaemia and certain adult lymphomas. However, in patients with non-haematological tumours, results were disappointing, with only partial responses of short duration. Attempts at retreatment met with either diminished response or frank resistance, while increased drug doses led to unacceptable toxicity.

The introduction of *combination chemotherapy* (several drugs administered in combination) for childhood acute lymphocytic leukaemia in the early 1960s marked a major turning point in the

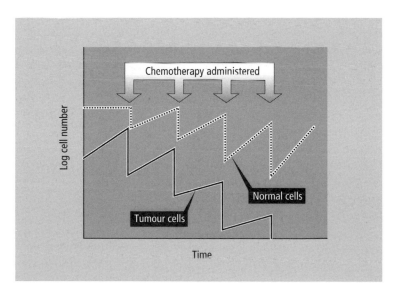

Fig. 30.5 Fraction cell kill hypothesis. Chemotherapy is administered intermittently to allow normal tissues to recover from drug-induced damage.

Table 30.1 Classification of major groups of chemotherapy agents and their mechanism of action

Group name	Examples of drugs	Mechanism of action	Cell cycle effect
Antimetabolites			
Nucleic acid	5-Fluorouracil Cytosine arabinoside Mercaptopurine	These agents resemble natural substrates within the cell and by virtue of chemical similarity, interfere with the utilization of the natural substrate e.g. methotrexate	S Phase specific
Folic acid	Methotrexate	inhibits the enzyme, dihydrofolate reductase; 5FU is metabolized to a substrate which inhibits the enzyme, thymidylate synthase. Inhibition of these enzymes reduces the availability of DNA precursors, so preventing DNA synthesis	S Phase specific
Alkylating agents	Cyclophosphamide Melphalan Chlorambucil Busulphan Nitrogen mustard	Bind to and cross-link DNA	Cycle (non-phase) specific Cell cycle non-specific
Natural products			
Mitotic inhibitors	Vincristine Vinblastine	Prevent polymerization of the mitotic spindle tubules required for mitosis	M Phase specific
	Epipodophyllotoxin	Binds to the enzyme, topoisomerase II, stabilizes it and produces double-strand breaks in DNA	M Phase specific
	Taxanes (e.g. taxol)	Bind to mitotic tubules, stabilizing them and preventing mitosis	M Phase specific
Antibiotics	Doxorubicin Daunorubicin	Topoisomerase II-dependent DNA fragmentation plus free radical formation	Cycle (non-phase) specific
	Bleomycin Mitomycin C	Bind to and cross-link DNA	
Random synthetics	Nitrosoureas Platinum complexes	Bind to and cross-link DNA	Cycle (non-phase) specific
Hormonal compounds			
Hormone antagonists	Tamoxifen Aminoglutethamide Cyproterone acetate	Probably bind to specific cytosolic receptor complexes, which are translocated to the nucleus, where DNA synthesis is inhibited	Hormonal compounds are non-cycle specific, *cytostatic* agents (inhibit cell division without killing cell)
Hormones	Cortisone Progestagens		

effective treatment of malignancy. Combination chemotherapy is now standard for the treatment of most advanced cancers. An example of an established drug combination is 'CAF' in the treatment of advanced breast cancer. This regimen combines cyclophosphamide, doxorubicin and 5-fluorouracil (5FU), each drug having a different mechanism of action and toxicity profile. Response rates of around 30–40 percent, obtained by treating patients with a single agent, are increased to around 60 percent when these drugs are administered in combination.

Drug resistance and therapeutic efficacy

As already alluded to, cancer cells are by no means equally sensitive to all chemotherapy agents. A major limitation of treatment, and the most common reason for treatment failure, is the existence of both intrinsic and acquired cellular drug resistance. *Intrinsic* (or primary) resistance is characterized by no initial response to chemotherapy. *Acquired* (or secondary) resistance develops after an initially successful period of therapy and is often due to the outgrowth of drug-resistant subclones.

Extensive laboratory studies have identified a wide range of resistance mechanisms including: decreased drug uptake; enhanced intracellular detoxification; inadequate drug activation; upregulation of DNA repair systems; and increased drug efflux. Although the precise clinical relevance of these mechanisms is unknown, it is clearly important to choose non-cross-resistant drugs when designing a combination schedule or deciding on a second line of therapy.

A more recent approach to the problem of resistance is to combine chemotherapy with drugs which can modify resistance. This is exemplified by chemical manipulation of the P-glycoprotein efflux pump.

P-glycoprotein and multidrug resistance

When malignant tissue culture cell lines are made resistant to a single chemotherapy drug by stepwise incubation in increasing amounts of the drug, some lines are found to become resistant to a number of non-structurally related drugs. This phenomenon is termed *multidrug resistance* (MDR). Cells that display the MDR phenotype are generally resistant to anthracyclines, vinca alkaloids, epipodophyllotoxins and taxanes.

MDR is associated with decreased intracellular drug accumulation as a result of a plasma membrane-associated glycoprotein (*P-glycoprotein*) which is not present in drug-sensitive cells. P-glycoprotein acts as an energy-dependent drug efflux pump with a number of drug-binding sites.

Certain drugs, such as calcium channel blockers, can compete with specific chemotherapeutic agents to bind to P-glycoprotein and so block the pump and reverse the resistant phenotype. Verapamil has already been tested in clinical trials as a potential MDR-modifying agent. Although this drug has been shown to enhance response to chemotherapy, unacceptable cardiotoxicity prohibits its further use in humans. A number of other inhibitors of P-glycoprotein are currently being investigated for clinical use.

Ionizing radiation in cancer therapy

A variety of sources of ionizing radiation—both electromagnetic and particulate—may be used in the treatment of malignant disease. DNA is considered to be the major intracellular target of ionizing radiation. Thus, as already described for chemotherapy, a major drawback of treatment is the concommitant damage to normal tissue. Radiotherapy is therefore confined to the treatment of localized disease in tumour types found to be empirically radiosensitive, either alone or as an adjunct to surgery or chemotherapy. In patients with disseminated disease, radiotherapy plays an important role in symptom control, particularly with regard to pain relief, spinal cord compression and superior vena caval obstruction.

Immunotherapy as an experimental approach

At the turn of the century, Ehrlich coined the term, 'magic bullet' to describe antibodies which he thought could be used to destroy specific cellular targets in the body responsible for a disease. Antibody-targeting in cancer therapy would seem attractive, since a variety of tumour-associated antigens (Table 30.2) have been shown to be expressed by cancer cells. Such a treatment could, in theory, be specific for a tumour, while also avoiding the toxic side effects recognized with conventional chemotherapy.

The development of monoclonal antibodies in

Table 30.2 Tumour-associated antigens with clinical relevance

Tumour type	Tumour antigen	Comment
Gastrointestinal (colorectal, pancreas, stomach)	Carcino-embryonic antigen (CEA)	May be expressed by other epithelial tumours, including breast, liver, lung, head and neck, bladder cervix and prostate, as well as normal tissues
Prostate	Prostate-specific antigen (PSA)	Specific for prostate tissue, but not for prostate cancer
Ovary	CA 125 Mucins: MUC1, MUC2	Elevated CA 125 may occur in pregnancy, pelvic inflammatory disease, endometriosis and other gynaecological cancers
Breast	CA 15-3, CA 549, CAM 26, CAM 29, CA 26.27, MCA, CEA	CA 15-3 Is the most sensitive and specific marker of breast cancer, but may be expressed in benign breast disease or hepatitis
Leukaemia/lymphoma	Human leucocyte differentiation (CD) antigens Immunoglobulin heavy/light chains	Extremely useful in diagnosis and classification, but negligible success with therapeutic antibodies
Melanoma	Ganglioside antigens: GD2, GD3, p97 glycoprotein	Experimental setting only

the 1970s led to a myriad of monoclonal anti-tumour antibodies being conjugated to conventional cytotoxic agents as well as to other toxins including: *radio-isotopes*; *diphtheria toxin*; *ricin*; and *abrin* which could kill cancer cells, both effectively and selectively, *in vitro*. However, to date, *in vivo* experience has been less impressive. In retrospect, this is understandable, since we now know that tumour-associated antigens are neither tumour specific, nor are expressed by all tumour cells.

Scientists continue to look for more specific tumour antigens with which to design antibodies with therapeutic potential. Meanwhile, other approaches to immunotherapy are being explored. For example, the concept of immune surveillance has been previously described (see Chapter 28). There is evidence to suggest that tumours are able to grow by escaping surveillance, the body's immune system becoming either tolerant or overwhelmed by the cancer cells. Active immunization of patients has been attempted, using tumour cells or tumour-cell extracts to elicit an immune response capable of eliminating or retarding tumour growth. Early clinical trials employing this technique have so far proved disappointing.

With the advent of recombinant DNA technology, attention has now turned to developing more selective *immunomodulators*, including the interferons, interleukins and retinoids. The place of these agents in the oncologist's armamentarium is currently being determined.

Summary

The ability of cancer cells to invade and metastasize often means that patients present with disseminated disease. This prevents effective surgical intervention aimed at curing the disease. Conventional chemotherapy, although systemic in its effects, has a number of drawbacks which include the toxicity of the agents employed and the development of drug resistance. Understanding the nature of the invasive and metastatic processes might enable us to design rational approaches to prevent the spread of cancer.

Key points

1 Malignant tumours are characterized by their ability to invade surrounding tissues (invasion) and to spread to distant sites to form secondary growths (metastasis).

2 The process of metastasis involves a number of distinct steps which include: tumour cells leaving the primary tumour; invasion of local tissues; dissemination via the bloodstream or lymphatics; and entry to and growth within a distant tissue.

3 Tumours are composed of heterogenous populations of cells with varying metastatic potentials. Experiments show that there are subpopulations of tumour cells within a primary tumour which have tissue-specific metastatic potential.

4 Chemotherapy is a systemic treatment approach which relies upon the fraction cell kill hypothesis. Since normal cells are affected to varying degrees many chemotherapeutic regimens are associated with toxicity. Toxic effects include bone marrow suppression and gastrointestinal disturbances.

5 Systemic toxicity, most often bone marrow suppression and gastrointestinal disturbance, limits the amount of drug that can safely be administered.

6 Combination chemotherapy involves the administration of several chemotherapeutic agents each having different mechanisms of action and toxicity profiles.

7 Drug resistance is a major obstacle to effective treatment using chemotherapy. Drug resistance may be either intrinsic or acquired.

Further reading

DeVita Jr. V.T., Hellman S. & Rosenberg S.A. (1993) *Cancer: Principles and Practice of Oncology*, 4th Edn. Lippincott, Philadelphia.

Gottesman M.M. (1993) How cancer cells evade chemotherapy: 16th Richard & Hinda Rosenthal Foundation Award Lecture. *Cancer Res.* **53**: 747–54.

Case Studies

31.1 Easy bruising, weight loss and abdominal discomfort

Clinical features

A 57-year-old woman presented to her family doctor with shortness of breath, weight loss, and abdominal discomfort of 2 months duration. She had also noticed bruising after minor trauma. On examination she was pale and had marked *spleno-megaly* (enlargement of the spleen), which was the cause of her abdominal discomfort. The heart rate was regular, 96 beats per minute, and the patient was *normotensive* (blood pressure was normal).

Investigations

The results of laboratory investigations are shown in Table 31.1.1.

The total and differential white cell counts are clearly abnormal. There is an absolute increase in all cells of the granulocyte and monocyte series. Immature cells of the myeloid series (blast cells, myelocytes and metamyeloctes) are present (Fig. 31.1.1). These immature haemopoietic cells are normally found in bone marrow, but are not usually seen in peripheral blood. This blood picture is consistent with a diagnosis of either leukaemia or leukaemoid reaction (see later).

Other investigations included the following two tests.

1 Neutrophil Alkaline Phosphatase (NAP) score: 6 (reference range 20–100).

2 Cytogenetic studies showed a reciprocal trans-location involving chromosomes 9 and 22: t(9q+;22q−).

Diagnosis

The patient is mildly anaemic with a very high white cell count, far in excess of that usually encountered as a result of infection or tissue damage. The differential leucocyte count, showing a range of cells from immature blast cells to relatively mature myelocytes and metamyelocytes, is consistent with a diagnosis of chronic myeloid leukaemia (CML) and this is supported by the reduced NAP score. CML is confirmed by cytogenetic investigations showing the chromosomal translocation, t(9q+:22q−) (see later).

Diagnosis: chronic myeloid leukaemia (also referred to as chronic granulocytic leukaemia or CGL).

Discussion

The leukaemias are a group of neoplastic disorders affecting haemopoietic tissue. Typical features of all leukaemias include: anaemia; *neutropenia* (low neutrophil count); and *thrombo-cytopenia* (low platelet count) due to bone marrow infiltration by leukaemic cells. Infiltration of other organs and tissues with leukaemic white blood cells is another typical finding. Sweating and weight loss also occur, due to an increase in basal metabolic rate.

Leukaemia is classified on the basis of the following two factors.

1 The maturity of the proliferating cells, which determines whether the disease is termed acute or chronic. In acute leukaemias, large numbers of immature (blast) cells proliferate in the bone marrow and also appear in the peripheral blood.

Table 31.1.1 Investigations performed

Analyte	Value	Reference range
Blood		
Total white cell count	$98.6 \times 10^9/l$	4.0–11.0
Red cell count	$3.40 \times 10^{12}/l$	3.8–5.8
Haemoglobin	11.0 g/dl	11.5–15.5
Haematocrit	0.335	0.37–0.47
Mean cell volume	98.5 fl	82–92
Mean cell haemoglobin	32.35 pg	27.0–32.0
Platelets	$110 \times 10^9/l$	150–400
Vitamin B_{12}	1150 ng/l	200–900
Serum folate	3.0 ug/l	1.9–14
Urea	6.5 mmol/l	2.5–6.7
Urate	0.44 mmol/l	0.12–0.36

Blood film
White blood cell differential:

Neutrophils	50%
Lymphocytes	5%
Monocytes	4%
Eosinophils	4%
Basophils	3%
Metamyelocytes	10%
Myelocytes	21%
Blast cells	3%

In chronic leukaemias the majority of cells in the peripheral blood have differentiated to form relatively mature cells.

2 The cell type involved, which determines whether the disease is classified as myeloid or lymphoid in origin. Myeloid leukaemias are those in which the proliferating cells are derived from myeloid progenitor cells, and lymphatic leukaemias are those in which the predominant cells are derived from lymphoid progenitor cells (see Chapter 20).

Thus, there are four major classes of leukaemia.

1 Acute myeloid (or myeloblastic) leukaemia (AML).

2 Acute lymphatic (or lymphoblastic) leukaemia (ALL).

3 Chronic myeloid (or granulocytic) leukaemia (CML or CGL).

4 Chronic lymphatic (or lymphocytic) leukaemia (CLL).

There are further subdivisions of leukaemia, particularly of the acute forms.

There are a number of conditions which have many of the features of the leukaemias, but which are not themselves regarded as true leukaemias. These include the *myeloproliferative disorders* and *leukaemoid reactions*. Leukaemoid reactions are unrelated conditions which produce a blood picture resembling that of leukaemia. It is essential to differentiate these disorders from true leukaemias because treatment and prognosis differ.

Differentiation of leukaemia from myeloproliferative disorders and from leukaemoid reactions depends on further clinical and laboratory investigations. The estimation of neutrophil alkaline phosphatase (NAP) activity within granulocytes by cytochemical methods is particularly useful in the diagnosis of CML. In leukaemoid reaction and myeloproliferative disorders, enzyme activity is normal or increased, whereas in CML it is invariably low.

The incidence of CML is approximately 1 per 100 000 of the population per year in the UK. CML is characterized by proliferation of large numbers of relatively mature cells of myeloid origin. The excessive *myelopoiesis* (white blood cell formation) which is a feature of CML usually causes a reduction in the rate of erythropoiesis and thrombopoiesis resulting in low numbers of circulating erythrocytes and platelets respectively. However, this is not always the case and red cell count and platelet counts may be normal or raised in some patients with CML.

CML is a neoplasm derived from myeloid stem cells (see Chapter 28) and is characterized by a chromosomal abnormality which is present in all neoplastic myeloid cell lines (myelomonocytic, megakaryocytic and erythroid). This chromosomal abnormality is a translocation involving chromosomes 9 and 22, giving rise to a small chromosome 22 (22q−) called the *Philadelphia chromosome*. As a result of this translocation, the oncogene c-*abl* becomes transferred from chromosome 9 to combine with the *bcr* gene on chromosome 22. The result is the production of a fusion gene (*bcr*–*abl*) which, when transcribed, produces a 210 kDa protein which has greatly increased tyrosine kinase activity compared to the normal c-*abl* protein (see Chapter 29).

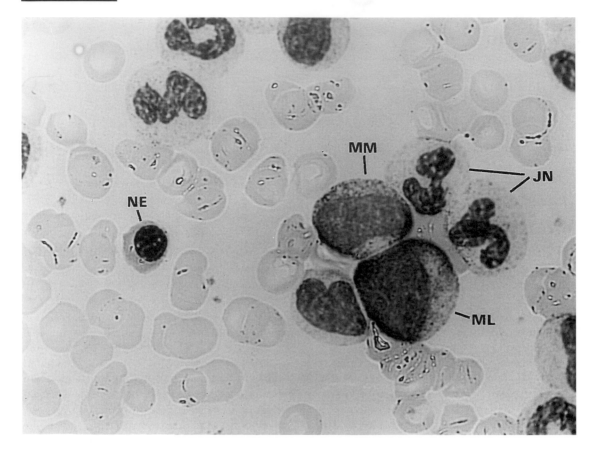

Transformation of CML to 'blast crisis' (see later) is associated with the development of other chromosomal abnormalities and with defects in oncogene and tumour-suppressor gene activity, notably those involving the p53 gene (see Chapter 29).

Fig. 31.1.1 Photomicrograph of a blood film from a patient with chronic myeloid leukaemia. The majority of cells are normal non-nucleated red blood cells with some platelets scattered in between. The large nucleated cells are myelocytes (ML), metamyelocytes (MM) and juvenile neutrophils (JN). A nucleated erythrocyte precursor (NE) is also present.

Treatment and prognosis

Treatment of CML aims to reduce the leucocyte count to normal and to prevent progression to its more aggressive terminal stage (blast crisis). This is usually achieved using alkylating agents or other cytotoxic drugs (see Chapter 30). Allopurinol is also useful if plasma urate concentration is high. Some patients remain in a stable chronic phase of the disorder for many months or years (median survival is 3–4 years), but most

patients with CML eventually undergo 'blast transformation', in which a distinct change in the population of leukaemic cells occurs. In the chronic phase most of the proliferating cells are relatively mature whereas after transformation the majority of the cells in the peripheral blood are myeloblasts, lymphoblasts or other primitive cells ('blast crisis'). At this stage, the disease has many of the features of acute leukaemia and is much more resistant to treatment than when in the chronic phase. Survival after blast transformation is typically 1–3 months. For this reason some patients are considered for potential cure by bone marrow transplantation at an early stage after diagnosis of CML, while the disease is still in the chronic phase.

1 What is the significance of the raised concentration of plasma urate?

Answer: plasma urate is derived in part from the breakdown of *adenine* and *guanine*, the purine bases present in nucleic acids, and in part from dietary sources. *Hyperuricaemia* (raised concentration of blood urate) occurs in CML due to a very high rate of nucleic acid breakdown resulting from increased cell turnover. When treatment commences, the rate of cell destruction can be so high that treatment of hyperuricaemia is essential.

2 Why are serum vitamin B_{12} concentrations typically very high in CML?

Answer: proliferation of large numbers of granulocytes and their precursors is a feature of CML. These cells produce transcobalamin I, a vitamin B_{12}-carrying protein, which is released into the plasma. High levels of transcobalamin I in the plasma are associated with raised vitamin B_{12} concentrations.

3 What is the relationship between myeloproliferative disorders and CML?

Answer: myeloproliferative disorders are low-grade neoplastic disorders characterized by proliferation of neoplastic clones of cells derived from haemopoietic stem cells. Examples include primary proliferative polycythaemia (formerly called polycythaemia rubra vera) and myelofibrosis, neither of which are regarded as true leukaemias. Cytochemistry helps to differentiate these conditions from CML, since the NAP score is usually high in myeloproliferative disorder and low in CML. However, a myeloproliferative disorder may transform to leukaemia, often initially to CML, but sometimes directly to an acute form.

31.2 *Fever and cervical lymph node enlargement*

Clinical features

A 23-year-old woman with a history of renal transplantation for chronic renal failure secondary to thrombotic thrombocytopenic purpura (see Chapter 21), was admitted to the hospital with new onset *cervical lymphadenopathy* (enlarged neck lymph nodes) and renal failure. At the time of transplantation, the patient had been started on prednisone and azathioprine immunosuppression to prevent rejection of the allograft. However, 3 weeks later the serum creatinine rose and a percutaneous renal biopsy yielded a diagnosis of acute rejection. This was treated by increasing the immunosuppression with an intravenous infusion of OKT3 (a mouse monoclonal anti-T lymphocyte antibody). Eleven days after the monoclonal antibody infusion, the patient developed pharyngitis, cervical and submandibular lymphadenopathy, and fever.

On examination the patient was mildly hypertensive (blood pressure: 170/95) and febrile (temperature: 38.5°C). The tonsils were enlarged and there was pharyngeal erythema (redness). There was bilateral submandibular and cervical lymphadenopathy, and hepatosplenomegaly (enlarged liver and spleen).

Investigations

Laboratory investigations included those shown in Table 31.2.1.

The clinical features and laboratory results suggest a systemic infection. Systemic infection is supported by pharyngitis, fever, lymphadenopathy, and hepatosplenomegaly. This syndrome is suggestive of Epstein–Barr virus (EBV)—associated infectious mononucleosis (glandular fever) typically characterized by: pharyngitis; fever; cervical lymphadenopathy; hepatosplenomegaly; and a leucocytosis (increased white cell count) with atypical lymphocytes. Other infections, including: cytomegalovirus; herpesvirus-6; human immunodeficiency virus infections; and toxoplasmosis, can produce similar or overlapping syndromes with lymphadenopathy and systemic symptoms. However, pharyngitis is not part of the constellation of symptoms in these diseases and is typical of EBV-associated infectious mononucleosis. The depressed white blood cell count and absence of atypical lymphocytes in this patient is unusual in infectious mononucleosis but may reflect treatment with the *myelosuppressive* (bone marrow-suppressing) and lympholytic agents employed (azothioprine, prednisone and OKT3). Detection of an IgM antibody titre to the EBV viral capsid antigen (VCA) is diagnostic of a recent EBV infection and is consistent with this interpretation.

In addition to infectious mononucleosis, a second diagnosis must be considered: post-transplant lymphoproliferative disease. Patients who are immunosuppressed, particularly with respect to T cell function are at risk for developing uncontrolled proliferation of EBV-infected B lymphocytes. This disease process may occur with or without an infectious mononucleosis-like syndrome. Lymphadenopathy in the post-transplant setting must always raise this concern.

A submandibular lymph node was biopsied and a proliferation of large activated B lymphocytes (B immunoblasts) was diagnosed. Nephrectomy of the transplanted kidney was per-

formed and showed focal proliferation of B immunoblasts as well as acute rejection. *In situ* hybridization showed the presence of Epstein–Barr virus within the immunoblasts in both tissues. Southern blot hybridization using an immunoglobulin heavy chain probe showed a clonal population of cells in the submandibular lymph node and a distinct clonal population in the kidney. No chromosome translocations were detected by conventional cytogenetics.

Diagnosis

The diagnosis of post-transplant lymphoproliferative disease is confirmed by study of the biopsied lymph node and the nephrectomy specimen showing proliferation of B immunoblasts. This syndrome is virtually always associated with Epstein–Barr virus. Any potential confusion with the benign lymphoid hyperplasia that may accompany infectious mononucleosis is eliminated by the demonstration of monoclonal populations of cells and the identification of the Epstein–Barr virus within virtually all of the B immunoblasts. The presence of one or more distinct clonal B cell populations and the absence of chromosomal translocations is characteristic of post-transplant lymphoproliferative disease.

Diagnosis: B cell lymphoproliferative disease in an organ transplant recipient.

Discussion

Epstein–Barr virus-associated B cell lymphoproliferative disease is recognized in patients with congenital immunodeficiencies (such as the X-linked lymphoproliferative syndrome), HIV infection, and in organ transplant recipients. In organ transplant recipients, the incidence of the disease seems to be a function of the particular immunosuppressive regimen used to prevent organ rejection. Patients receiving cyclosporine A or anti-T cell antibodies are at highest risk. The

Table 31.2.1 Investigations performed

Analyte	Value	Reference range
Blood		
Urea	17 mmol/l	2.5–6.7
Creatinine	1112 μmol/l	70–150
White blood cell count	1.8×10^9/l	4.0–11
VCA-IgM titre	1:128	–

pathogenesis of the disease is thought to be related to the ability of EBV to immortalize human B lymphocytes. EBV-immortalized B lymphocytes will proliferate indefinitely *in vitro* and will grow as tumours in mice with *severe combined immunodeficiency* (SCID mice). However, in the presence of memory T cells, *in vitro* or *in vivo*, the EBV-induced lymphoproliferation is suppressed. In immunosuppressed patients, the inadequate T cell response allows the outgrowth of EBV-infected B cells. Histologically, these tumours may have features of benign hyperplasia or frank malignancy.

A tendency to involve extranodal sites is characteristic of these opportunistic lymphoproliferative diseases and involvement of the allograft itself is particularly common. Although the disease may mimic a viral illness or be entirely asymptomatic at presentation, and may appear to be histologically benign, the lymphoproliferation will result in the death of the patient in most instances unless appropriate interventions are undertaken.

Treatment and prognosis

When immunosuppressive agents are discontinued, tumours will resolve in approximately half of cases. When the graft is involved by tumour and can be sacrificed without endangering the patient, as is the case with renal transplants, the graft is generally removed. If these measures fail, other interventions including antiviral agents to inhibit further spread of viral infection, interferon, anti-B cell antibodies, or combination chemotherapy have all been reported to be of benefit in some patients.

Questions

1 This patient's lymphoma was associated with Epstein–Barr virus. Are other viral infections associated with lymphomas?

Answer: human T lymphotropic virus-1 (HTLV-1)

infection is associated with adult T cell leukaemia and lymphoma and is found within the tumour cells. HIV infection is associated with aggressive B cell lymphomas but the viral genome is not found in the tumour cells and its role may be limited to bringing about immune dysfunction (see Chapter 8).

2 This patient was deliberately immunosuppressed in order to prevent graft rejection. This immunosuppression allowed the development of EBV-associated lymphoma. Is immunosuppression associated with a global increase in risk for all kinds of malignancy?

Answer: no, immunosuppression is associated with an increased risk of developing certain tumours but not others. For example, the increased risk of common solid tumours such as lung, breast, or colon cancer is small or non-existent.

31.3 Hoarseness and weight loss

Clinical features

A 71-year-old retired plumber attended his family doctor's surgery regularly for monitoring of his diabetes (which was controlled by dietary restriction) and his hypertension. On one visit, his doctor noticed that he had lost about 10 pounds in weight and was about to commend his efforts at dieting when she noticed how hoarse his voice sounded. The patient had noticed this symptom for approximately 6 weeks but since there was no pain in his throat had thought little of it. He put it down to the strain of his smoker's cough. In fact he had coughed so hard recently that he had brought up flecks of blood.

The patient had smoked at least 20 cigarettes daily since serving in the army during the war. On questioning, he admitted to being rather short of breath for a few months and feeling rather wheezy at night.

On examination the patient was pale and was mildly breathless at rest. He was not blue (which would indicate hypoxia) but his fingers were club-shaped, which is often a sign of heart or lung disease. There was a pronounced wheeze localized to the left upper lung but no evidence of infection or fluid around the lung. There was no lymphadenopathy (enlargement of lymph nodes) and the liver was not palpable. Urgent investigations were arranged.

Investigations

The laboratory investigations shown in Table 31.3.1 were performed.

The results show a mild normocytic normochromic anaemia (see Chapter 20) and a raised erythrocyte sedimentation rate. The total leucocyte count is high, the majority of cells being neutrophils. A blood film showed the presence of immature leucocytes and nucleated red blood cells. This finding (known as *a leuco-erythroblastic blood picture)* is similar to a leukaemoid reaction and is suggestive of bone marrow infiltration by tumour which replaces normal haemopoietic cells (see Case Study 31.1).

A chest radiograph showed a large opacity in the left lung. The patient was referred urgently to the chest clinic and bronchoscopy was performed. He was found to have a tumour in the left main bronchus. Histological analysis of a biopsy specimen taken at bronchoscopy showed an undifferentiated carcinoma. Closer examination of his chest X-ray revealed the presence of several metastases in his ribs.

Diagnosis

The clinical features and laboratory data confirm the presence of a tumour in the left lung. Histology showed this to be an undifferentiated carcinoma. The presence of metastases in the ribs and the blood film results suggest significant involvement of bone marrow. The absence of any lymphadenopathy, hepatomegaly (enlargement

Table 31.3.1 Investigations performed

Analyte	Value	Reference range
HAEMATOLOGY		
Haemoglobin	10.7 g/dl	13.5–17.5
Red cell count	3.84 × 10^{12}/l	4.5–6.5
Haematocrit	0.325	0.40–0.5
Mean cell volume	84.6 fl	80–98
Mean cell haemoglobin	27.9 pg	27.0–33.0
Mean cell haemoglobin concentration	33.0 g/dl	32.0–36.0
Erythrocyte sedimentation rate	84 mm/hour	0–10
White cells	13.58 × 10^9/l	4–11.0
Neutrophils	82.8% 11.24 × 10^9/l	2.2–7.5
Lymphocytes	8.80% 1.20 × 10^9/l	1.2–4.0
Monocytes	7.20% 0.98 × 10^9/l	0.2–1.0
Eosinophils	1.00% 0.14 × 10^9/l	Up to 0.5
Basophils	0.30% 0.04 × 10^9/l	up to 0.15
Platelet count	258 × 10^9/l	150–400
Blood picture	Neutrophilia with some toxic granulation Occasional nucleated red blood cells and myelocytes present	
BIOCHEMISTRY		
Urea	8.4 mmol/l	2.5–6.7
Creatinine	134 µmol/l	70–150
Urate	0.3 mmol/l	0.12–0.36
Glucose	8.0 mmol/l	3.5–8.9
Phosphorus	1.25 mmol/l	0.8–1.4
Total bilirubin	15.2 µmol/l	2–16
Alkaline phosphatase	86 U/l	30–135
Alanine aminotransferase	7 U/l	0–40
Aspartate aminotransferase	18 U/l	5–40
Gamma glutamyltransferase	13 U/l	2–50
Total proteins	77 g/l	60–80
Albumin	35 g/l	34–48
Globulin	42 g/l	16–37
Cholesterol	2.47 mmol/l	3.6–6.7
Triglycerides	0.85 mmol/l	0.8–2.0

of the liver) and the normal values for the enzymes alkaline phosphatase, alanine aminotransferase and aspartate aminotransferase suggest there was no metastatic spread to the lymph nodes or liver.

Diagnosis: undifferentiated carcinoma of the left lung.

Discussion

This patient's carcinoma was almost certainly a result of his cigarette smoking. This type of bronchial neoplasm is uncommon in non-smokers. Over the last 80 years the incidence of this disease has closely paralleled cigarette smoking patterns. In the mid-1970s it was estimated that cigarette smoking was responsible for 95 percent of all lung neoplasms in men.

Populations in which smoking has been reduced or low tar preparations favoured, have experienced a decline in the incidence of the disease. Women, who tended not to smoke before the 1940s, are increasingly victims of the disease. Other possible environmental carcinogens are asbestos, coal smoke, radon (in certain areas such as Cornwall) and other atmospheric pollutants. All the available evidence suggests that these account for only a small minority of cases.

The anaemia present in this case was almost certainly due to infiltration of bone marrow by tumour which had displaced normal haemopoietic tissue (see Chapter 20).

Treatment and prognosis

The patient's tumour was inoperable but he was given palliative deep X-ray treatment and improved symptomatically.

Three weeks later his wife rang the doctor for advice. The patient was complaining of thirst and constantly going to pass urine. He was rather confused and was complaining of nausea, abdominal pain and constipation. The doctor suspected deterioration of his diabetes but analysis of his urine and blood glucose screen were normal. However, his serum calcium was found to be high at 3.3 mmol/l (reference range: 2.2–2.6). He was admitted to hospital and treated with rehydration and corticosteroids followed by calcitonin to control the hypercalcaemia (raised blood calcium levels).

Questions °

1 Was the patient's hoarseness caused by his tumour?

Answer: yes, the hoarseness was caused by the tumour spreading outwards and pressing on the recurrent laryngeal nerve which lies near the left main bronchus on its way to supply the larynx. This is an example of a local effect of a tumour.

2 Can you explain the hypercalcaemia observed in this patient?

Answer: there are two possible causes of hypercalcaemia in malignant disease: (a) when malignant cells metastasize they damage the tissues in which they settle. Hypercalcaemia can be caused by metastatic destruction of bone leading to the release of calcium; and (b) some tumours can influence distant sites in the body by producing hormones or their analogues. For example, some types of lung cancer can make antidiuretic hormone (ADH) causing water retention. Similarly, hypercalcaemia can be caused by secretion of parathyroid hormone or an analogue by the tumour cells. Other remote effects of tumours are less easy to understand, for example abnormalities in peripheral nerves (*neuropathy*) or muscle (*myopathy*). The clubbing of the patient's fingers was a remote effect of his lung disease but the mechanism is not understood and certain non-malignant conditions can also cause this.

Part 9
Psychiatric Disorders

An Introduction to Biological Psychiatry

Introduction

Elucidating the biology of mental illness is one of the major challenges facing medical science. It is now widely accepted that biological mechanisms have a role in the onset of the major psychoses and other mental illnesses and that in some disorders they may be the most important factors. The term *biological psychiatry* acknowledges this influence. However, the biological approach does not deny the role of adverse life events and the effects of other psychological and social factors in ill health.

The purpose of this chapter is to introduce some important topics in biological psychiatry by way of a consideration of the biology of selected psychiatric disorders. Certain of these themes are developed further in Chapter 33.

Types of mental illness

Some disorders of mental function have a well defined basis in physical illness (*psychiatric organic states*), whereas in others there is no discernable pathology (*functional psychiatric disorders*). Functional psychiatric disorders have traditionally been classified mainly as either *neuroses* or *psychoses*, although the distinction between the two groups is not always obvious. Some regard neuroses as clinically milder than psychoses, and it is often said that patients with neurosis have some insight into their condition whereas those with psychotic illness do not, although this is not invariably the case. One view of the neuroses is that they represent an exaggeration and prolongation of normal reactions to psychological stress. Psychosis, on the other hand, is characterized by bizarre behaviour with such distortion of reality that patients' mental experiences are well beyond the range of normality.

Most people have experienced some of the symptoms associated with neurosis (for example anxiety or depression), albeit perhaps rather more mild and shortlived, and usually with an obvious external cause. This contrasts with the abnormal thought processes of psychotic illnesses, such as schizophrenia, which are completely alien to the majority of people.

From the viewpoint of biological psychiatry, the classification of mental illness on the basis of symptoms is of less importance than the search for its biological mediators. This chapter reviews some of what is known of the biology of affective disorder, schizophrenia and dementia, and briefly considers some physical factors contributing to psychiatric organic states.

Affective disorders

Affective illnesses are disorders of mood characterized by recurrent periods of depression with or without episodes of mania. The term *bipolar* affective disorder is reserved for those patients who have experienced at least one manic episode, and *nonbipolar* and *unipolar* affective disorder for those who have experienced depression but no manic episodes.

Depressed patients feel gloomy, helpless and hopeless. They usually also experience sleep disturbance: problems in falling asleep; waking early; and difficulty in resuming sleep again once they are awake. In contrast, mania is characterized by: uninhibited restless activity; excitement; apparent happiness or euphoria; and generation of a succession of ideas, often behaving impulsively or irrationally.

In bipolar disorder, the transition from depression to mania and vice versa can occur in regular cycles lasting from less than one day in some patients to months or years in others. However, bipolar disorder is relatively rare, affecting approximately 1 in 1000 of the population in Western societies. Unipolar depression is much more common, with up to 5 percent of the population experiencing depression at some time in their lives. Family, twin and adoption studies have supported the influence of genetic factors in affective disorders. Research has indicated at least two subgroups of bipolar affective disorder, one X-linked and another transmitted on chromosome 11, though these studies are not conclusive and genes on other chromosomes may be involved.

Biological changes in affective disorder

The search for biological indicators of depression has revealed two procedures which are claimed to help to distinguish *endogenous depression* (which cannot be solely explained by life events) from *reactive depression* (following, for example, bereavement).

In the *dexamethasone suppression test*, the administration of the drug dexamethasone suppresses adrenal release of cortisol in both normal subjects and in those with reactive depression. In endogenous depression there is no suppression of cortisol release by the drug. The second indicator is the speed of entry to *rapid eye movement* (REM) sleep: those with endogenous depression enter this phase of sleep much more rapidly than normal subjects or those with reactive depression. These functional differences, though not completely reliable or consistent, support the view that biological factors contribute to endogenous depression.

It has been shown that depression is associated with several other biological abnormalities, which range from hormonal deficiencies to a relative inactivity of the left hemisphere of the brain. In addition, research has indicated the possibility that viruses or other infectious agents may be linked to a small proportion of cases of depression. However, most research has focused on well recognized alterations in neurotransmitters in mental illness, although it is recognized that such changes may be secondary to other factors.

Neurotransmitters in depression

The discovery that mood can be influenced by pharmacological agents which alter neurotransmission adds weight to the theory that the affective disorders have a biological basis. Depressed patients tend to have abnormal transmission at noradrenaline, dopamine or serotonin (also known as 5-hydroxytryptamine) synapses, though the precise causes of these abnormalities have not yet been fully explained. However, the common anti-depressants ('tricyclic' drugs and monoamineoxidase inhibitors) are known to prolong the synaptic effect of catecholamines and serotonin (see Chapter 33), although their clinical effect often takes some time to become evident.

Lithium in bipolar affective illness

Lithium salts are used prophylactically in the long-term management of bipolar affective disorder and research into the mode of action of lithium has provided much impetus to the search for biological factors in this illness. Lithium is of particular interest because, at therapeutic doses, it exerts a range of diverse physiological and biochemical effects. However, its precise mode of action in controlling mood swings in manic depressive illness has yet to be elucidated, though it is likely that lithium modulates intracellular signalling mechanisms. One hypothesis proposes that lithium exerts its effect through intracellular cyclic AMP and phosphatidyl-inositol metabolism to induce adrenergic and cholinergic balance. However, of the vast array of theories that have attempted to explain the pharmacological action of lithium, none has yet withstood the test of time.

Schizophrenia

Schizophrenia affects around one percent of the

population in most 'developed' countries. There are no reliable physiological or biochemical tests for the disorder, diagnosis of which relies on psychiatric evaluation. The symptoms of schizophrenia are described as 'positive' (for example, delusions and auditory hallucinations) or 'negative' (for example, withdrawal, blunted emotions and lack of motivation). In certain patients either positive or negative symptoms predominate, but it is unclear whether these are manifestations of different syndromes or whether they represent different points in the spectrum of a single disorder. There is some evidence that structural abnormalities of the brain are more closely associated with negative symptoms, yet the positive symptoms appear to respond more satisfactorily to anti-psychotic drugs.

Biological features

The aetiology of schizophrenia remains obscure, though research has indicated the following four features in the majority of cases – a genetic influence; seasonal differences; CNS abnormalities; and involvement of dopamine receptors.

A genetic component

It has long been recognized that schizophrenia is more prevalent in some families. However, this does not necessarily imply a genetic basis to the disorder, since social, cultural and environmental factors are all shared within families. Support for the hypothesis that genes contribute to the aetiology of schizophrenia comes from adoption and twin studies, with concordance of 40–50 percent demonstrated between monozygotic twins. It is likely that several genes are involved, and that they are partially, but not necessarily fully, responsible for most cases of schizophrenia.

Season of birth

It has been shown that patients with schizophrenia are more likely to have been born in the winter months. The increase is slight (5–10 percent), but statistically significant. The significance of this finding is not clear, but could indicate the involvement of either an infectious agent acquired early in life, or seasonal factors affecting ambient temperature, diet, pregnancy, or complications in childbirth.

CNS abnormalities

Structural abnormalities in the brains of schizophrenic patients have been demonstrated by a variety of techniques. Evidence of *cerebral atrophy* (reduction in cerebral mass) in schizophrenia has been demonstrated by *computed tomography* (CT) scans, which have revealed enlargement of the cerebral ventricles of obscure aetiology.

Left temporal lobe dysfunction has been suggested as a contributing factor in schizophrenia. *Magnetic resonance imaging* (MRI) has demonstrated reduced tissue volume in the left temporal lobe in schizophrenic patients. This finding is supported by a reduction in the thickness of the left temporal cortex in *post mortem* brains from schizophrenic patients.

Other brain structures, particularly the hippocampus and amygdala have been shown to have reduced numbers of neurones, and evidence of neural disorganization, in schizophrenia. Increased concentrations of dopamine in the left amygdala have also been demonstrated in schizophrenia.

Measurements of blood flow and energy metabolism have indicated the frontal cortex as another possible site of neural dysfunction in schizophrenia. *Single photon emission computed tomography* (SPECT) has demonstrated that, in schizophrenic patients experiencing auditory hallucinations, blood flow was significantly increased to *Broca's area* in the frontal lobe of the left cerebral cortex (the area of the brain involved in producing language). The same patients were later investigated when they were free of this symptom, and this time the activity in Broca's area was not significantly increased.

Positron emission tomography (PET) has shown the pre-frontal cortex to have reduced activity in schizophrenia. This was particularly apparent in patients exhibiting the negative symptoms of the disorder. The significance of the diverse and inconsistent CNS abnormalities observed in schizophrenia is currently subject to speculation. However, they indicate the extent to which the biology of the disease is, as yet, poorly understood.

Involvement of dopamine receptors

Neuroleptic drugs, (drugs with an antipsychotic action), block dopamine synapses in the brain and relieve the positive symptoms of schizophrenia. However, the pharmacological reduction in dopaminergic neurotransmission occurs much more rapidly than the alleviation of symptoms, so anti-psychotic drugs are assumed to exert some of their effects indirectly. The synaptic effects of dopamine antagonists are covered in more detail in Chapter 33.

A possible abnormality in glutamate neurotransmission

Abnormalities which will eventually lead to the development of schizophrenia have been suggested to arise early in the development of the brain, perhaps during the second trimester of pregnancy. It is thought that the migration of neurones to their designated sites in the developing brain could be disrupted, leading to abnormal development of the cortex and faulty connections with the limbic system. If such damage occurs, it could be due to genetic or environmental factors, perhaps also involving abnormalities in glutamate neurotransmission. Glutamate is a neurotransmitter released by axons connecting the cortex with the limbic system and it is known that glutamate receptors are involved in the differentiation and migration of young neurones in the developing brain.

Other research has indicated that, in *post mortem* brains from schizophrenic patients there is a reduction in glutamate receptors, particularly in the left temporal lobe. The activity of dopamine synapses is thought to inhibit the release of glutamate, so pharmacological reduction in dopaminergic neurotransmission may gradually increase glutamate activity. If this is demonstrated to be the case, it could explain the delayed clinical response to anti-psychotic medication in schizophrenia.

The dementias

Alzheimer's disease

Alzheimer's disease, the most common cause of pre-senile and senile dementia, is associated with degenerative changes in cortical association areas, particularly those of the hippocampus and the temporal, frontal and parietal lobes. The degenerative changes include *plaque* and *tangle* formation (Fig. 32.1), with loss of somatostatin- and glutamate-containing cell bodies in the cerebral cortex. The distribution of lesions suggest that the degenerative process spreads along glutamate-containing association neurones within the cortex. The discovery that plaques contain a high concentration of aluminium, and epidemiological data linking exposure to high levels of aluminium in drinking water and the formation of tangles, suggest that aluminium may have a role in the pathogenesis of Alzheimer's disease. In addition, there is a strong genetic element in many cases of Alzheimer's disease, possibly involving a gene on chromosome 21 (see Chapter 33).

Other forms of dementia

It is possible that infectious agents are responsible for certain other forms of dementia: the pathogenesis of *Jakob–Creutzfeldt* disease in humans has some similarities to that of *scrapie* in sheep and *bovine spongiform encephalopathy* (BSE) in cattle, both of which have been demonstrated to be due to infectious agents known as *prions* (see Chapter 6). HIV can also infect the brain, where it is associated with the occurrence of distinctive multinucleate giant cells. The condition may progress to cause psychotic symptoms or intellectual deterioration. Other causes of dementia include: *cerebral artery atherosclerosis* (resulting in cerebral ischaemia);

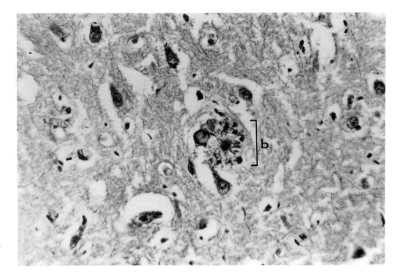

Fig. 32.1 Alzheimer's disease is characterized histologically by the presence of neurofibrillary tangles and of plaques (P) containing amyloid protein.

demyelination (as in multiple sclerosis); and neoplasia.

Mental illness and organic disease

Despite the undoubted advances in understanding disease processes in mental illness, it is essential to appreciate that physical illness can also produce psychiatric symptoms. For example, confusional states have a number of possible causes including inflammation, infection, *uraemia* (retention in the blood of waste products including urea), or drug intoxication. Less dramatically, the tiredness and lethargy of anaemia can present as depression, and many patients with thyroid disorders exhibit psychiatric symptoms ranging from depression in hypothyroidism, to anxiety in hyperthyroidism.

Psychological and social factors in disease

There is often a psychological component to many other physical illnesses, particularly those associated with prolonged incapacity or social isolation such as rheumatoid arthritis. Conversely, specific psychological states of mind are thought to predispose to certain disease states: Type A behaviour (excessive ambition, hostility and time urgency) and its proposed link with coronary heart disease is one example. More controversial is the claim that certain psychological traits and behavioural characteristics are associated with a higher prevalence of malignant disease. It is postulated that feelings of depression, hopelessness and other psychological stressors adversely affect the immune system, which in turn influences susceptibility to cancer.

Finally, despite the emphasis in this chapter on the biology of mental illness, it is important not to overlook the influence of social factors on mental health. Poverty, unemployment and poor housing all impact on self-image, particularly in societies where expectations are high. It has been estimated that a high proportion of primary medical consultations are for symptoms associated with anxiety and depression, some of which can be attributed to biological factors and others to social and environmental influences or adverse life events.

Summary

The purpose of this chapter has been to introduce the reader to some important topics in biological psychiatry and to set the scene for the chapter

Key points

1 The precise biological mechanisms underlying the functional psychiatric disorders have yet to be fully elucidated.

2 There is some evidence that endogenous and exogenous forms of depression can be differentiated by biological markers.

3 Abnormalities of catecholamine and serotonin synaptic neurotransmission are a feature of depression.

4 The mode of action of lithium in controlling bipolar affective disorder is not yet understood, but may involve intracellular signalling mechanisms.

5 Schizophrenia is characterized by genetic factors, CNS changes, and abnormalities in dopaminergic neurotransmission.

6 Degenerative changes in Alzheimer's disease, the cause of which is unknown, include plaque and tangle formation in the CNS. Certain other forms of dementia are due to infection, demyelination or ischaemia.

7 Physical illness can cause psychiatric symptoms. Conversely, many physical symptoms may have an emotional basis and certain disease syndromes are recognized to have a strong psychological component.

which follows. Comprehensive coverage of the biology of mental illness is not possible in the space available but Chapter 33 expands on, develops and criticizes certain of these concepts from a clinical viewpoint. Finally, the case studies in this section of the book give a flavour of the challenge of psychiatry in clinical practice.

Further reading

Brown P. (1994) Understanding the inner voices. *New Sci.* **143**, 26–31.

Helmchen H. & Henn F.A. (eds.) (1987) *Biological Perspectives of Schizophrenia.* Wiley, Chichester.

Kalat J.W. (1992) *Biological Psychology*, 4th edn. Wadsworth Publishing, Belmont.

Owen F. & Itzhaki R. (1994) *Molecular and Cell Biology of Neuropsychiatric Diseases.* Chapman and Hall, London.

Biology of Mental Illness

Introduction

The phrase 'biology of mental illness' would not please every psychiatrist. 'Biology' risks becoming a status word, for instance when used to refer to the physical symptoms of depression, implying that the other symptoms do not attain such a state of grace. Some have objected to the term being used exclusively for the physical when the psychological and the social have as strong a claim. To others the phrase may suggest the 'medical model' in a new guise, the three following aspects of which have been particularly criticized.

1 The importance attached to lesions in the concept of disease.

2 The assumption of necessary causes.

3 The actual (as opposed to the semantic) neglect of social and psychological factors.

In this chapter, the biology of mental illness is considered in the light of these objections. This leads to a consideration of the difference between weak and strong concepts of disease, to an account of some illustrative research findings and to a comment on the interpretation of such findings.

The concept of disease

Symptoms may be regarded as *natural phenomena,* but diseases are *concepts,* constructed as guides to treatment. A disease can only be inferred from its '*indicators*', that is, its symptoms and any objective features it might have. One objective feature, the *lesion*—a distinctive tissue abnormality—has played a key part in the concept of many diseases.

D. T. Campbell and D. W. Fiske (1959) made the point that the more diverse the domains of the indicators, the more convincing their joint delineation of the disease. For example chest pain, electrocardiographic abnormalities, and enzyme changes are collectively convincing delineators of myocardial infarction precisely because they are indicators from very different domains: three sightings from widely separate vantage points.

Progress in psychiatry has been seriously hampered because, for the most part, abnormal mental states have had to be defined solely as collections of symptoms which tend to occur together, and so constitute sightings from one vantage point alone. Such psychiatric disorders or syndromes are called 'functional', and the following is a brief account of the three most important functional mental illnesses.

Functional mental illness

There are two illnesses characterized by states of abnormal mood: mania and depression. In mania the patient is typically garrulous, exuberant, uninhibited, overbearing, distractible, irritable if not aggressive, and overconfident, in short, larger than life.

Depression, in most respects, is the opposite. There is lack of energy, of zest, of self confidence, and of the capacity for pleasure. The patients are dispirited, worried, tense, self critical, and mentally and physically sluggish. He or she often contemplates, and may commit, suicide. Curtailment of sleep is common to both states. Oddly enough, those prone to spells of mania are also prone to periods of depression, and are consequently said to have 'bipolar disorder' (see Chapter 32).

Schizophrenia, usually a chronic disease, has a very wide range of symptoms. Some, such as lack of motivation, of emotional warmth, of interest in fellow men and of ideas, are called 'negative'. The more distinctive, or 'positive', symptoms are auditory hallucinations, delusions, illogical thought, and a collection of experiences in which the normal perception of a boundary between the mind and the outside world, its 'pales and forts', breaks down. The patients then believe that their thoughts are public knowledge, that their minds and bodies are controlled from outside, and that neutral events have some special and usually menacing significance for them.

The quest for objective indicators

There has been a long-standing belief that the syndromes of depression and of schizophrenia encompass several distinct aetiologies, just as do the syndromes of heart failure and stroke. Heart failure and stroke are associated with objective indices which enable finer distinctions, relevant both to cause and management, to be made. Such prospects have motivated the search for objective indices in mental illness.

Over 30 years ago, the technique of *air encephalography* demonstrated cerebral ventricular enlargement in schizophrenia. This discovery has been largely confirmed by more recently developed techniques in computed tomographic and magnetic resonance imaging, although the enlargement is neither striking nor frequent. Currently, there is great interest in the possibility that the left temporal lobe and corpus callosum may be smaller than normal in schizophrenia, possibly through damage inflicted early enough to arrest development. There are some pointers to early brain damage in an increased incidence of obstetric and birth complications, and of maternal influenza in mid-pregnancy in those destined for schizophrenia, but these associations have not been found in all studies. Imaging techniques have been used less extensively to investigate mood disorders, although there is interest in the possibility that either generalized or focal cerebral atrophy might be associated with depressive illness in the aged.

There remain the other two criticisms of the medical model, namely that to speak, even if speculatively, of necessary physical causes of mental illness is both to ignore social and psychological factors and to give way to what Szasz has called 'the biological reductionist impulse'. These concerns may be laid to rest by considering the motor neurone. The motor neurone stimulates muscle, but is itself a point of convergence of many potential influences generated from throughout the nervous system. C.S. Sherrington (1947) designated this the 'final common path'. To assert that this common path is necessary to elicit a particular response, for example a kick at a passing cat, in no way denies the importance of the inter- and intra-personal tensions and the social stresses which compelled the kick. However, taking a military analogy, the hope in psychiatry is more of defiles (i.e. narrow passes) towards which battalions of causes converge, and then fan out to the wide array of symptoms so characteristic of mental illness — defiles where, it is hoped, the causes of mental illness will prove as vulnerable as soldiers to attack.

Depressive illness

The belief that there is such a defile in depressive illness arises from the sources outlined below.

1 Depression (and schizophrenia) runs in families, and there is evidence from twin and adoption studies that genetic inheritance is at least partially responsible.

2 There seemed to be a most encouraging precedent in the discovery of a deficiency of the neurotransmitter dopamine in the putamen of patients with Parkinson's disease, a discovery which led to the use of the dopamine precursor, L-DOPA, as a successful treatment. Equivalently, it was found that L-tryptophan the precursor of another neurotransmitter, 5-hydroxytryptamine (5-HT) was a weak antidepressant, whose potency could be increased by combination with drugs which conserved 5-HT at the synaptic cleft.

3 However, the main and initial expectation of a defile arose from three remarkable observations:

(a) in 1954, that the administration of the drug

isoniazid to treat tuberculosis caused some patients to become euphoric;

(b) in 1958, in trials of imipramine for schizophrenia, that this drug was an antidepressant; and

(c) in 1955, that reserpine, when used to treat hypertension, caused depression.

The collective significance of these last three observations is that both isoniazid and imipramine increase, but reserpine decreases the availability of the neurotransmitters 5-HT and of noradrenaline at the synaptic cleft. Isoniazid inhibits their main catalytic enzyme, monoamine oxidase (MAO), and imipramine inhibits their re-uptake into the presynaptic nerve. Reserpine, in contrast, hastens their destruction by MAO by preventing their entry into safe presynaptic storage sites. There is an echo here of the Campbell and Fiske principle: evidence from three divergent sources fortifies the suspicion that the CNS monoamine synapse might be a defile.

Efforts to find such defiles have taken the form of exploiting every new promising technique and almost every applicable new iota of knowledge about CNS monoaminergic neurones. In recent years this knowledge has increased considerably. It is now known that these neurones can release neurotransmitters not only focally at the synapse but broadcast from their long axons. Whole families of receptors have been defined. Some of the interactions between different receptor types within the same synapse are beginning to be understood. More is known about the molecular structure of the receptor and the sequence of events between the receptor stimulus and the consequences within the post-synaptic neurone. This new knowledge has dispelled some old hypotheses and increased the scope for new ones, which, given the nature of the problem, may in their turn succumb to the advance of neurophysiology. The reader is referred to Paykel (see 'further reading') for more on this large and difficult topic.

Schizophrenia

Work in schizophrenia has followed very much

the same lines as for depression and was inspired originally by these similar observations.

1 Many drugs effective in schizophrenia have in common that they are *dopamine (D2) receptor blockers*. A straight line relationship between the clinical potency of a large group of such drugs and their ability to block post-synaptic D2 receptors in the CNS has been demonstrated (more precisely, a straight line relationship between log mean therapeutic dose and log drug concentration required to displace 50% of haloperidol from D2-binding sites).

2 *Cis*-flupenthixol, a powerful D2 blocker, is effective in schizophrenia but its trans-isomer, which has little such effect, is not.

3 D-Amphetamine, which releases dopamine from intra-neuronal stores, is known to cause a psychosis not very different from schizophrenia.

An excess of dopamine was soon replaced by D2 post-synaptic supersensitivity as the prime suspect for schizophrenic symptoms. Both possibilities are now doubted since anti-psychotic drugs block D2 receptors very rapidly, yet relieve symptoms only after some 3 weeks. Furthermore, clozaril an effective drug for schizophrenia, is a relatively weak D2-blocking agent.

Estimates of D2 receptor density in living subjects using radioactive ligands detected with *positron emission tomography* (PET) and *single photon emission computed tomography* (SPECT) have given equivocal results, some finding increased density in never-treated schizophrenic patients, but others not so. Recent work has shown greater D2-receptor binding in the left striatum than in the right striatum in schizophrenic patients, but no such difference in controls. The effect was apparent in male patients only.

Problems of interpretation

Generally speaking, the search for physical factors in schizophrenia and in depression has given equivocal results. In evaluating reports it is worth considering a number of points. Extraneous or confounding variables (see Chapter 2) may give the false impression of a link between an illness and a phenomenon under study, or obscure any genuine link ('Type 1' and 'Type 2' errors respectively). For instance, there is a relationship between wrinkled skin and dementia almost certainly due to the shared link with the confounding variable, age. In experiments, the random allocation of the factors under study to experimental and control groups randomly disperses the influence of extraneous factors. However, the causes of mental illness are not inflicted at random. When confounding variables are known they can be eliminated by *matching* (e.g. for sex), or allowed for by analysis of *covariance* (e.g. for age); when they are unknown nothing can be done about them.

There is also the problem of knowing whether effects are *causative* or *secondary*. Investigations of genes have the strength that they begin at the beginning. Depressed patients are several stages removed from any beginning, and may be afflicted by a variety of attendant disabilities such as reduced food intake, weight loss, fear, curtailment of sleep; and occasionally alcohol abuse, any of which might be the source of secondary effects. However, regarding sleep disorder as 'attendant' is very much a clinician's perspective; some believe it to be of central importance and refer to the early appearance of the first rapid eye movement (REM) phase in the nights sleep, and the proportionate reduction of Stage 2 and 3 sleep as specific for depressive illness.

Finally, the CNS is so complicated that there is always the possibility of finding differences between mentally ill and control groups which had not been anticipated. Such differences may be very important, but since they are suggested by the data they require confirmation in a separate investigation dedicated to examining them alone. For instance in the SPECT study mentioned above, such a complex interaction as that reported (group $\times$ sex $\times$ laterality), would require confirmation if there had been no particular reason to anticipate it. Because the assumption is so specific, successful replication would be a strong reassurance of a real effect.

Dementia

Dementia is defined as: a chronic impairment of intellect, memory and personality. Indices in the form of structural abnormalities in the brain have enabled different types of dementia to be delineated.

An *infarct* denotes a portion of brain that has died as a result of inadequate blood supply. A succession of infarcts may do enough cumulative damage to the cerebrum to cause dementia, a condition referred to as *multi-infarct dementia*.

The *Lewy body*, a proteinaceous structure with radiating filaments, is found in the cytoplasm of neurone cell bodies. Lewy bodies are rare in the brains of people without neurological or mental disease. They are found in the cells of the substantia nigra in Parkinson's disease. In patients with Parkinsonism and dementia they may also be found in the cerebral cortex, this more general distribution defining *diffuse Lewy body disease*. Recently, it has been shown that the cortical Lewy body is an indicator of a relatively common cause of senile dementia in which antipsychotic drugs are particularly dangerous. Some regard this condition as a distinct entity and call it senile dementia of Lewy body type, but others consider it a variant of diffuse Lewy body disease.

In Alzheimer's disease (AD) the brain is shrunken and the cerebrum contains neurofibrillary tangles within neurones and extracellular plaques (see Fig. 32.1). Both amyloid and aluminium silicate have been identified in plaques and in tangles, amyloid having been found in plaques as long ago as 1927. There has been long debate as to whether the aluminium is 'passenger' or 'driver'. Epidemiological evidence linking aluminium concentration in tap water with the prevalence of AD suggests driver, and aluminium is known to cause an encephalopathy in patients on long-term dialysis. However, the epidemiological evidence has been questioned, and dialysis encephalopathy is not associated with either tangles or plaques.

The neurofibrillary tangle protein has been identified as *tau amyloid* and the plaque protein as *beta-amyloid*. The protein from which beta amyloid is derived is called *amyloid precursor protein* (APP) and one of the constituent peptides of this precursor is encoded by a gene on the long arm of chromosome 21. This location is of special interest because patients with Down's syndrome (see Chapter 26) have an extra chromosome 21 and are prone to AD, possibly because of over-expression of the APP gene. Furthermore, a point mutation at codon 717 of the APP gene, coding for glycine instead of valine, has been identified in affected members of a single family with a rare form of *familial Alzheimer's disease* (FAD). In two other families with early-onset AD, point mutations have also been found in this codon, in one family coding for isoleucine, and in the other for phenylalanine. Other discoveries have made it clear that AD is genetically heterogeneous. In some cases of early onset FAD the defective gene is on the long arm of chromosome 14, and on chromosome 19 in some cases of late onset FAD.

Recent work has shown that that an allele, E4, on chromosome 19 has a significantly higher frequency in a sample of patients with the senile, sporadic form of AD than in age-matched controls. The E4 allele codes for ApoE-4, one of the molecular variants of apolipoprotein E, a versatile protein which plays a part in clearing cholesterol from plasma and redistributing peripheral nerve cholesterol after damage. The pathogenic credentials of ApoE-4 are beginning to look interesting. It is found in senile plaques and in tangles, and binds tightly to beta-amyloid. Furthermore, E4 homozygotes are at high risk of developing atherosclerosis (see Poirier in further reading section).

Huntington's disease is an inherited autosomal-dominant condition which causes *chorea* (uncontrollable jerky movements) and progressive dementia. The dementia may antedate the chorea, either as a deterioration of personality or as an impairment of intellect. The responsible gene has been located on chromosome 4 in a linkage study on a large kindred group of Venezuelan lake-dwellers with a tendency to inbreed. This gene has now been identified by the Huntington's Dis-

ease Collaborative Research Group. It contains a nucleotide base triplet, *cytosine-adenine-guanine* (CAG), repeated between 38 and 100 times, whereas the repeat factor in the normal gene is 34 or fewer. It is remarkable that three other inherited disorders affecting the CNS: myotonic dystrophy; fragile X syndrome; and X-linked spinal and bulbar muscular atrophy are also caused by genes with abnormally long trinucleotide repeat sequences (see also Chapter 25).

Summary

These, amongst other discoveries, make it clear that the biology of mental illness is no longer just a set of expectations; there is now a fund of facts, small, but growing and very impressive. That there is also a welter of contradictory and puzzling research findings is not surprising since the topic is one around which, to quote Sir C. Sherrington again, 'the main interest of biology must ultimately turn'.

Key points

1 The 'biology of mental illness' is a convenient, but inaccurate shorthand for the belief that physical factors contribute to the aetiology of mental illness and for a set of findings which support this belief.
2 The concepts of mental illness are on the whole weak, and strengthening them is an important research priority.
3 The living human brain is, for many investigatory purposes, ethically out of bounds.
4 The brain is one of the most complex and diverse of all the organs and a commensurately difficult topic for research.
5 Despite these difficulties, there is now a fund of impressive discoveries, particularly in the genetics of mental illness.

Further reading

Curr. Opin. Psych. H.L. Freeman and D.J. Kupfer eds (1993) The Royal College of Psychiatrists, London.

Kendell R.E. & Zeally A.K. (1993) *Companion to Psychiatric Studies*. Churchill Livingstone, Edinburgh.

Paykel E.S. (ed.) (1992) *Handbook of Affective Disorders*. Churchill Livingstone, Edinburgh.

Poirier J., Davignon J., Bouthillier D., Kogan S., Bertrand P., Gauthier S., *Lancet* 1993; **342**, 697–699.

Rose N. (ed.) (1992) *Essential Psychiatry*, 2nd edn. Blackwell Scientific Publications, Oxford.

Case Studies

34.1 Neurotic symptoms following a road traffic accident

Clinical features

A 25-year-old woman complained of an inability to drive or travel by car, lack of concentration and distressing palpitations of the heart. A cardiologist had reassured her that nothing was wrong with her heart, and she had been told to 'pull herself together'.

The symptoms dated back 6 months, to when she had been injured in a car crash due to a tractor being carelessly driven out in front of her. Her head had impacted against the steering wheel and she was briefly knocked out; on recovering consciousness she had been terrified to discover that she was trapped in the wreck. On admission to hospital she was noted to have lost her memory for the first few minutes after impact (*post-traumatic amnesia*). A skull radiograph and neurological examination were normal, and she was discharged home the next day.

Two weeks after the car accident the family doctor was summoned as she had apparently become totally paralysed. Neurological examination was again completely normal and the family doctor diagnosed a 'hysterical reaction', noting that she was suing the tractor driver for compensation. Although the paralysis responded to strong reassurance, over the next few weeks other non-specific symptoms took its place. She complained of dizziness, short-temperedness and headaches (*post-concussional syndrome*). She was constantly tense (*generalized anxiety*). Attempting to drive made the anxiety worse, and at the sight of trac-

tors she would panic, her heart thumping uncontrollably (*phobic anxiety*).

The patient had always been a worrier, although at the same time this had made her a cautious driver with an excellent safety record. It was noted that 2 years previously she had been very upset when a friend had been permanently paralysed by a spinal injury.

Further enquiry disclosed that she came from a family of high achievers, some of whom had a personality trait towards anxiety. Her brother, a company director, had developed hypertension which was successfully treated by beta-blockers.

Investigations

Physical examination revealed a pale, tense woman with *tachycardia* (an elevated heart rate, usually defined as greater than 100 beats per minute), who was hyperventilating and tremulous. Blood pressure was normal at 120 mm systolic, 82 mm diastolic. Results of laboratory investigations are shown in Table 34.1.1.

Blood film examination showed a normal white cell differential count. Erythrocyte morphology revealed some microcytic hypochromic cells. This finding usually indicates early iron deficiency anaemia, but in patients of Asian or Mediterranean origin could also indicate a thalassaemia syndrome (see Chapter 20). Thyroid function tests and gammaglutamyl transferase concentration were normal.

Diagnosis

Diagnosis: anxiety neurosis with post-concussional syndrome.

Table 34.1.1 Blood investigations

Analyte	Value	Reference range
Total white cell count	$7.45 \times 10^9/l$	4.0–11.0
Red cell count	$4.26 \times 10^{12}/l$	3.8–5.8
Haemoglobin	11.2 g/dl	11.5–15.5
Haematocrit	0.338	0.3–0.4
Mean cell volume	79.5 fl	82–92
Mean cell haemoglobin	26.29 pg	27.0–32.0
Platelet count	$260 \times 10^9/l$	150–400
Erythrocyte sedimentation rate	12 mm/hour	0–20
Serum gammaglutamyl transferase	15 U/l	2–50
Free thyroxine	12.2 pmol/l	9–24
Thyroid-stimulating hormone	2.3 mU/l	0.3–4.0

Discussion

Unlike symptoms of physical disease, there is an unfortunate tendency for neurotic symptoms to be held to be the fault of the sufferers, who are told to 'pull themselves together'. This attitude is only partly based on prejudice, as even modern enlightened treatments presume that neurotics are capable of taking some responsibility for their difficulties, and tend to emphasize self-help and self-understanding.

Hysteria provides an example of symptoms mimicking organic disease, which on closer examination turn out to correspond to the patient's ideas or fears about what is wrong with him or her, rather than the actual physical pathology. Such fears may be suggested to the patient, in this case by her friend's injury. There is often an element of 'secondary gain', in the form of extra attention and sympathy, the avoidance of an intolerable situation, or (as here) financial compensation. However, it is characteristic that the hysteric, in contrast to the malingerer, is completely unaware of such motives.

These concepts, expounded by Freud at the turn of the century, have coloured our understanding of neurosis and delayed the appreciation of the biological aspects. In the case of closed head injury, sophisticated methods of brain-imaging (applied to boxers, for example), have demonstrated significant structural damage to the brain from relatively minor blows. Such diffuse damage may be insufficient to produce gross neurological signs, but may be manifest in the more sensitive area of emotional change. Here it probably contributed to the patient's post-concussional syndrome, and may have increased her vulnerability to develop a hysterical reaction. Another determinant of this reaction may have been her friend's injury. The glib assumption of financial compensation as the main cause should be viewed with caution, however.

The aetiology of this case is a typical combination of *heredity* (her worrying disposition) and *environment* (the accident). Genetic factors play a more prominent role than once assumed; note that they are expressed in her relatives as a beneficially high drive towards success, as well as a tendency towards hypertension.

Anxiety symptoms have *psychological* (fear, apprehension) and *physical* (tremor, tachycardia) aspects. Treatment should reflect this dual nature.

Treatment and prognosis

The patient was reassured that her post-concussional symptoms had a definite physical explanation and were not 'all in her imagination'. Her current difficulties in concentration, however, were caused by anxiety and not permanent brain damage, as she feared. Mild iron deficiency anaemia, which was confirmed by estimation of serum ferritin, is quite common in females of this age group (see Chapter 20), and was thought to be an incidental finding. This was treated with oral iron preparations.

Once it was explained to the patient that hyperventilation was worsening her anxiety, she felt more confident that she could overcome her symptoms by breathing control exercises. Instruction in relaxation techniques enabled her to contemplate tractors whilst remaining calm (*desensitization*). Prescription of the beta-blocker propranolol, also helped considerably, by preventing the sympathetic over-stimulation which had been causing her tremor and cardiac palpitations. Throughout, she was encouraged to practise driving rather than avoiding it (*exposure therapy*). After four months she was driving confidently again but it was some years before she was entirely comfortable as a passenger.

Neurotic symptoms following trauma were highlighted during both world wars (shell shock, battle fatigue). These days they are often labelled as *post-traumatic stress disorder*, and frequently feature in litigation following public disasters (e.g. Hillsborough Stadium, Kings Cross fire), as well as in personal injury claims.

This case illustrates the complex interplay between biological and psychological factors which makes the evaluation of neurosis so fascinating, and so controversial. Symptoms which appear explicable in psychological terms may also have a subtle biological basis.

Questions

1 Why were haematological investigations and thyroid function tests performed on this patient?

Answer: a routine full blood count and erythrocyte sedimentation rate are useful investigations to exclude physical causes of psychiatric symptoms. Thyroid function tests were performed because hyperthyroidism (overactivity of the thyroid gland) can produce agitation and anxiety (see also Chapter 32).

2 Why were gamma-glutamyl transferase (gamma-GT) levels measured?

Answer: an increase in serum gamma-GT concentration is a sensitive marker of acute liver cell damage. Gamma-GT concentration is usually raised in alcohol abuse (see Chapter 17). Alcohol withdrawal could produce anxiety symptoms.

34.2 *Depressive illness in pregnancy*

Clinical features

A 23-year-old female was referred for a psychiatric opinion when 30 weeks pregnant. She was suffering from the typical features of a severe depressive illness (see Chapter 33), including agitation and insomnia. She ruminated for most of the day and well into the night on a number of morbid ideas. The most distressing of these was that she had wanted members of her family killed to attract attention to herself.

The patient had a history of depression. She had previously been prescribed fluoxetine, a specific presynaptic 5-hydroxytryptamine uptake inhibitor, which had been discontinued when she became pregnant.

Investigations

Full blood count and routine tests of thyroid, liver and renal function were performed. All were normal. Laboratory investigations have no special role in establishing the diagnosis of depressive illness (see Chapter 33) but simple screening tests to exclude systemic physical illness should be done in all psychiatric inpatients; they are essential if electroconvulsive therapy (ECT) is to be used.

Diagnosis

Diagnosis: severe depressive episode with psychotic symptoms.

Treatment and prognosis

Two ways of treating her depression were discussed with the patient: *antidepressant drugs* and *electroconvulsive therapy (ECT).* Initially she was treated with doxepin, a tricyclic antidepressant drug which inhibits presynaptic uptake of both noradrenaline and 5-hydroxytryptamine. It also has sedative and hypnotic properties, useful in this case, because of the patient's agitation and insomnia.

After 5 days on this treatment the patient was still deeply depressed and pleaded for ECT. Five days is not long enough for tricyclic antidepressants to relieve symptoms, but 'in view of her serious suffering' (to use a phrase from the Mental Health Act, 1983), she was given a course of ECT.

The patient required a course of five treatments for full recovery. After the first application she enjoyed a respite from her distressing ideas which then gradually returned before the next treatment. With successive treatments the period of respite from depressive symptoms lengthened.

Discussion

One of the reasons for believing that depressive illness is 'biological' is its remarkable response to ECT. A course of ECT consists of a succession of electrically induced fits given between two and three times a week. Patients vary in the number of fits required, a few recovering after three or so but most needing six to eight; it is rarely worth giving more than 12. The fit is induced by an electrical stimulus consisting of a rapid succession of very brief unidirectional pulses applied between the temples. The electrical impedance of the human skull varies considerably between individuals. Modern ECT machines adjust the voltage accordingly to ensure that peak current is near-constant.

Strictly speaking ECT is a misnomer, because there is no convulsion, only muscle-twitching. Succinyl choline, a muscle relaxant, is given to prevent convulsions. It does so by briefly depolarizing the muscle end-plate, making it unresponsive to its neurotransmitter, acetylcholine. A brief-acting anaesthetic, methohexitone, is also given to render the patient oblivious, not to ECT,

itself an anaesthetic, but to the respiratory paralysis induced by the succinyl choline. ECT is safe in the third trimester of pregnancy, but it is important to ensure adequate muscle relaxation. Using modern apparatus the incidence of adverse effects during or following ECT is very low. There may be some impairment of memory for events occurring during a short period before ECT and some difficulty in registering new information for a variable period after ECT. It has been shown that ECT actually improves memory in depressed patients probably by relieving the lack of concentration and mental retardation caused by the illness.

Questions

1 Why should caution be exercised when treating patients with drugs during pregnancy and lactation?

Answer: many drugs cross the placenta or may appear in breast milk. In the first trimester of pregnancy some are *teratogenic*, that is, they may cause fetal malformation. Later in fetal development and in early life, drugs may cause serious physiological disturbance. Doxepin was chosen for this patient because it is the least able of all the tricyclic antidepressants to cross the placental barrier. However, it is secreted in breast milk and should be replaced during lactation by imipramine.

2 What are the clinical indications for ECT?

Answer: the value of ECT in the treatment of depressive illness has now been established in a number of double-blind trials in which the control group has been given muscle relaxant and anaesthetic but no ECT.

ECT is most effective in severe depressions in which there is marked retardation or agitation, or when some of the ideas are delusional. A *delusion* is a false belief, not amenable to reason and not shared by people with a similar educational and cultural background. *Retardation* is a slowing of the mind and a reduction in activity; when severe there is no speech and long periods of near-immobility, a state referred to as *stupor*.

ECT may also be used to treat patients who are dangerously suicidal, who choose it, or for whom other measures such as drugs have failed. Depressive illness may relapse after a course of ECT, but the risk is reduced by treatment with an antidepressant drug in maintainance dose during the succeeding 6 months.

Index

Page numbers in **bold** type refer to tables; those in *italics* to figures.